Hospital Performance in Brazil

Hospital Performance in Brazil

The Search for Excellence

Gerard M. La Forgia
Bernard F. Couttolenc

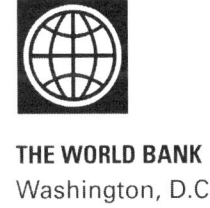

THE WORLD BANK
Washington, D.C.

© 2008 The International Bank for Reconstruction and Development / The World Bank
1818 H Street, NW
Washington, DC 20433
Telephone 202-473-1000
Internet www.worldbank.org
E-mail feedback@worldbank.org

1 2 3 4 :: 11 10 09 08

This volume is a product of the staff of the International Bank for Reconstruction and Development / The World Bank. The findings, interpretations, and conclusions expressed in this volume do not necessarily reflect the views of the Executive Directors of The World Bank or the governments they represent.

The World Bank does not guarantee the accuracy of the data included in this work. The boundaries, colors, denominations, and other information shown on any map in this work do not imply any judgment on the part of The World Bank concerning the legal status of any territory or the endorsement or acceptance of such boundaries.

ISBN: 978-0-8213-7358-3
eISBN: 978-0-8213-7359-0
DOI: 10.1596/ 978-0-8213-7358-3

Library of Congress Cataloging-in-Publication Data has been applied for.

Contents

Figures

Tables

Boxes

Foreword

Health care poses a conundrum for all countries, and hospitals are the most important, most critical, and most costly components of any health care system. In low- and middle-income countries, hospitals are the central focus of all health care. Even in the poorest countries, hospitals provide the training ground, the referral, and the benchmark for the health system at large. In these countries, hospitals are the engine behind sound health care. Yet in much of the developing world, hospitals have been systematically neglected.

The range of services provided by hospitals, from high-tech clinical care to complicated surgeries, from intricate accounting to basic hotel services, make their management costly and complex and their oversight and control profoundly challenging. Gaining control of such complicated entities requires depth and breadth of expertise to understand all the components of a hospital and effectively integrate them, while tracking performance and use of resources requires reliable, updated information—all of which can be difficult to come by in the developing world. As a result, in countries where hospitals are central and a significant proportion of all health spending goes to running them, hospitals can become expensive "black boxes" that eat up resources while providing an uneven and unmeasured set of outputs.

This book combines a comprehensive overview of the Brazilian hospital sector with in-depth analyses of the key elements of interest in promoting and ensuring excellence in hospital performance. It does so in an accessible manner and within the organizational and financial context of Brazil. Thus, the book can offer specific recommendations that go to the heart of the problem, as well as suggest what kinds of approaches work in that context. The recommendations themselves are based on what works in Brazil while drawing on international experiences relevant to the Brazilian context to broaden the policy options. But the authors go a step further by providing recommendations on implementation, specifically highlighting the need to strengthen governance arrangements, improve accountability, and sharpen resource management.

One of the major challenges of Brazilian health care is making sense of the highly creative but random experiments in health care management that proliferate across Brazil. Having been ahead of much of the world in financing hospitals by a form of diagnostic related groups (a fixed amount of reimbursement per diagnosis), the system failed to adequately evaluate the effectiveness of the implementation or adapt to a rapidly changing environment. As a result the full benefits of such ideas have not been realized.

Similarly, Brazil has pioneered innovative ways to hold public hospitals accountable. An important example is the São Paulo experiment in making public hospitals more autonomous and holding directors accountable for good performance, offering both incentives for good performance and flexibility in implementation. This represents an important breakthrough, not only because of its creative framework, but also because it was enforced—a critical factor, since many hospitals making similar experiments are restricted in their ability to make decisions, which lessens their autonomy. This book has brought together a wealth of experience and evidence that will inform federal, state, and municipal governments as well as private hospitals about successful efforts, such as in São Paulo, in raising hospital efficiency and quality.

This book offers important guidance for interested policy makers in Brazil, but it has lessons for other middle-income countries facing similar problems in assessing their hospitals and finding effective and creative solutions to difficult problems. The linkages between organization arrangements, management and performance are universal problems, and new ideas may be transferable if they are carefully evaluated and understood. Indeed, the OECD countries continue to search for improvements. The single biggest challenge across the richest countries is how to maintain quality and contain costs at the same time.

The ideas presented here provide valuable suggestions to the twin problems of quality and savings. It should be read by policy makers and hospital administrators and planners in both the public and private sectors. It is a guide for better health care, something we can all agree is a global good and a public priority.

Maureen Lewis
Chief Economist, Human Development
World Bank

Acknowledgments

This volume was commissioned by the World Bank and received additional financial support from the U.K. Department for International Development (DfID)/Brazil. The authors are grateful for this support. Gerard M. La Forgia, Human Development Sector Management Unit, Latin American and the Caribbean Region, World Bank, conceptualized and coordinated the work. Collaborators in Brazil included the Ministry of Health (Ministério da Saúde, MS), the National Agency for Sanitary Surveillance (Agência Nacional de Vigilância Sanitária, ANVISA), the Fundação Oswaldo Cruz (FIOCRUZ), and the National Accreditation Organization (Organização Nacional de Acreditação, ONA). The volume draws heavily on background papers prepared for the World Bank and its partners by the following principal investigators:

Nilson Costa, Escola Nacional de Saúde Pública (ENSP)/FIOCRUZ

Bernard Couttolenc, Interhealth Ltd, and Universidade de São Paulo (USP)

Afonso José De Matos, Planejamento e Organização de Instituições de Saúde (PLANISA)

Leni Dias, Planejamento e Organização de Instituições de Saúde (PLANISA)

Flavia Freitas, ANVISA

Fábio Gastal, ONA

Marcos Kisil, USP

Adélia Marçal dos Santos, ANVISA

Jose Mendes R., ENSP/FIOCRUZ

Eugenio V. Mendes, independent consultant

Luis Fernando Rolim Sampaio, independent consultant

April Harding was a coauthor of the concluding chapter and also provided valuable comments on other chapters. James Allen assisted in the drafting of chapter 7. Maureen Lewis, Loraine Hawkins, André Medici, and Toomas Palu provided very helpful peer review comments. We also would like to thank Kathleen A. Lynch for her rigorous editing and Marize Fatima de Santos, Carla Zardo, and Adriana Paula Sales Correa for assistance in formatting the volume.

About the Authors

Gerard (Jerry) M. La Forgia is a lead health specialist at the World Bank, currently working out of São Paulo, Brazil. He has worked in Argentina, Colombia, Ecuador, El Salvador, Guatemala, India, México, Nicaragua, Panamá, and Uruguay. His recent work includes an edited World Bank Working Paper, *Health System Innovations in Central America: Lessons and Impact of New Approaches* (2005) and an Economic and Sector Report (no. 36601) on the governance and quality of spending in Brazil's Unified Health System (2007). He formerly was a research associate at the Urban Institute and a senior health specialist at the Inter-American Development Bank. He holds a Sc.D. in health service administration from the Graduate School of Public Health, University of Pittsburgh (U.S.).

Dr. Bernard Couttolenc holds a PhD in Health Economics from the Johns Hopkins University (Baltimore, U.S.) and a Master's degree in Health Care Management from Fundação Getúlio Vargas (Sao Paulo, Brazil). He has accumulated over 20 years of experience in consulting in health economics, health care management and planning, economic evaluation, and health sector reform. He has worked extensively in developing countries, including Brazil, Angola, Dominican Republic, Lao PDR, and Belize. He is a professor and researcher in health economics at the University of São Paulo, Brazil.

Policy Summary

Hospitals are at the center of the health care universe in Brazil and are critical to the health of the Brazilian people. When ill, many Brazilians go straight to the hospital, for want of a family doctor or primary care network. Hospitals are a critical part of the government's budget, absorbing nearly 70 percent of public spending on health. Hospitals influence the ebb and flow of politicians' careers, when hospital mishaps hit the headlines or the limelight falls on high-performing facilities. Hospitals are at the forefront of policy discussions in Brazil. These discussions reflect hospitals' promise as centers of technological innovation and medical advances, as well as widespread concern about their cost and quality. Brazilian hospitals are thus important to many people for many different reasons. What makes hospitals important is easy to understand. What makes hospitals deliver quality care efficiently—or not—is much harder to grasp.

Challenges to Brazil's Hospital System

Brazil's hospital system is pluralistic. An array of financial, ownership, and organizational arrangements is found in both the public and private sectors, and there is a long tradition of public financing of private facilities. The system is also highly stratified. A few hospitals are world-class centers of excellence, and they serve the well-off minority. But most hospitals—the ones serving Brazilians who cannot pay out of pocket or afford private insurance—are best described as substandard. These hospitals, many of them dependent on public financing, deliver inefficient, poor-quality care, judging from the available data.

Although hospitals are the de facto health care delivery system in Brazil, until recently they have received scant attention as health care organizations from either policy makers or researchers. Since the mid-1980s, the development of health policy in Brazil has focused on decentralizing service delivery, reducing financial disparities, and achieving universal access to basic care. Issues of hospital performance, however defined, have been left mainly to the individual facility.

In 2004 a publication by the Ministry of Health (Ministério da Saúde, MS) on hospital reform sounded the call for change. It was the first MS document to focus entirely on the hospital sector, and it opened a national discussion on hospital problems, performance, and potential. The broad policy directions outlined there are aligned with the policy recommendations contained in this book. The MS called on research and hospital communities to collaborate with it to strengthen analysis of hospital performance and help develop a vision and strategy for hospital reform. It is in this spirit of collaboration that this book has been written.

Brazil's challenge is not unique. Implementing hospital reform policies is notoriously difficult, and it is more problematic still when hospital ownership, governance, and payment mechanisms take as many different forms as they do in a federal state like Brazil. Yet the pluralistic nature of these arrangements is also a strength of the Brazilian hospital sector. As is shown throughout this volume, Brazil does not lack approaches, ideas, innovations, and initiatives for addressing the shortcomings of underperforming facilities. The foundations for change aimed at raising performance are present throughout the country's hospital system. Whether these ideas and innovations will be generalized and woven into the fabric of the system is the question.

Can Brazil improve the performance of its hospitals? The evidence presented in this volume suggests that the answer is, yes. However, it will take strong leadership, coordinated efforts by federal, state, and municipal governments, direct engagement with the private health sector, and systematic and continuous vision, policies, and actions. Such enabling factors have been generally weak or absent in the Brazilian health system. Promising initiatives have often been gutted or scrapped after changes of government.

The Main Policy Messages

This book emphasizes the following policy messages that are important for improving hospital care in Brazil.

- Government needs to enhance the autonomy and accountability of public hospitals.
- Government and private payers of hospital care need to wield their funding power so as to influence hospital behavior.
- Coordination among hospitals and between hospitals and other types of providers needs to be improved.
- The quality of all hospitals must be raised to acceptable standards.
- The absence of reliable information about the quality, efficiency, and costs of hospital services underlies all issues and hampers any effort to improve performance.

Enhancing the Autonomy and Accountability of Public Hospitals

Any efforts to improve the quality and efficiency of public hospitals will rely on increasing the motivation and proactivity of hospital managers. Under current conditions, even the best-motivated and trained managers will have a tough time improving performance. Too many key decisions are made outside the hospital, and rigid constraints on management undermine efforts to increase accountability. To bring autonomy to the great majority of public hospitals, it will be necessary to develop strategies for converting hospitals to autonomous organizational arrangements and to test those strategies against Brazilian and international experience. Although autonomy is a necessary ingredient in reform, it alone cannot drive performance in public hospitals. Also needed are service contracts, contract enforcement, performance-based financing, flexible human resource management, and a robust information environment.

Wielding Funding Power so as to Influence Hospital Behavior

Government and private payers of hospital care are not using funding to its fullest potential to influence hospital behavior. In some cases, funding arrangements hamper performance. Most funding is not linked to performance and gives no incentive for cost consciousness.

Although no payment system is perfect, many countries have linked payments to treatment costs on the basis of diagnosis, adjusted for severity. In the United States the diagnosis-related group (DRG) payment system has been found to improve efficiency and control costs.

Brazil's Authorization for Hospitalization (Autorização de Internação Hospitalar, AIH) mechanism can serve as a foundation for a DRG-based hospital payment system. In moving toward DRGs, the first order of business is to align AIH rates with costs. Developing a robust DRG-based payment mechanism would also reduce distortions arising from the fragmentation of payment systems, if private and public payers switched to the same payment basis. But accountability for hospital performance requires more than performance-based funding (or autonomy). Contracting arrangements are needed to define the content of funding arrangements and thereby link funding to performance. Moreover, successful hospital contracting requires contract management and enforcement. Global budgeting efforts combined with contracting are under way in a handful of states and municipalities. These promising initiatives have been shown to raise performance.

Improving Coordination among All Providers

Coordination—among hospitals and between hospitals and other providers—is critical to improving quality. It will also raise efficiency and broaden equity by rationalizing the supply of hospital beds and expensive medical technologies. Coordination is handicapped in Brazil by the decision-making and financial independence granted to states and municipalities, the absence of ties with private providers outside the Unified Health System (Sistema Único de Saúde, SUS), fragile public administration, and the general ineffectiveness of coordinating instruments such as Integrated and Negotiated Programming (Programação Pactuada e Integrada (PPI). Considering the monetary and quality costs of this fragmentation, Brazil would benefit greatly by applying mechanisms to enhance coordination related to hospital services. Coordination can be pursued by setting up funding-based contractual arrangements, by pooling funding and creating regional command structures with decision-making authority over resource allocation across municipalities, or by tightening regulations governing relations among providers. Some states and municipal consortia are already experimenting with one or more of these mechanisms, and these experiences can provide the basis for effective coordination. To reduce duplication and waste of infrastructure and equipment, two final elements are needed, a policy-based investment strategy, and a system for vigorous technology assessment and allocation.

Raising Service Quality to Acceptable Standards in All Hospitals

Government is responsible for ensuring quality in all hospitals, public and private alike. Quality standards already exist, in the form of licensure requirements and government-sanctioned accreditation systems, but their implementation has been meager. To promote compliance, the SUS and private health plans could institute time-bound funding conditionality and link financing to licensure and accreditation, following the example of a number of countries that use the power of the purse in this way.

Achieving standards, however, does not in itself guarantee quality. Many critical actions needed to improve the quality of hospital services take place at the hospital level under the leadership of hospital management. They include the establishment of continuous quality improvement programs that involve performance assessments, effective teamwork, use of information technologies, incorporation of evidence into practice, development and use of clinical guidelines, and coordination of care within the hospitals, as well as with providers at other levels. Hospitals acting alone may not get far with these elements. Continuous quality improvement requires a systematic approach backed by a solid national support system that includes policies and strategies for enhancing quality; support for systematic research on patient satisfaction and evaluation of clinical practices; and the creation through public-private partnerships of institutions for measuring, monitoring, and benchmarking quality and for providing guidance and support to individual hospitals. Finally, there is a need to address the low quality of some medical schools and to strengthen institutional capacity to address medical malpractice.

Improving the Reliability of Basic Managerial Information

The absence of reliable information about the quality, efficiency, and costs of hospital services underlies all issues and hampers any effort to improve performance. Without this information, policy makers, as well as public and private payers, are flying blind. This situation is untenable. There is an urgent need to develop and install standardized systems to measure costs and quality. These systems should focus on essential information for decision making and should be designed with the needs of the local manager in mind. At the same time, the systems should be based on standards to allow cross-hospital and cross-state benchmarking.

The rest of this summary elaborates on these five main messages. The evidence and analysis that support the messages and the diagnosis of the underlying problems are described in this volume. The close linkages among the themes (highlighted in chapter 9) make some overlap unavoidable. Because of these linkages, a specific policy may not work as intended on its own.

Analyzing or evaluating hospitals, especially public hospitals, is difficult. The literature gives little guidance on appropriate methodologies. What studies do exist usually come from the United States and a handful of European countries, and the findings may not be applicable to low- and middle-income countries with fewer health resources. The findings and recommendations in this volume are based on available evidence in Brazil, drawn from a mix of sources. Limitations related to the availability and quality of data and the use of small sample sizes restricted the breadth and depth of some of the analyses reported in this volume.

Problems in Brazil's Hospital Sector and Action Recommendations

This section examines the main problems in Brazil's hospital sector. For each, short- and medium-term actions to remedy the shortcomings are suggested.

Rigid and Unaccountable Hospital Governance: Hospital Types and Performance

Incentives given by payment mechanisms, contracts, and regulations clearly influence provider behavior. But hospitals do not all respond the same way to similar incentives. A hospital's response to incentives depends on its organizational form. The evidence presented in this volume indicates that organizational arrangements make a difference to hospital performance.

A range of distinct hospital types has emerged in the past 50 years in Brazil, particularly in the public and nonprofit subsectors. The direct administration form dominates the organizational landscape in the public sector, representing over 97 percent of all public hospitals. These are the most poorly performing hospitals across the board. Some public hospitals, operating under autonomous organizational models, display higher production, efficiency, and quality than direct administration facilities; indeed, their efficiency rivals that of for-profit private hospitals (figure 1). They also appear to achieve greater gains in efficiency and quality over time than do nonautonomous facilities.

Some characteristics of the organizational forms involved suggest reasons why this should be so. Hospitals under direct administration display a rigidity that is inherently at odds with modern hospital management. Given the existing organizational rules, even motivated and committed managers can make only limited improvements. Hospital managers who do not have the authority to manage staff, reorganize departments, or reconfigure services, are simply not able to make the changes that could substantially improve their operations. Many managerial functions are rule-based and are centralized in higher administrative levels within municipal and state health, finance, and administrative secretariats. In addition to being far removed from the front line of service provision, most central-level managers lack the know-how, motivation, or information to manage hospitals. Excessive centralization of managerial functions, combined with rigid civil service rules, political interference, and lack of information, spawn an organizational environment that deprives facility managers of the means to manage and improve performance.

Deficient governance practices and organizational arrangements contribute to low performance in many private hospitals, as well. But the nature of these hospitals' problems is qualitatively different from those of public facilities. Because of lack of information, the relation between performance and governance arrangements in private facilities remains unknown, but it is probable that overlapping and informal governance and management

FIGURE 1
DEA Efficiency Scores, by Organizational Arrangement and Ownership, Hospitals with More Than 50 Beds, 2002
(N = 248)

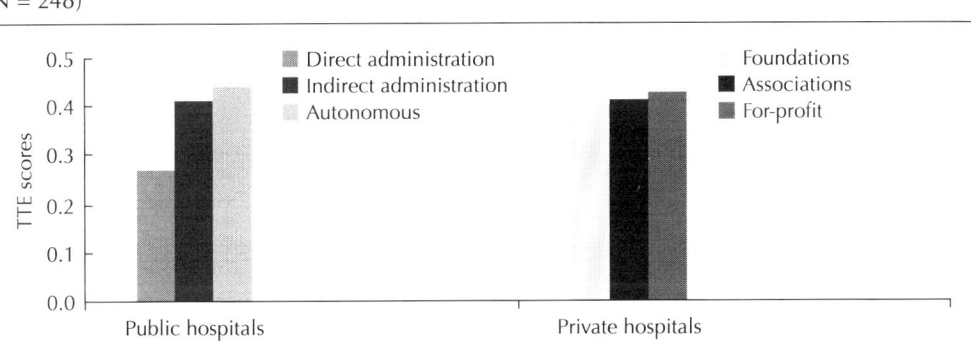

Source: Table 5.7, chapter 5 in this volume.

functions (as seen in table 1), together with lax monitoring and a weak information environment, may compromise performance. This is especially true in the small, nonprofit facilities that account for most SUS-financed private hospitals. The weakness of contract pressures and the lack of competition mean that the hospitals have few incentives to perform and therefore to address organizational shortcomings. An undetermined number of hospitals appear to serve the interests of their medical professionals rather than the broader health system.

Policy Priority: Enhance Hospital Autonomy and Accountability

- Develop a strategy, regulatory framework, and implementation plan to convert direct and indirect administration facilities to alternative organizational arrangements that offer autonomous authority and flexible human resource management.
- Formulate an investment policy that promotes the application of autonomous organizational arrangements in any new public hospital.
- Establish public-private mechanisms to strengthen governance arrangements in private hospitals under contract with the SUS, including regulatory reform and enforcement, strengthening of contracting, and stimulation of competition.

The most promising arrangement for public hospitals is a model based on experience with health social organizations (*organizações sociais em saúde*, OSSs) in São Paulo state. As table 2 shows, OSSs have proved more productive and efficient providers of higher quality care than comparison facilities under direct administration, and they also give better value for money. The elements of the OSS model therefore merit policy makers' attention. The findings suggest that OSSs benefit from an accountability arrangement that includes five key elements: autonomy, flexible human resource management, strategic purchasing, contract enforcement, and a robust information environment. These elements should be building blocks in any reform strategy for the Brazilian hospital sector. A recent MS proposal (2007) to create a new institutional form for public hospitals, state foundations (*fundações estaduais*), contains all these elements and represents a promising step forward.

TABLE 1
Executives Responsible for Nonprofit Hospital Management, by Hospital Size and Type, 2002
(percent)

	Individual facilities		
Type of executive	Small (N = 69)	Large (N = 15)	Facilities operated by conglomerates (N = 80)[a]
Hospital-based executive	49	33	99
PCO statutory executive	22	33	0
PCO executive director and statutory executive	29	33	0
Total	100	100	100

Source: Barbosa et al. 2002.
Note: Small: mean = 67. Large: average = 576 beds. Conglomerates: average = 136 beds. PCO, philanthropic or charitable organization. Columns may not sum to 100 percent because of rounding.
a. Eleven conglomerates with a total of 80 hospitals. Data were unavailable for one facility.

TABLE 2
Comparison of Selected Quality and Efficiency Indicators, Hospitals under OSS and Direct Administration Arrangements, São Paulo State, 2003

Indicator	OSS hospitals (N = 12)		Direct administration hospitals (N = 12)[a]	
	Mean	Range	Mean	Range
Quality (mortality rate)				
General[b]	3.3	2.7–5.8	5.3	3.2–9.1
Surgical[b]	2.6	1.7–4.8	3.6	0.9–10.3
Clinical	11.6	9.5–14.0	12.0	10.7–14.1
Pediatric	2.8	1.7–4.2	2.6	1.1–4.9
Allocative efficiency (hours: full-time equivalent)[c]				
Physician[d]	143	95–273	203	90–339
Nurse	54	24–100	41	7–64
Auxiliary	234	78–385	257	89–391
Efficiency: descriptive statistics				
Bed turnover rate[e]	5.2	3.7–7.6	3.3	1.9–4.8
Bed substitution rate[e]	1.2	0.1–3.8	3.9	1.7–9.7
Bed occupancy rate[d]	81	52–99	63	38–76
Average length of stay (ALOS)[d]	4.2	3.8–5.6	5.4	4.1–8.1
ALOS surgery[b]	4.8	3.0–5.7	5.9	2.3–7.7
Technical efficiency (discharges/bed)				
General[e]	60	43–94	46	32–73
Surgical[d]	71	24–103	44	27–84
Clinical[d]	86	25–198	53	17–101
GYN/OB(N = 20)[b]	96	34–169	58	24–80
Annual spending (R$ thousands)				
Expenditures/bed	177	116–279	187	149–227
Expenditures/discharge[d]	2.9	2.3–3.9	4.3	2.9–7.0

Source: Costa and Mendes 2005.
a. For allocative efficiency and descriptive statistics, N = 10.
b. $p < .10$.
c. Full time equivalent = total hours/40.
d. $p < .05$. e. $p < .01$.

Autonomy appears to be the critical feature of the organizational models. Policies to enhance the autonomy of public hospital management are a prerequisite for addressing most of the performance issues in public hospitals discussed in this volume. Many of the current policy discussions focus on expanding resources and improving skills. None of these changes will have the desired effect, however, if hospital managers are not given enough flexibility to make needed changes. Various implementation strategies can be explored; some countries have implemented sectorwide organizational changes in public hospital governance, while others have phased in governance reforms.

Mandating organizational changes in new hospitals—as in the case of the OSSs—is an important first step, but it will have no effect on the hospitals where most patients are treated. The recent MS proposal to convert public hospitals into independent state foundations incorporated under private law would establish a robust policy and legal framework for autonomous management of public facilities. In any event, it seems clear that an implementation and transition strategy must be developed for existing hospitals. Actions are needed to develop hospital conversion strategies and test them against Brazilian and international experience. Because of the thorny human resource and financial issues involved, conversion will require leadership and a strong policy push. Tinkering at the margins is unlikely to improve organizational arrangements.

Weak governance is not limited to the public sector. Although private hospitals do not suffer from the rigidities and lack of decision-making authority seen in public facilities, informality and the absence of clear lines of authority contribute to deficiencies in their performance. Action is needed to strengthen regulations specifying governance arrangements and functions in nonprofit hospitals and to enforce these provisions. Additional measures include strengthening contracting and promoting competition for public contracts. These measures will increase pressures to perform, which would stimulate efforts to correct governance shortcomings. In some cases the governance arrangement will require modification so that the facility can be held accountable for pursuing health system objectives.

Passive, Distorted, and Diluted Funding: Flaws in the Payment Mechanisms Used in Brazil

The term *provider payment mechanism* (PPM) refers to the way in which purchasers compensate health care providers for their services. Through incentives, PPMs shape hospital behaviors and therefore their performance. PPMs are powerful levers that purchasers, including government and private insurers, can use to make providers responsive to policies and priorities such as improving quality, raising efficiency, expanding access, and containing costs.

In Brazil payment mechanisms are little used as policy instruments for supporting policy priorities and stimulating performance. Most PPMs used in Brazil are deficient; they are not linked to costs, they are unrelated to diagnoses, and they are not adjusted for case severity.

Some payment mechanisms such as line-item budgets (the predominant form in public hospitals) contribute to inefficiencies and higher costs. Line-item budget allocations are based on historical input and spending patterns, with no rewards for quality or cost consciousness. Budgets provide few incentives to raise productivity, adopt managerial innovations, stimulate managerial flexibility, decrease excess capacity, or establish a sound information environment. Because of the limitations of this mechanism, most high-income countries that once used line-item budgets to pay hospitals are replacing them with more sophisticated systems that contain vigorous performance incentives.

In contrast, in recent years the SUS has expanded line-item budgets as the main payment mechanism for public hospitals. This step responds to the increased use by the federal government of direct transfers (*fundo-a-fundo*) to states and municipalities, which, in turn, convert these transfers into line-item budgets. Since the transfers themselves are unlinked to performance, subnational entities have few incentives to develop and implement performance-enhancing PPMs for hospitals.

The AIH payment mechanism, consisting of a predefined fee schedule linked to outputs (in the form of procedures), is used to pay private hospitals under contract with the SUS and in principle could promote more efficient resource use. But as currently applied, it contributes only modestly to cost control because the payment rates are seriously distorted. For most inpatient care, AIH payment rates are much below cost, whereas they are substantially over cost for a few treatments and procedures, mostly high-complexity care (see figure 2). The result is overemphasis on a few "profitable" services and not enough provision of money-losing but high-volume services. This imbalance seriously undermines patient access to needed services and cost-effective use of public resources. It is also a major driver of the well-publicized financial crisis in the nonprofit hospital sector, which is heavily dependent on SUS funding. Moreover, it may drive hospitals to provide overlapping services or submit fraudulent coding to raise revenues; to specialize in lucrative treatments; and to seek (and depend on) lump-sum bailouts from local governments to make ends meet.

SUS-imposed expenditure ceilings set an overall limit on spending but do not drive behaviors that result in efficient resource use at the facility level. The ceilings themselves are based on historical trends and therefore perpetuate inefficiencies that have become embedded over the years; in addition, they are adjusted depending on government tax revenues during the fiscal year. Moreover, hospitals often reduce service supply near the end of the fiscal year as they approach their assigned ceilings and then exert political pressure for additional budgetary transfers, or they may reduce planned outlays for equipment maintenance and material inputs. In general, financial planning and management, along with efforts to improve the efficiency of resource use so as to stay within expenditure limits, are rare. The passive and nonstrategic utilization of SUS funds for hospital care is striking because in pluralistic hospital systems public funding is usually the most influential instrument for pursuing efficiency and quality.

FIGURE 2
Mean Ratio, SUS Schedululed Payments to Cost by Complexity of Procedure, 2002
(N = 107)

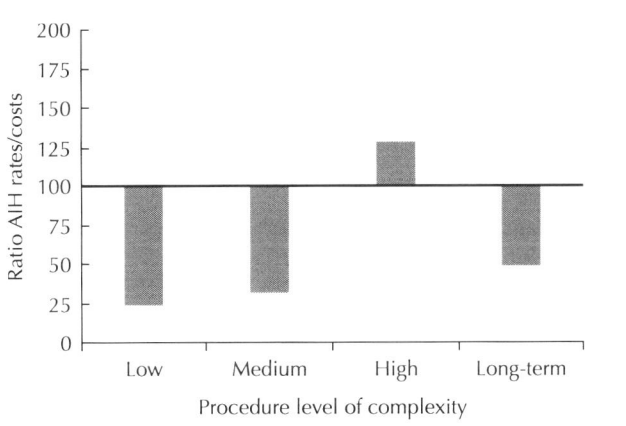

Source: Dias, Couttolenc, and de Matos 2004.

Payment systems in the private sector also encourage providers to increase production of services, sometimes leading to oversupply of the most lucrative services and to unnecessary, and higher costs. Most private insurers and health plans pay for hospital care through a pre-defined fee schedule negotiated between the plans and hospitals. The payment systems based on fee schedules that are used by private insurers are associated with more efficient use of resources, but this may be because private facilities usually treat less complex and less severe cases than do many public facilities and enjoy far more managerial autonomy. Rate setting has little to do with costs or with resource use, partly because of the absence of reliable information on costs and a lack of cost consciousness among providers and insurers alike. As in the case of the SUS, discrepancies between rates and costs in the private sector have not been systematically analyzed, but the disputes over rates between insurers and providers (e.g., hospitals and physicians) that are often aired in the press suggest that fee schedules are not aligned with costs. The impact of discounted fee schedules on cost containment appears modest at best because private facilities, like SUS-funded hospitals, have an incentive to overprovide better-reimbursed treatments.

The multiple payment systems confronting the typical hospital manager dilutes the impact of the incentives in any single mechanism (see figure 3). Incentives for improving efficiency and quality or controlling costs in one PPM may be offset by disincentives in another. Discrepancies in payment rates may contribute to systemwide distortions. For example, lower-rate payers such as the SUS may drive hospitals to skimp on quality, shift costs to higher-rate payers, or transfer complex cases to public facilities that do not depend on production-based payment but are bound to treat everyone. Increasing numbers of private hospitals cater to patients covered by private health plans, which pay higher rates than the SUS and cover higher-income patients. This contributes to stratification in the hospital system.

The financial relationship between payers and hospitals often involves contracting. Contracts are part of many payment mechanisms because they specify the terms and conditions of the payment. Although the SUS has a long history of contracting private hospitals to deliver hospital services, it applies a passive instrument, the *convenio*, which does not specify functions, define outputs, or indicate performance targets in return for funding. Convenios

FIGURE 3
Hospital Funding, by Payment Mechanism, 2002
(N = 428)

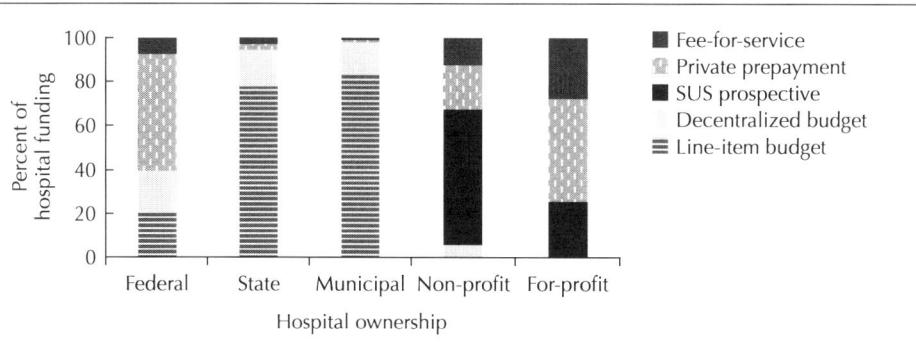

Source: Couttolenc et al. 2004.

are essentially legal instruments for distributing budget to private providers traditionally linked to the public system. The convenio, as a contracting tool, is devoid of accountability and is not used to create production or efficiency incentives.

What Can Be Done?

Enhance Leverage of Funding Flows to Increase Efficiency, Cost Consciousness, and Quality

- Enhance leverage of public funding (SUS) flows by
  1. Implementing alternative payment systems, such as global budgets linked to performance, for public hospitals to replace line-item budgets and build in strong incentives for quality and efficiency enhancement
  2. Improving contractual arrangements by applying instruments that specify volume and type of services and priority targets, linking a proportion of payment to performance, and enforcing compliance with agreed targets
  3. Upgrading the AIH/SIA system, aligning payment with costs, and gradually converting to a DRG-like system.[1]
- Initiate regulatory reform that will improve private funding flows (to constrain cost shifting and enhance cost containment and fiscal discipline), foster payment system consistency, and generate incentives for efficiency for hospitals and managers.]

Use of a global budgeting system by all public hospitals would impel improvements in performance. A few states and municipalities have already introduced global budgeting systems that feature resource ceilings and link a portion of payment to performance. Equally important, these funding arrangements leave hospital managers sufficient flexibility to allocate funding across expenditure categories in ways that will improve productivity and quality. The available evidence suggests that when combined with measures such as greater autonomy and strategic contracting (discussed below), global budgets would improve accountability and performance.

True accountability for hospitals requires more than governance arrangements and performance-based funding. It requires clear delineation of the roles and responsibilities of public hospitals and their managers so that what must be done to meet those obligations is clearly understood. Straightforward delineation of performance expectations makes it easier to identify and correct shortcomings.

Clarity can best be achieved through strong contractual arrangements that define the content of funding agreements. Such arrangements with SUS-funded public and private hospitals should establish clear performance-related goals, including specific outputs and results, as well as the resources for achieving them. Contracts should also specify the portion of funding linked to the achievement of the goals, as suggested above.

Changing the content of the funding agreements between the SUS and hospitals is necessary but not sufficient: the process of the relationship must also change. As demonstrated by experience with the OSSs and in many member countries of the Organisation for International Co-operation and Development (OECD), the funder's capacity to manage the contracting process and to monitor and enforce contracts, once established, contributes critically to outcomes. Most successful hospital contracting initiatives have included a contract management capacity-building program in the initial phase.

The contractual relationship must also minimize opportunities for bias in public contracting with public facilities. In organizational arrangements such as direct administration, facilities are essentially budgetary arms of the funding agency, and this creates a conflict of interest. Some countries have achieved an "arm's-length" relationship by implementing reforms that separate the public payer from providers. In others, where a number of public hospitals remain under direct administration, external bodies have been set up to oversee the contracting process and fulfillment of the contracted provisions. The latter option was used in São Paulo state to ensure transparency and fairness in the implementation of the OSS contracts.

If the payment system is to motivate all hospitals to improve performance, the system for paying nonprofit hospitals under the SUS must be changed, as well. It is critical that the funding arrangements provide reimbursement that covers costs, to ensure the financial stability of private hospitals and the achievement of minimal levels of quality. Once reimbursement rates are adjusted to cover costs, it is equally important to move toward using contracts to motivate improvements in quality and efficiency. Where capacity is sufficient to deliver certain services among multiple hospitals, the introduction of selective contracting and competition for these services should be initiated. In a competitive environment in which hospitals face the loss of money-generating services, they would naturally shift toward a more proactive strategy with respect to quality enhancement and cost containment.

Although no payment system is perfect, many countries have adopted case-adjustment methods such as DRGs to pay hospitals directly or to strengthen global budgeting systems. The main rationale for adopting DRGs has been to improve the efficiency of hospital care and to control costs. Although DRGs are not without problems, they have stimulated efficiency and cost containment in hospital services. Unlike the AIH system, which is based mainly on procedures—that is, services provided—and hospital characteristics (teaching vs. nonteaching), DRGs also reflect patient characteristics, such as diagnosis and age, and costs (relative use of resources). Thus, a DRG-based system is more effective than some others in linking resource allocation to disease patterns, risks, and costs.

The AIH system represents a building block for developing DRGs. DRG development, however, would require, in addition to the elimination of distortions in available AIH data on procedures, strengthening of data collection on diagnostics, to facilitate case adjustment, and the introduction of systematic and standardized collection of cost data.

A well-formulated DRG-based payment mechanism would contribute to another policy recommendation—reducing fragmentation in the payment systems—if private payers could be motivated through regulation or other means to utilize a common payment basis. In the current situation of multiple and often poorly designed payment systems, hospital managers face a mix of often-contradictory incentives and inequities in payment that leads to under- or overfunding of specific services, depending on the payer and the mechanism applied. A first step toward correcting this situation would be to study international experience in designing uniform payment systems. In any event, achieving uniformity of payment will be impossible without a solidly designed payment mechanism, such as DRGs, that can be used by the SUS, as well as by private payers.

Weak Coordination and Distorted Capacity Configuration

Delivery of hospital services requires close coordination within the hospital and with other providers (specialists, diagnostics, or primary care services). For health systems to work well, and for people to get good care, providers need to coordinate in myriad ways: with each other (e.g., sharing patient information to ensure quality of care and follow up); with the public health system (e.g., regarding reportable diseases for surveillance); with regulatory and self-regulatory bodies, for quality control (e.g., reporting medical errors, adverse events, and practice statistics to identify problems); and with funders and planning and regulatory bodies (e.g., obtaining approval to buy high-cost equipment or expand capacity).

By and large, publicly funded hospitals in Brazil do not coordinate with one another or with other care providers on patient care, referral, or follow-up. Even hospitals and other providers controlled or financed by the same entity, such as a municipality, do not work together effectively. Coordination between SUS and non-SUS private hospitals is nonexistent. This is not because the people involved do not care but because no mechanisms are in place to motivate and enable such coordination. And even in the best of circumstances, coordination is hard to accomplish, partly because of Brazil's federal structure, which grants state and municipal governments considerable independence. Coordination is further compromised at the subnational level by often fragile public administration, weak capacity to manage public hospitals, ill-defined responsibilities across subnational levels, precarious referral systems, and the absence of ties with non-SUS private providers. The situation has resulted in a blame game between federal, state and municipal authorities over financing, responsibilities, and results that is often played out in the hospital sector. Furthermore, most of the municipalities—which directly administer more health care delivery than the other actors—cover too small a catchment area. In the absence of regional or intermunicipal coordination, scale economies are not realized, and cost shifting takes place.

Problematic Scale and Location

Evidence from data envelopment analysis (DEA) presented in this volume shows that hospital size is the single most important driver of efficiency (figure 4). Many hospitals in Brazil are in the wrong places and are too small to operate efficiently or to ensure quality. About

FIGURE 4
DEA Efficiency Scores, by Bed Size
(N = 428 with 25+ beds)

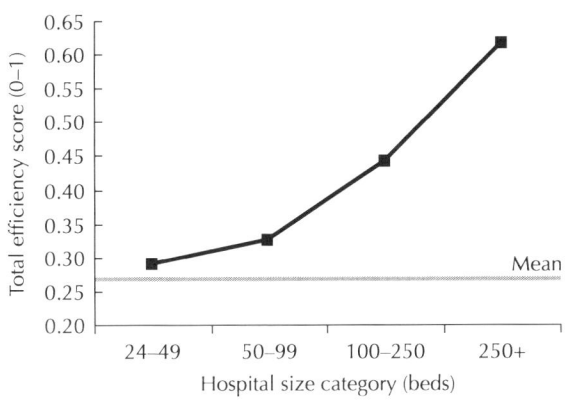

Source: Couttolenc et al. 2004.

60 percent have fewer than 50 beds, whereas international evidence suggests an optimal size of between 150 and 250 beds. Worse, small hospitals are severely underutilized, suggesting that demand for their services is limited. Despite low efficiency and utilization, many small hospitals survive through subsidies ("public donations") from state and municipal governments. These funds are generally secured politically and represent an additional outlay not often registered in subnational health accounts.

Small scale also contributes to higher spending and lower quality. For example, Minas Gerais state estimated that it was spending excessive sums of money treating low-complexity conditions in hospitals instead of at the more affordable primary level. In 2002 these conditions represented 40 percent of admissions and 25 percent of hospital spending in hospitals with fewer than 50 beds but only 13 percent of admissions in hospitals with more than 200 beds.

Higher volume is known to be associated with better outcomes, particularly for complex procedures, and Brazil is no exception. Higher mortality rates for coronary bypass surgery were found in facilities that performed fewer surgeries (table 3). As noted above, patient volume is closely associated with facility size.

In Brazil too much high-cost equipment is located in some areas and too little in others. Oversupply, underuse, misplaced allocation (in small, low-volume hospitals), and inequitable concentration of medical equipment exacerbate access problems and undermine efficiency This distortion of hospital capacity makes services much costlier than necessary and compromises quality. All levels of government, and many nongovernmental entities, own hospitals in Brazil, and so all these hospital "owners" make important decisions about equipment investments largely in isolation from one another.

Capacity Distortion, Lack of Networks, and Fragmented Management

Investment financing further complicates and often impedes coordination. The location, scale, and service configuration of hospitals strongly influence the cost of services, and therefore governments throughout the world guide the development of hospital capacity. In Brazil funding mechanisms for capital replacement are inconsistent and susceptible to political pressure. The current system sets priorities for public investments, but not on the basis of a rigorous needs assessment. The system is ineffective in blocking additional, and often politically driven, investments unrelated to stated priorities. For example, many small municipal facilities have been financed through this mechanism, usually to fulfill a mayoral campaign promise. Another important weakness in investment policies is that investment decisions are

TABLE 3
Coronary Bypass Surgery, Brazil, 1995

Surgeries per hospital	Number of hospitals	Total operations	Total deaths	Mortality rate (%)
1–9	22	93	12	12.9
10–49	31	681	86	12.6
50–149	43	2,947	264	10.0
150–299	23	8,077	509	6.3
300+	5	4,269	228	5.2

Source: Noronha et al. 2003, WHO 2003a.

not, as a rule, linked to provisions for recurrent costs. Consequently, health facilities are built and equipped but remain unused for long periods for lack of budgetary resources to cover personnel and operating costs.

Investment financing is rarely included in annual budgets or hospital payment mechanisms. Instead, hospital investment relies on ad hoc finance mechanisms that do not encourage rational decision making and planning. For example, a significant source of investment funding is international lending by multilateral development agencies. This lending is sporadic and is usually designated for specific areas. Another, more common, mechanism is legislative riders or amendments (*emendas parlamentares*) supported by individual legislators for special projects in their electoral districts. The MS has attempted to offer guidance for these investments to make them compatible with health policies and priorities, but it has not always been successful. In contrast to other systems with pluralistic hospital sectors such as Germany and France, no roadmap guides the development of independent hospital capacity to meet the people's needs and demands.

The Brazilian health system, and particularly the hospital sector, is organized mostly to provide acute care at stand-alone facilities. Network arrangements, in which various providers come together to formalize arrangements to manage and provide health care, are rare. The current organization is inappropriate for handling the high and increasing incidence of chronic diseases, which require integrated and continuous treatment arrangements across provider settings.

What Can Be Done?

Systematically Pursue Service Coordination and Capacity Configuration

- Develop and implement state-level master plans for care coordination and establishment of regional networks.
- Strengthen the national strategy for rationalizing hospital supply, including the transformation or closure of small hospitals, and improvement of primary care coverage and quality.
- Strengthen policy-based investment financing for hospitals on the basis of regulatory approval or investment master plans.
- Develop a national system for technology assessment and allocation.

Difficulties crop up in coordinating across political jurisdictions in highly decentralized systems, such as Brazil's, in which local governments own hospitals. In these instances, where the political jurisdiction is much smaller than the catchment population served by the facility, local governments must establish coordination mechanisms with each other, as well as with private providers. In Brazil this means that hospital planning and operation must be coordinated across multiple government levels and providers.

At least three forms of service coordination can be identified. (1) Where there is joint ownership of providers, and therefore administrative linkage, provider behavior is coordinated on the basis of hierarchical or employment relations. In the public sector this usually involves regulatory provisions or service norms. This is the current modus operandi for public providers in Brazil, and it has been unsuccessful, partly because of the constraints discussed above. (2) Corporations (public and private) that own a wide network of providers are another example of ownership-administrative coordination. (3) "Contractual coordination" operates through funders' contracting procedures and coordination requirements for contracted providers.

Government bodies do not directly control private hospitals, and given the constraints on norm-based coordination, administrative approaches to enhancing coordination are not feasible. Funding-based coordination through contractual arrangements may offer the best chance of success, but it will have to be complemented by pooling of funding and authority across municipalities. Resource pooling would mean putting federal, state, and municipal resources into a single pot to pay for all services and programs for a defined population-based network that comprises a number of municipalities.

Coordination across providers will be impossible unless there is a command structure with real decision-making authority over a defined catchment area, as well as a network of SUS-funded primary care units, diagnostic centers, and hospitals, including nonprofit facilities. To enable pooled financing and oversight, a coordinating body would probably require a governance structure involving municipal consortia or state-affiliated but autonomous foundations. An executive arm would manage the network. Although governance and management arrangements can be highly context specific, coordinating bodies need sufficient authority to allocate resources, including human resources, within the network (e.g., to distribute pooled funds to providers within a specified region that includes multiple municipalities); to make strategic decisions regarding capital investment, service configuration, and technology acquisition; and to direct or provide incentives for hospital strategic development—but not to direct day-to-day activities.

Much more needs to done regarding the oversupply of small hospitals and the inequitable distribution of technological resources. The current MS strategy regarding small hospitals does not go far enough toward reducing the unnecessary waste of scarce resources in these facilities. A more comprehensive policy is required—one that questions the need for any facility with fewer than 100 beds. Clearly, some small facilities are warranted in remote rural areas. Over the last 20 years, however, improvements in the road network have considerably expanded people's access to bigger and better facilities. All investments should be policy based and part of coordinated investment plans linked to service networks. Resource pooling could reduce the problems associated with too small hospitals.

The cost of having the wrong hospitals in the wrong places is an expense Brazil cannot afford much longer, in terms of both costs and quality. Significant gains can be made by guiding the capacity of the hospital sector toward a better geographic distribution, more economical scale, and better configuration of services across facilities. The best response to fragmented and politically driven investment is a policy-based investment strategy and funding mechanism. Either a sectorwide direct regulatory constraint via a certificate of need or an enforced master plan linked to public funding could work for Brazil. Both approaches have proved workable in pluralistic hospital systems elsewhere, with capital investments being undertaken by a wide range of actors, both governmental and nongovernmental. Policy-based (and enforced) allocation of investment funds precludes the construction of unneeded hospitals or hospital wings or the procurement of expensive equipment. The allocations can also be used to ensure that new capacity is located in places where the population is growing. In systems with pluralistic delivery a master plan is developed that contains medium-term plans for hospital capacity development. Only facilities and departments whose capacities are included in this master plan are reimbursed with public funds. Hence, if a municipal government builds a facility not included in the master plan, there is no assurance that any services will be paid for with public funds.

Although the MS has been discussing mechanisms to foster vigorous technological assessment, these initiatives have been timid. To reduce duplication, waste, and inefficiency, a strong national system for assessment and allocation of technology is needed. Such a system requires not only the design and implementation of a technology assessment methodology but also the training of sufficient specialists to apply and interpret assessment results. Above all, it requires mechanisms for enforcing the system's recommendations or decisions. Enforcement can be achieved through funding mechanisms (by allocating public funding only to technologies proved cost-effective—the preferred approach in the SUS sector); through regulation (the feasible approach in the private, nonpublicly funded sector); or by both means. Internationally, many of the successful initiatives in this area have established strong national independent bodies with broad stakeholder participation.

Lack of Systematic and Continuous Programs to Enforce Standards and to Measure and Ensure Quality

"Quality" is an abstract notion, easy to describe but difficult to operationalize. "Good health care" is difficult to define and often depends on country-specific standards set by regulatory agencies. Brazil does have some world-class facilities, but the evidence suggests that many hospitals are simply unsafe, with serious shortcomings in structure, process, and results. In addition to jeopardizing the health of individuals, low quality generates large, needless costs that undermine the affordability of the health system. Poor quality results in higher health spending due to overuse, underuse, errors, adverse events, lost information, repeated diagnostics and procedures, and readmissions.

Quality improvement has been mentioned in nearly every government health policy statement over the last 15 years, but few strategies and actions have been put in place to address quality issues in public hospitals systematically. The situation is similar in the private sector. The press seems to do a better job of monitoring quality than do system stakeholders such as the SUS, insurers, or providers. The media is not, however, the best means of monitoring quality of care. Despite widespread recognition that data on quality are essential for assessing and improving hospital care, the surveys and literature reviewed in this volume suggest that measuring and comparing quality is not a priority topic for analysis.

A commonly used measurement of structural quality involves the state of buildings and infrastructure within a hospital complex. Facility inspections by several state and national groups found disturbingly few facilities in compliance with licensing registration (table 4).

TABLE 4
Physical Conditions in São Paulo Hospitals, by Ownership, 2003

(N = 743)

	Public			Private			
Physical area	All	State	Municipal	All	Nonprofit	For profit	Total
Adequate (%)	50.0	45.7	46.5	44.0	30.3	62.8	45.4
Inadequate (%)	47.6	51.4	50.5	53.9	68.8	33.3	52.5
No information (%)	2.4	2.9	33.0	2.1	0.9	3.9	2.2
Number (total)	164.0	35.0	101.0	579.0	337.0	231.0	743.0

Source: CREMESP 2004a.
Note: Qualification standards are based on licensure legislation.

In other countries these hospitals would be deemed unsafe and forced to meet standards or close their doors. Reviews of patients' medical records showed that clinical management is also deficient (table 5).

Not enough is being done to pursue quality—although the actions that have been taken have been partially effective. Brazil has been a pioneer in the Latin American region in the development of hospital accreditation programs, but these standards are neither applied nor enforced in most hospitals. Only 55 of the more than 6,500 hospitals in Brazil were accredited in 2003; most of them earned the Level 1 accreditation of the National Accreditation Organization (Organização Nacional de Acreditação, ONA), which is essentially basic licensure. Evidence is emerging that accredited or externally certified hospitals surpass unaccredited facilities in quality and efficiency. In 2005 Control of Hospital Quality (Controle de Qualidade Hospitalar, CQH), a hospital certification program based in São Paulo, conducted a comparative analysis of hospitals participating in its Seal of Quality program between 1999 and 2003. Certified facilities far outperformed their uncertified counterparts on nearly all the efficiency and quality indicators selected for the study.

Hospitals that participate in accreditation programs have been found to develop and implement continuous quality improvement programs. Accreditation forces hospitals to examine their competencies, assessing and comparing the care they provide against the standards. Thus, compliance with the standards becomes the driver for a quality improvement process throughout the organization. Unfortunately, hospitals appear to have few external incentives to complete the requirements for accreditation. Accreditation is not yet on the policy agenda of the SUS, despite MS support for the founding of the ONA, nor do private purchasers place much emphasis on it.

When it comes to professional competence and behavior, surprising degrees of attention and neglect coexist. For example, Brazil recently implemented mandatory physician recertification but has no system for certifying the competence of medical school graduates. As to physician malpractice, although Brazil has regulations and institutional mechanisms to protect its citizens, the mechanisms have no teeth. Partly because of physician self-interest, regional and federal boards rarely pull medical licenses and are more likely to issue a confidential warning or censure (table 6). Lines of accountability in the Regional Medical Councils appear diffuse because neither the public nor the government is represented.

TABLE 5
Adequacy of Record Keeping in Hospitals in São Paulo State, by Ownership

(N = 743)

	Public			Private			
State of record keeping	*All*	*State*	*Municipal*	*All*	*Beneficent and philanthropic*	*For-profit*	*Total*
Patient records appropriately filled out (%)	31.7	42.9	23.7	16.6	10.7	23.4	19.9
Records incomplete (%)	55.5	42.9	62.4	71.8	80.7	60.2	68.3
No information (%)	12.8	14.2	13.9	11.6	8.6	16.4	11.8
Number	164.0	35.0	101.0	579.0	337.0	231.0	743.0

Source: CREMESP 2004a.

TABLE 6
Disciplinary Actions against Physicians in Brazil and the United States, 2001–5

Country or state, and action	2001	2002	2003	2004	2005
Brazil					
Cases (number)	141	184	239	231	344
License suspension, 30 days (%)	4	3	3	4	8
License revocation (%)	4	8	4	4	2
United States					
Cases (total number)	4,758	4,946	5,342	6,261	6,213
License restriction (%)	25	25	25	21	22
License revocation (%)	35	36	34	34	32
California					
Cases (state number)	495	569	572	651	624
License restriction (%)	26	25	29	24	23
License revocation (%)	34	33	36	33	35
New York					
Cases (state number)	503	461	508	534	534
License restriction (%)	19	21	28	38	29
License revocation (%)	51	49	46	42	39

Source: Brazil: Conselho Federal de Medicina 2006; United States: Federation of State Medical Boards 2006.

The countless isolated efforts to improve quality in Brazil have yet to coalesce into a national movement for quality improvement. Few systematic and continuous efforts have been made to measure and improve the quality of care in Brazilian hospitals. Generally absent are national policies, programs, and systems to support measurement and evaluation of quality, quality performance review and comparison, capacity building in quality improvement, dissemination of evidence-based research, and public disclosure. Furthermore, there is no institutional infrastructure for developing, coordinating, and implementing such policies. A few promising MS and regional initiatives, as well as facility-based quality improvement programs that are organizationwide and continuous, but their suitability for replication is unknown because they have not been evaluated. Without a concerted policy and an institutional effort to address quality concerns, any real progress will remain elusive.

What Can Be Done?

Raise Quality Standards in All Hospitals

- Develop and implement a three-pronged national strategy for quality assessment and improvement founded on three building blocks: system support, accountability mechanisms, and organizational development (see figure 8.1 in chapter 8).
- Institute a rigorous national licensing exam for medical school graduates.

No sick person entering a Brazilian hospital should face unnecessary treatment-associated risks. National leadership is sorely needed to establish policies and institutional arrangements that support quality improvement systemwide, but particularly in hospitals. Broad stakeholder involvement is required to formulate a national quality strategy and establish the institutional infrastructure to measure and monitor quality, to conduct quality-based evaluation research, and to provide technical support to facilities seeking to develop continuous quality improvement programs.

Another priority is to rapidly raise all hospitals operating in Brazil to the minimum quality standards prescribed in the licensure requirements. All hospitals should be required to meet these standards immediately. In most countries minimum standards are usually achieved through regulation—for example, by withholding or revoking operating rights for noncompliant hospitals. In Brazil such regulatory provisions are in place, but they are not enforced. Many facilities do not comply with licensure legislation on minimal structural standards and would be forced to close if compliance were enforced.

In any case, because most licensing standards pertain to only to structural quality, compliance with them is unlikely to have sufficient impact on the quality of care. Therefore, at the same time Brazil needs to expand accreditation to motivate hospitals to monitor and improve care processes and outcomes. Here, too, Brazil possesses well-designed accreditation programs, but their uptake is mostly limited to a few hospitals of and for the elite.

For both licensure and accreditation, an alternative strategy is necessary. The best implementation strategy is probably a gradual reduction of reimbursement rates (or maintenance of the rates at current levels) for unlicensed and unaccredited hospitals and the use of the savings to increase reimbursement for compliant hospitals. This measure should be part of a strategic purchasing framework in both the SUS and the private sector aimed at fostering compliance with licensing requirements and promoting accreditation. In several countries accreditation is broadly implemented via public funding criteria. For example, in the United States the Medicare program does not reimburse unaccredited hospitals. Accreditation is also required for hospitals to receive public funding in Spain (Catalonia) and Belgium. The funding reforms discussed above should incorporate financial incentives for hospitals to achieve accreditation.

Improving quality involves changing the behavior of frontline teams and cultivating within the organization an enabling environment to facilitate their work. A minority of hospitals have implemented continuous quality improvement (CQI) programs that target changes in the process or the environment in which quality problems arise. Basic tenets of the CQI approach in health consist of leadership, systematic assessment of performance, effective teamwork, proactive change, use of information technologies, a focus on improving all care processes, incorporation of evidence into practice, and coordination of care across different provider settings. CQI needs to be expanded to all hospitals.

These critical actions must take place at the hospital level under the leadership of hospital management. A range of policies is required to promote such changes. Managers need to be highly motivated to improve quality. Such motivation can be enhanced in Brazil via management hiring practices, incentives in hospital funding arrangements, and clarity concerning management responsibility and performance expectations in contracting arrangements. Even if such policies lead managers to be highly motivated, it is also necessary to give public hospital managers latitude to take action, as outlined in the discussion of governance reforms, above.

Hospital managers will need significant technical and capacity-building support from national structures to acquire the know-how to develop, introduce, and maintain quality improvement programs. Continuous quality improvement requires a systematic approach with a robust national support infrastructure. Major elements include formation of national policies or strategies to enhance quality; establishment of institutions (public or private) to measure and monitor quality, provide guidance to health care organizations, and strengthen their capacity; and provision of support for systematic research on patient satisfaction and evaluation of clinical practices. Recent policy initiatives in Australia, the United Kingdom, and the United States put quality on each country's policy agenda and precipitated an array of activities that, together, can be viewed as the foundation for national structures and institutions specializing in quality performance evaluation, monitoring, and capacity building. Such experiences can provide important lessons and guidance for developing similar initiatives in Brazil.

The quality of education in a number of medical schools is weak. Voluntary assessments of recent graduates suggest that some medical schools do not adequately train their students for medical practice. Although an exam will not directly improve quality, it may put pressure on medical schools to improve the quality of instruction. Publishing each medical school's results will enable future students to better select a school and thereby exert pressure on the low performers.

Lack of Information for Decision Making

The absence of useful information about the quality, efficiency, and cost of hospital services underlies all issues. At every level, critical information on which to base decisions is absent or incomplete. For example, hospital quality in Brazil is often based on subjective assertions and marketing strategies claiming "prestige," "trust," or possession of the "latest technology." Without data on processes and outcomes, such claims are difficult to evaluate. Perhaps the most worrisome finding in this volume is that the quality of care provided in most hospitals is unknown and is nearly impossible to measure because information is lacking. Worse, almost nothing is being done to measure and assess quality performance systematically.

Shortcomings of Hospital Information Systems

The absence of systematic and reliable information on costs, volume, outcomes, and patient characteristics impedes the design of robust hospital payment mechanisms. Payers such as the SUS and private plans constantly clash with hospitals over funding levels, but the debate lacks substance because of the absence or unreliability of cost information on treatments and procedures (figure 5).

Without systematic data collection, progress on quality, outcomes, efficiency, and costs cannot be monitored, analyzed, or compared. Any data available are often unreliable or not comparable because of variations in the definition and measurement of variables. The limited availability of sound data and the high cost of collecting primary data at the facility level compel Brazilian researchers to undertake small-scale, affordable, but often ungeneralizable studies. This situation limits the volume and usefulness of policy-relevant research on hospital performance.

Federal, state, and municipal policy makers are forced to make key decisions about resource allocation without having even minimal information about the quality, cost, or value of services. Nor do hospital managers have the information they need to spot pressing quality problems or to reconfigure staff and other resources to raise quality and productivity. Decision makers are flying blind as they seek to take steps to improve Brazil's hospitals.

FIGURE 5
Financial Information Available at Health Facilities, 2003
(N = 49)

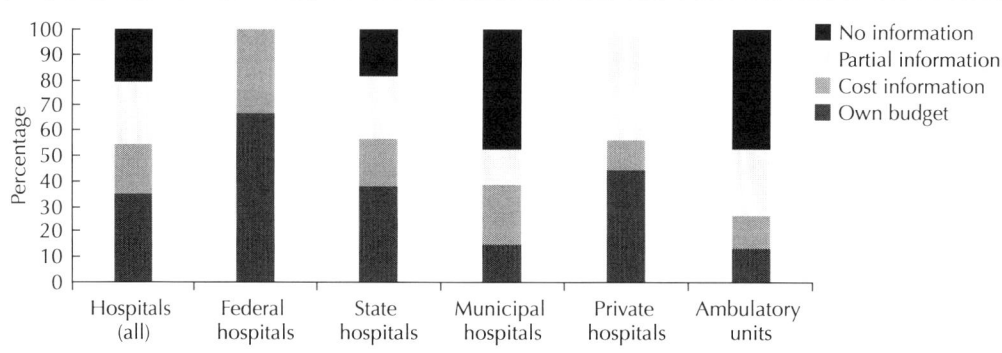

Source: World Bank 2007.

What Can Be Done?

Strengthen the Institutional Environment for Resource Use and Performance Management

- Promote the effective use of information technologies to support performance and outcome measurement, cost collection and analysis, access to clinical information, clinical decision making, and coordination across medical care organizations and teams.
- Support modernization of management structures and practices in public and SUS-financed private hospitals.
- Develop nationwide benchmarking and a public report card system focused on efficiency and quality.

Hospitals need information systems that allow quality to be assessed, problems to be identified, and remedial actions to be taken. These systems need to generate both quality-related information and cost- and efficiency-related information. To be useful for policy makers, the systems must be standardized across all SUS-funded hospitals. Standardized reporting, analysis, and presentation of information will enable insurers and patients to make knowledgeable decisions about where to seek care, and their choices can, in turn, put pressure on hospitals to make improvements. The federal government should develop standards to allow cross-hospital and cross-state benchmarking. Conditionality for receiving SUS-funding or bonuses should be used to motivate hospitals to use these standardized information systems.

Global budgeting systems were recommended above as a mechanism for funding public hospitals. These systems, however, do not always generate critically needed information about service costs; they must be tailored to support the establishment of a meaningful information base. Eventually, it will be possible to base hospital payment on realistic service costs.

For any of the initiatives described here to work, Brazil's hospital managers need modern hospital management skills—and few have them. Hospital directors, lacking these skills, function as passive administrators. A significant effort must be made to build the capacity of new and current managers to function as proactive, strategic leaders.

Three additional and desirable features of these information systems should be considered:

- *Selectivity.* The systems should collect and generate essential information useful for decision making. Considerable amounts of data are routinely collected in the SUS, but they are often irrelevant and are not used for decision making.
- *Utility.* Information systems should be designed with the needs of local managers in mind, so that they can actually use the information to monitor and evaluate the services managed.
- *Standardization.* Cost information systems should be designed for pricing specific treatment procedures, cases, and diagnoses. The data generated will provide input for a DRG-like databank and payment system.

Notes

1. SIA stands for Sistema de Informação Ambulatorial, the Ambulatory Information System.

Acronyms and Abbreviations

ABC	activity-based costing
ACERP	Associação de Communicação Educativa Riquette Pinto [Riquette Pinto Education Communication Association]
ACSC	ambulatory care–sensitive condition
AIH	Autorização de Internação Hospitalar [Authorization for Hospitalization]
ALOS	average length of stay
AMB	Associação Médica Brasileira [Brazilian Medical Association]
AMS	Assistência Médico-Sanitária [national survey of health facilities]
ANS	Agência Nacional de Saúde Suplementar [National Agency for Health Insurance]
ANVISA	Agência Nacional de Vigilância Sanitária [National Agency for Sanitary Surveillance]
BTR	bed turnover rate
CBA	Consórcio Brasileiro de Acreditação [Brazilian Accreditation Corsortium]
CLT	Consolidação das Leis do Trabalho [private labor regime]
CMI	case-mix index
CNES	Cadastro Nacional de Estabelecimentos de Saúde, Health Facility Registry, Ministry of Health
CONASEMS	Conselho Nacional de Secretários Municipais de Saúde, Board of Municipal Health Secretaries
CONASS	Conselho Nacional de Secretários de Saúde [National Council of Secretaries of Health]
CQH	Controle de Qualidade Hospitalar [Control of Hospital Quality (hospital certification program based in São Paulo)]
CQI	continuous quality improvement
CR	*centro de regulação* [screening and appointment center)]
CREMESP	Conselho Regional de Medicina do Estado de São Paulo [Regional Medical Council of São Paulo State]
CREMERJ	Conselho Regional de Medicina do Estado de Rio de Janeiro [Regional Medical Board of Rio de Janeiro State]
CRS	constant returns to scale
CT	computed tomography
CV	coefficient of variation
DALYs	disability-adjusted life years
DEA	data envelopment analysis
DRG	diagnosis-related group
EP	*empresa pública*, public enterprise
EPNL	*entidade privada não lucrativa* [nonprofit private organization]

ESE	*empresas sociales del estado* [state social enterprises, Colombia]
FA	*fundaçãõ de apoio,* private support foundation
FBH	Federação Brasileira de Hospitais, Brazilian Federation of Hospitals
FIDEPS	Fator Incentivo ao Desenvolvimento de Ensino e Pesquisa em Saúde [payment to university hospitals for teaching and research]
FIOCRUZ	Fundação Osvaldo Cruz, Osvaldo Cruz Foundation
FTE	full-time equivalent
FUNASA	Fundação Nacional de Saúde [National Health Foundation]
FUNDACOR	Fundação Pró Coração [Pro-Heart Foundation]
GDP	gross domestic product
HI	hospital infection
HMO	health maintenance organization
HU	hospital universitário [federal university hospital]
IBGE	Instituto Brasileiro de Geografia e Estatística [Brazilian Census Bureau]
ICU	intensive care unit
IDSM	Instituto de Desenvolvimento Sustentável Mamirauá [Mamirauá Sustainable Development Institute]
IMPA	Instituto Nacional de Matemática Pura e Aplicada [National Basic and Applied Mathematics Institute]
INAMPS	Instituto Nacional de Assistência Médica da Previdência Social [Social Security Medical Institute]
INCL	National Cardiology Institute of Laranjeiras
INSS	Instituto Nacional de Seguridade Social [Social Security Institute]
IOM	Institute of Medicine (United States)
IVH	Indice de Valorização Hospitalar [Hospital Incentive Index]
JCAHO	Joint Commission on Accreditation of Healthcare Organizations (United States)
LOS	length of stay
MAC	medium- and high-complexity (payment mechanism)
MDC	major diagnostic category
MF	Ministério da Fazenda [Ministry of Finance]
MPAS	Ministério de Assistência e Previdência Social [Ministry of Social Welfare and Social Assistance]
MRI	magnetic resonance imaging
MS	Ministério da Saúde [Ministry of Health]
NCD	noncommunicable disease
NICE	National Institute for Health and Clinical Excellence (United Kingdom)
NOAS	Normas Operacionais de Assistência à Saúde [Health Care Operational Norms]
NOBs	Normas Operacionais Básicas [Basic Operational Directives]
OECD	Organisation for Economic Co-operation and Development
ONA	Organização Nacional de Acreditação [National Accreditation Organization]
OR	occupancy rate

OS	Organizaçõ Social [social organization as defined by federal law]
OSCIP	*organização de sociedade civil de interese público* [public interest social organization]
OSSs	*organizações sociais de saúde* [health social organizations (São Paulo state)]
PAB	Piso de Atenção Básica [Basic Care Grant
PAS	Plano de Atendimento à Saúde [Health Care Plan (São Paulo municipality)]
PCO	philanthropic or charitable organization
PLANISA	Planejamento e Organização de Instituições de Saúde [Planning and Organization for Health Care Institutions, consulting firm]
PNAD	Pesquisa Nacional por Amostra de Domicílios [National Household Survey]
PNASH	Programa Nacional de Avaliação dos Serviços Hospitalres [National Hospital Services Assessment Program]
PNASS	Programa Nacional de Avaliação de Serviços de Saúde [National Health Service Assessment Program]
PPI	Programação Pactuada e Integrada [Integrated and Negotiated Programming]
PPM	provider payment mechanism
PPP	public-private partnership
PROAHSA	Programa de Estudos Avançados em Administração Hospitalar e de Sistemas de Saúde (a teaching and research program)
PROHOSP	Programa de Fortalecimento e Melhoria da Qualidade dos Hospitais [Program to Improve Quality of Hospital Care]
PSF	Programa de Saúde da Família [Family Health Program]
RTS	returns to scale
SAMPHS	Sistema de Assistência Médico Hospitalar da Previdência Social [Social Welfare Hospital Assistance System]
SIA	Sistema de Informação Ambulatorial [Ambulatory Care Information System]
SIH	Sistema de Informação Hospitalar [Hospital Inpatient Information System]
SIOPS	Sistema de Informações sobre Orçamentos Públicos em Saúde [Information System for Public Budgets in Health]
SIPAC	Sistema de Informações para Procedimentos de Alta Complexidade [Information System for High-Complexity Procedures]
SSA	*serviços sociais autônomos* [autonomous social services]
SUS	Sistema Único de Saúde [Unified Health System]
SVS	Secretaria de Vigilância em Saúde [Health Surveillance Secretariat, MS]
TCU	Tribunal de Contas [Federal Comptroller General]
TTE	total technical efficiency
UNIDAS	União Nacional das Instituições de Autogestão em Saúde [National Association of Self-Insured Health Plans]
UNIMED-BH	(cooperative health plan, Belo Horizonte, Minas Gerais)
USP	Universidade de São Paulo [São Paulo State University]
VRS	variable returns to scale
WHO	World Health Organization

1

Introduction

Hospitals are at the center of the health care universe in Brazil, accounting for two-thirds of health spending and a huge share of services. They are major employers of doctors, nurses, and many other health care professionals. They are the institutional leaders of the health sector, and their professionals occupy leadership positions in that sector. Hospitals are the centers of professional training and the main developers and adopters of new technologies.

Unlike the situation in most countries, Brazil's hospital system is highly pluralistic, consisting of an array of financial, ownership, and organizational arrangements that encompass both the public and private sectors. Brazil is also unusual in that it has a long tradition of public financing of private facilities.

Brazil is like many other counties, however, in that its system is highly stratified. A small number of hospitals are world-class centers of excellence, but despite the country's universal health system, these facilities tend to serve the well-off minority. Most hospitals can best be described as substandard. These hospitals, which are dependent on public financing, serve the great majority of Brazilians who cannot pay out of pocket or afford private insurance.

What is most interesting about the Brazilian hospital system is its dynamism. There is no shortage of ideas, innovations, and initiatives for addressing the shortcomings of under-performing facilities. The foundations for change aimed at raising performance are present throughout Brazil's hospital system.

Hospitals have an ambivalent relationship with Brazilian society. They are praised, yet distrusted; revered, yet feared. For physician specialists, they are centers of treatment breakthroughs, technological innovation, and scientific advancement. For public health professionals, hospitals represent a kind of evil empire, biased toward high-technology medicine and consuming large amounts of resources while contributing little to the public's health.

Most Brazilians value hospitals. Rightly or wrongly, they consider the hospital the first stop for treating a sickness deemed to require medical attention. They tend to pass judgment on the broader health system according to the perceived quality and timeliness of care received in hospitals.

Politicians embrace hospitals as favorite sites for photo ops alongside a new wing, a rehabilitated emergency room, or the latest equipment. Their behavior shifts to avoidance when the adverse results of hospitals' shortcomings appear on the front pages of local newspapers. For the press, hospitals are a reliable source of newsworthy material—medical innovations and miraculous cures, together with adverse events and avoidable injuries and deaths. In recent years a constant stream of negative press stories—usually, reporting on individual cases—has led to the general impression that many hospitals are unsafe. Some of the criticism is unfair. It is not the hospital's fault when patients in advanced stages of life-threatening conditions—pregnant women with high blood pressure or seizures, severely dehydrated infants, or stroke victims with poorly managed blood pressure—end up in hospital emergency rooms suffering the consequences of lack of access to primary care, where potential complications could be managed at an earlier stage.

Why This Book?

Hospitals, although arguably the main component of Brazil's health care delivery system, have received relatively scant attention, as health care organizations, from either policy makers or researchers. Since the mid-1980s, the development of health policy in Brazil has focused on decentralizing service delivery, reducing financial disparities, and achieving universal access to basic care. Issues of hospital performance, however defined, have been left mainly to the individual facility.

But as costs have escalated in the health sector, government financial authorities have become increasingly concerned. Calls for cost containment and for enhanced value for money spent on health care are growing. The share of health spending in gross domestic product (GDP) has surpassed 8 percent. Meanwhile, in 2006 the shares in GDP of Brazil's public debt (46 percent), public spending (over 40 percent), and tax burden (35 percent) are all significantly higher than in most middle-income countries. Because hospitals are the big spenders in the Brazilian health system and nearly 60 percent of hospital spending is publicly financed, curbing the growth of hospital spending has become an important policy issue for all levels of government.

Yet hospitals persistently complain about the insufficiency of resources. Stakeholders representing hospital interests pressure the government to raise hospital budgets and reimbursement rates, buy medical equipment, and upgrade physical plant.[1] Other groups, inside and outside government, lobby for significant increases in funds for primary care and essential drugs, salary raises for health workers, and reductions in interregional inequities. Municipal governments, which supported "municipalization" of federal hospitals in the 1980s and 1990s, are finding hospitals increasingly unaffordable. Indeed, burdened by the soaring costs of formerly federal hospitals, some hard-pressed municipalities now want to give them back to the central government—hospital recentralization.

In a climate of frustration bordering on hostility, it is convenient to blame lack of resources for the inadequate conditions evident in the hospital sector. Absent from the debate over sufficiency of resources, however, is any discussion of the costs and the efficiency of hospital services. Is lack of resources a main driver of low performance? How aligned or unaligned are reimbursement rates and costs? Are efficiency gains possible, and if so, how can they be achieved? Through in-depth comparative analysis of hospital costs and efficiency, this volume attempts to shed light on these questions.

Mirroring the social divisions in contemporary Brazil, a tiered system of hospital care has become increasingly evident. A small minority of hospitals, particularly large private facilities and public facilities affiliated with universities, have developed and introduced organizational arrangements, modern management techniques, and quality enhancement practices aimed at making these facilities centers of excellence that rival the best hospitals in high-income countries. These hospitals also lead the way in pioneering biomedical and clinical research. Most have been accredited by national or international accreditation programs. The organizational culture of these facilities allows for ready adoption of changing treatment patterns and technologies. Some of these institutions have recorded impressive achievements, as evidenced by international recognition of their quality of care. This volume attempts to cull the lessons learned from such high-performing institutions, particularly with respect to organizational structure and quality management.

In by far the greatest number of Brazilian hospitals, however, performance lags. This is particularly true of facilities that serve poor populations. These are the facilities where information is lacking, low quality of care makes headlines, production is plagued by inefficiency, and accountability is diffuse. Most are out of compliance with Brazilian facility licensing legislation. These facilities have difficulty adapting to change, often applying outmoded practice patterns and managerial arrangements. Under what conditions will these hospitals become higher performers? Or will they continue to limp along as second- or even third-rate facilities? This volume tries to answer these questions through a comparative assessment of high- and low-performing Brazilian hospitals.

As is the case with hospitals everywhere, the evidence increasingly points to wide variations in quality, production, and costs in Brazilian facilities. In light of this evidence, demand is mounting among policy makers and stakeholders to understand the factors underlying these differences, the incentive structure driving them, and, most important, viable solutions for correcting the shortcomings. This volume seeks to fill analytical gaps concerning what has gone right and wrong. It also aims to provide evidence of effective and workable changes, drawn from Brazilian and international experience, that can drive a hospital reform strategy and a long-term program of hospital development.

Finally, Brazilian policy makers increasingly face questions about the configuration of the hospital subsystem, facility size, the role of hospitals in the overall health care delivery system, and the complexity of the treatments provided. In Brazil, as in higher-income countries, chronic conditions are the main causes of morbidity and mortality. Chronic care is best provided through organized networks that coordinate care among providers and medical organizations at different delivery levels. Yet (mostly) independent acute care facilities dominate the Brazilian hospital landscape. Formal network or care coordination arrangements among different levels are rare, even among public providers. Partly because of the weakness of the primary care system, an unacceptable number of admissions are for conditions that can be more effectively and affordably treated at an ambulatory level. In addition—although it is internationally recognized that hospitals should have between 100 and 200 beds (Posnett 2002) to achieve economies of scale and scope and allow for sufficient volume to drive quality gains for specific procedures—most hospitals in Brazil have fewer than 50 beds. Using available evidence, this volume attempts to review the trends in the structure and conformation of the hospital system, with special focus on the above issues.

Objectives, Approach, and Conceptual Framework

This volume has three objectives: to contribute to the development of a medium-term hospital reform strategy; to develop viable options for improving the performance of hospitals that serve low-income populations; and to build consensus on hospital reform among policy makers and major stakeholders. To meet these objectives, the report draws, to the extent possible, on evaluations and research that apply robust methodologies.

Brazilian policy makers have watched the continuous expansion of hospitals over the last few decades, but few have questioned the role of hospitals in an effective health care delivery system. As in most other countries, persistent problems related to the financing, efficiency, and quality of hospital care are compelling government and private purchasers to consider policies for systematically addressing these shortcomings. Not surprisingly, the desire to rationalize hospital supply, improve efficiency in the use of resources, and raise the quality of care will drive hospital reform in Brazil. The articulation of a strategic vision of the reforms needed to improve performance will be crucial. Such a vision should encompass a set of policy elements that together can drive changes in the organization and behavior of hospitals. Although evidence is still emerging regarding the exact combination of policies that will foster change, analyses of trends and strategies in hospital care and hospital restructuring in developed and developing countries suggest a conceptual framework consisting of the three analytical dimensions that shape system performance:[2]

- *External environment.* The external environment consists of the policies, regulations, market settings, and payment mechanisms that together are important determinants of the hospital's incentive regime.
- *Organizational environment.* The set of structures and governance arrangements that enable the hospital to respond to incentives from the external environment shapes its organizational environment.[3] These elements include the structure and formality of accountability mechanisms, the scope of decision-making authority, the degree of market exposure, and financial discipline.
- *Internal environment.* It is in the internal environment that hospital behaviors respond to the external and organizational environments, and that resources are converted into care delivery. Important behavioral elements include resource management practices (personnel, procurement, clinical, financial, and so on); structural characteristics of the health care setting such as plant, equipment, and manpower; and treatment processes.

Together, these environments directly affect results, as measured by patient outcomes, quality of care, equity, efficiency, and patient satisfaction. Figure 1.1 depicts the conceptual framework.

This study addresses elements of each of the three analytical dimensions by separating them into six policy dimensions that are key elements for crafting a coherent and viable strategy for hospital reform: the structure and trends of the hospital subsystem; allocation and use of resources within hospitals; hospital payment mechanisms; organizational and governance arrangements; management practices; and regulation and quality.

The Hospital Subsystem: Structure and Trends

Hospitals are part of broader policy, market, and financial environments. It is difficult to understand the current situation of Brazilian hospitals without first understanding the health policy and reform environment, the supply and demand characteristics that structure the hospital system, the finance and resource allocation systems on which hospitals depend, and the historical spending trends and patterns that have often developed in response to these environments. These themes are discussed in chapter 2. Specific questions addressed in that chapter include the following: How do hospitals fit into the broader and ongoing health system reform

FIGURE 1.1
Conceptual Framework for Hospital Performance

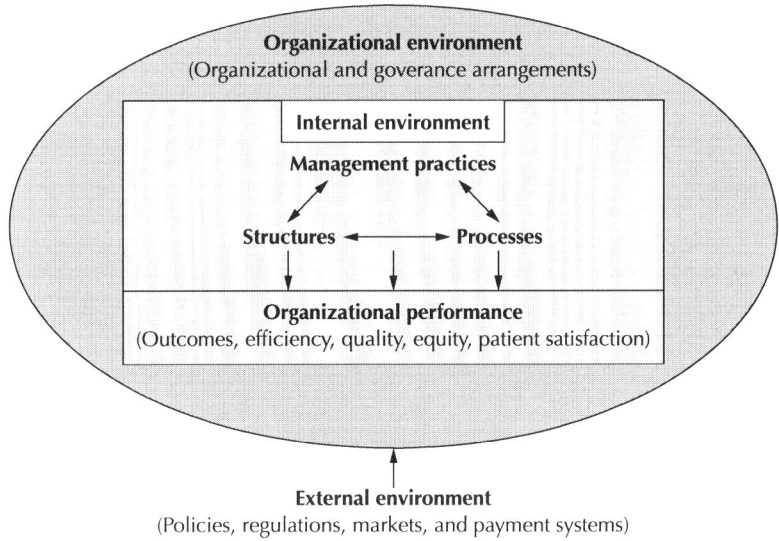

Source: Authors' elaboration.

process that gave birth to Brazil's Unified Health System (Sistema Único de Saúde, SUS)? How much does Brazil spend on hospital care, by source, payment mechanism, type of facility, and ownership? Who are the main buyers of hospital care, and how do they allocate resources?

Resource Allocation and Use within Hospitals

How well hospitals use the resources allocated to them to produce treatments and other clinical and nonclinical activities is an important determinant of performance. Poor use of resources prevents efficient service delivery, compromises quality, and results in higher costs. In chapter 3 the use of resources in Brazilian hospitals is analyzed from various perspectives: *technical efficiency* (to what extent hospitals obtain the maximum output for a given set of inputs); *allocative efficiency* (whether hospitals use inputs in the optimal proportion for a given price and technology); and *scale efficiency* (whether hospitals are operating at optimal returns to scale). Other questions addressed in the chapter are the following: What drives the variations in efficiency observed in Brazilian hospitals? What are the characteristics of efficiently operated facilities?

Hospital Payment Mechanisms

Payment mechanisms are features of the external environment that determine hospital behaviors. They create incentives that drive the organizational arrangements and internal management practices that contribute to efficiency, equity, and quality. Brazil has a mosaic of often overlapping payment mechanisms that together blur the incentives intended by each one. Chapter 4 examines the hospital payment systems applied in Brazil and their impact on costs, efficiency, and quality. Key questions include, How do costs relate to the reimbursement rates paid by the SUS and private purchasers? How do payment systems affect managers' decisions regarding the allocation and use of resources? What are the options for hospital payment systems and rate-setting formulas that would more realistically reflect costs, account for case severity, and provide incentives for efficient resource use for the delivery of services?

Organizational and Governance Arrangements

Incentives derived from payment systems and from market and policy environments affect hospital behaviors, but hospitals under different ownership and organizational arrangements respond differently, often depending on the extent of their independence, accountability, and market exposure. These organizational arrangements have much to do with the ability of hospital management to act on external incentives. Chapter 5 examines the various organizational forms present in Brazilian hospitals and how these forms are linked to behaviors and performance. Questions addressed include, What alternative organizational arrangements and innovative management techniques have been introduced in publicly financed hospitals, and what have been their comparative effects on efficiency, quality, and patient satisfaction? What are the leading and trailing practices of governance arrangements, and what are their effects on accountability to the community and to facility owners? What best practices related to the design and implementation of alternative organizational arrangements, particularly in public hospitals, can be identified?

Management Practices

Management practices are organizational behaviors that respond to incentives embedded in organizational arrangements, payment systems, and the policy environment. Management consists of a wide range of clinical and nonclinical functions. Particularly important for performance are functions related to human resource management, procurement, financial management, and contracting. Chapter 6 examines these functions in public and private hospitals in Brazil and their linkages to organizational structures. The chapter attempts to answer the following questions: How are managerial practices related to organizational forms? How does the link between managerial practices and organizational arrangements contribute to performance? Can management, acting alone, systematically improve performance without first modifying organizational structures? How can public hospitals with low-performing organizational arrangements and management practices be converted to high performers?

Regulation and Quality

Quality of care is an issue increasingly at the forefront of national attention in Brazil, as elsewhere. Although difficult to define and even more difficult to operationalize, quality is generally accepted as the determining factor in judging hospital performance. Quality improvement involves three kinds of intervention: creating a quality-enhancing environment through financial incentives and regulation; establishing systemwide infrastructure to support quality; and inducing frontline health workers in hospital emergency rooms, operating theaters, and wards to change their behaviors. Chapter 7 describes the current state of quality in Brazilian hospitals, while chapter 8 analyzes regulatory mechanisms and quality improvement initiatives aimed at raising the quality of care in Brazilian hospitals. Research questions include the following: What major quality problems and clinical errors occur in Brazilian hospitals? What approaches toward systematically measuring quality and ensuring quality in hospitals work in Brazil? What lessons can be drawn from these experiences? What approaches internal to the hospitals have been successful in identifying errors and modifying clinical practice? What has been the impact of the unified accreditation system initiated by the Ministry of Health (Ministério da Saúde, MS) in 1997? How can accreditation be expanded to more facilities?

Audience and Policy Environment

The audience for this volume is federal, state, and municipal authorities responsible for financing, purchasing, and managing hospital care. Private sector purchasers, facility owners, and managers make up another important constituency. Brazil's hospital sector exhibits a diverse mix of financial, ownership, and organizational arrangements—public ownership and management; public ownership and financing with private management; public financing with private ownership and management; and private financing and ownership. Other countries will have at least one of these arrangements, and so a secondary audience is the international community interested in issues of hospital performance and policies for driving hospital reform.

The policy environment is very favorable for a systematic review of major issues affecting hospital performance in Brazil. There is a recognized need to develop a coherent policy framework that will address both the external and internal contexts of hospitals with the aim of facilitating efficient resource use and improving quality of care and patient satisfaction while raising overall system effectiveness. Brazil's Finance Ministry and Treasury have called for greater efficiency in the organization and delivery of social services. Enhancing the efficiency and effectiveness of public spending, especially in the social sectors, is a major strategic objective supported by the government (World Bank 2006b).

For its part, the MS has taken some modest steps to put hospital performance on the policy agenda. In late 2004 the ministry published a proposal for hospital reform that included an assessment of hospital shortcomings.[4] Six major problems were highlighted: irregular supply of beds, with oversupply in some regions and undersupply in others; deficient management practices; lack of information on efficiency and quality; distortion-inducing hospital payment mechanisms; lack of network arrangements linking hospitals to ambulatory care; and high variation in the volume and quality of services across hospitals (MoH 2004c). This volume provides greater in-depth analysis of these problems.

The MS proposal contained a long list of recommendations for improving the management, financing, efficiency, and quality of hospital services. The ministry has acted, however, on only a handful of the recommendations: promoting the voluntary reduction of beds in small hospitals (fewer than 30 beds) or the conversion of these hospitals to ambulatory centers; implementing performance agreements with university hospitals and linking a portion of financing to a subset of negotiated indicators; establishing norms for certifying "day-hospital arrangements"; and creating epidemiological surveillance centers in hospitals.

Unfortunately, little information is available on the extent to which these measures have been implemented. The proposal has sparked an ongoing debate on hospital issues at the federal, state, and municipal levels. A number of the recommendations proposed for improving hospital autonomy, streamlining and consolidating payment mechanisms, establishing organized networks, and measuring and improving quality are major themes addressed in this volume.

The National Agency for Health Insurance (Agência Nacional de Saúde Suplementar, ANS), the government's regulatory body for private health insurance, in coordination with private insurers and prepayment plans, has organized a working group and has held a series of workshops on policies and practices for improving the efficiency and quality of hospitals under contract with these private purchasers. An important theme under discussion is the provision of financial incentives to improve quality of care. Private sector initiatives to improve performance are a subject of this study.

In 2006 the MS launched a set of reforms, collectively known as the Health Covenants (*pactos pela saúde*). These reforms represent the first steps in an important shift in federal-subnational relations in the health sector. Unlike previous regulations that normatively specified a one-size-fits-all delivery structure, the *pactos* aim to give subnational entities the flexibility to design and organize their delivery systems to fit the local context. In Brazil the federal government cofinances health care mostly through a grant-based financial subsystem, and states and municipalities are responsible for service delivery. The pactos specify performance targets to be negotiated with each level of government and specified in intergovernmental management contracts (*termos de compromisso*).[5] The idea is that future increases in federal financing will be linked to compliance with performance indicators stipulated in the contracts.[6] The policy also collapses more than 80 earmarked grants into six block grants. Although still a work in progress, the pactos establish the foundation for a stronger federal orientation toward results.

Finally, in early 2007 the MS developed a legislative proposal to convert public hospitals directly managed by government to independent foundations incorporated under private law. The proposal involves the establishment of governance boards that would be granted decision-making authority over all resources. As of this writing (December 2007), the legislative bill is pending congressional review.

Chapter Summaries

For the convenience of readers who may wish to focus on only parts of this book, detailed summaries of the chapters are presented here.

Chapter 2. The Brazilian Hospital Sector: Structure, Financing, Spending, and Outcomes

Chapter 2 provides background information on Brazil's health sector, as well as an overview of the hospital sector—its structure, financing, spending, and outcomes. Both the health sector and its hospital subsector are shaped by the configuration of the decentralized and publicly funded SUS and by a vigorous private insurance industry. The resulting system is pluralistic and large, with nearly 7,400 hospitals and 67,000 ambulatory facilities. It encompasses a complex mix of public and private funding streams, governance and ownership arrangements, and payment mechanisms that are difficult to coordinate, monitor, or evaluate. In the health sector reform that led to the creation of the SUS (which formally occurred in 1988), most responsibilities for health care delivery were decentralized to municipalities and, to a much lesser extent, to the states. Decentralization is financially supported in part by direct federal transfers to municipalities and states. The federal, state, and municipal governments retain complementary and often competing functions.

Brazil spends more on health than other middle-income countries: 8.2 percent of GDP (US$753 per capita in purchasing power parity dollars) in 2006, with 45 percent of the total coming from public sources. Yet it gets only average results. This is also true of the hospital subsector, with nearly one half million beds and 20 million admissions. Private providers predominate, accounting for 70 percent of all beds, but most hospital care is funded by the SUS through a variety of transfer and payment mechanisms that are being consolidated and streamlined.

Hospital emergency rooms, by default, are the gateway to the health care delivery system in Brazil. The country relies heavily on hospitals for 70 percent of emergency care, 27 percent of ambulatory care, and all inpatient care. Hospitals employ 56 percent of health personnel and receive 67 percent of all health spending. Given the "hospital-centric" nature of the delivery system and the emphasis on hospital-based care for acute cases, Brazil appears unprepared for the rising incidence of chronic illnesses, which require coordinated care across a number of medical care providers.

Since the founding of the SUS, a tacit policy of promoting public hospital network expansion to improve access has resulted in the proliferation of small hospitals: 60 percent of all facilities have fewer than 50 beds. This development has had important implications for efficiency and the quality of care. Despite the expansion, important regional disparities persist, especially in referral and high-complexity services. The disparities also suggest inefficiencies, with many metropolitan areas showing higher equipment densities than those observed in industrial countries. The abundance of expensive high-technology services, for which Brazil is a strong international benchmark, contrasts with a poor record on basic indicators such as maternal and neonatal mortality. These issues of efficiency and quality, together with their underlying factors, are taken up in the remaining chapters.

Chapter 3. Comparative Analysis of Costs and Efficiency

Chapter 3 analyzes hospital efficiency and its implications for costs and cost containment. It begins with a comparative analysis of hospital procedure costs and cost variations within and between hospitals. To help understand the relation between costs and efficiency, findings from data envelopment analysis (DEA), benchmarking, and regression analyses are reported for a large and representative sample of Brazilian hospitals.

The cost analysis disclosed wide variations in costs for the same procedures, both across cases and across facilities. The main contributing factors are large variations in clinical practice (attributable to a very low use of clinical protocols), as observed in medical records; the type of procedure (e.g., greater variation in clinical than in surgical cases); differences in case mix across hospitals; other hospital characteristics such as teaching status and ownership; differences in length of stay, associated with individual case severity or with efficiency of resource use; lack of standardization in costing methods; and weak patient information systems. After adjusting for case mix and length of stay, significant cost variations remain, even for the same procedure performed in the same hospital. The findings suggest that the cost variation is driven by lack of standardization in clinical practice patterns, giving rise to differing input use.

The data envelopment analysis estimated relative efficiency scores for the sampled hospitals and compared mean efficiency scores across hospital groups to identify sources of inefficiency. The mean total technical efficiency score (on a scale of 0 to 1) was .34, revealing a gaping chasm between most facilities and the few highly efficient performers. Efficiency was greatly affected by scale, with most hospitals operating below optimal size. Public hospitals operating under an autonomous organizational arrangement and private hospitals were more efficient than the typical public hospital.

Benchmarking also indicated wide variation among hospitals by ownership (federal, state, municipal, private for-profit, and private nonprofit). The average bed occupancy rate was low, below 40 percent, and was much lower than international standards, especially in smaller hospitals. Both DEA findings and personnel per bed ratios indicated excessive use of personnel in comparison to the best performers. Personnel represented a major source of inefficiency; the personnel per bed ratio is much higher than international averages. Other productivity and resource use indicators confirmed the inefficiencies detected in the DEA and benchmarking analyses. Regression analysis found that facility size, bed turnover, and the ratio of emergencies to inpatient discharges had a positive and highly significant effect on efficiency, as measured in DEA scores.

A high proportion (30 percent) of inpatient admissions was found to be treatable in ambulatory care. Such admissions could be avoided if the primary care network were more effective. No conclusive evidence was found that greater efficiency hurt the quality of care.

Finally, nonexistent or undeveloped national investment policies result in an oversupply of hospital infrastructure and high-technology diagnostic equipment in some metropolitan areas. Meanwhile, more remote areas lack such infrastructure and resources.

Chapter 4. Hospital Provider Payment Mechanisms and Contracting Arrangements

Chapter 4 takes up the issue of hospital provider payment mechanisms (PPMs). Brazil uses a variety of PPMs to direct funds to hospitals. Most private hospitals and a growing number of public hospitals receive funds through multiple channels, resulting in unclear or conflicting incentives for hospital managers. Both the SUS and the private sector are currently debating the appropriateness of these payment mechanisms, and a number of proposals for change have been aired.

The different types of PPM used by the SUS and private funders are critically reviewed in the chapter, and their advantages and disadvantages are assessed. A comparison of SUS payment rates with actual costs for a sample of inpatient procedures shows that, on average, the SUS pays well below costs. Furthermore, the incentives embedded in payment rates are distorted. High-complexity procedures such as cardiac surgery and organ transplants are paid well above costs, and basic, low-complexity procedures are paid at less than 30 percent of cost, on average. This distorted incentive structure helps explain the oversupply of high-complexity equipment and services and the increasing specialization of private hospitals in such lucrative procedures. The chapter also shows that below-cost payment patterns have contributed to the financial crisis of nonprofits, which are heavily dependent on the SUS for revenues. These facilities are increasingly seeking and receiving ad hoc public bailouts to make ends meet. Such bailouts provide few incentives for efficiency.

Payment mechanisms are shown to affect hospital efficiency and costs. Public hospitals funded through the traditional line-item public budget are the least efficient, whereas those funded through global budgets and other decentralized budget modalities perform on a par with private providers funded mainly by prepaid health plans. Private hospitals treat patients for less, but cost differentials nearly disappear once adjusted for differences in case mix. Private hospitals that depend on (greatly underreimbursed) SUS payments achieve good efficiency scores but exhibit low quality, suggesting that SUS underpayment of private providers is detrimental to the quality of care.

Contracting experience in the SUS is also reviewed. Although the SUS has a long history of contracting private hospitals and outsourcing both medical and nonmedical services in hospitals, contracts are generally passive instruments that lack service specification and output definition. Performance (if specified) is unrelated to financing, pricing is unrelated to costs, and contract management and monitoring by public purchasers are lax.

Overall, the chapter shows that the incentives embedded in payment mechanisms are diluted by their sheer diversity and are inappropriate because they are unrelated to service cost. The absence of systematic and reliable cost information, the lack of adjustment for case severity, and the distortions in the SUS case-based payment system lend further urgency to the need for a reform of hospital PPMs in Brazil. Any reform should also consider linking payment mechanisms to results through performance contracting.

Chapter 5. Organizational Arrangements and Performance of Brazilian Hospitals

Chapter 5 examines organizational arrangements in Brazilian hospitals and their relation to performance. The analysis focuses on three types of organizational arrangement in the public sector: direct administration, indirect administration, and autonomous administration. Although direct administration is the dominant modality in the public sector, accounting for 97 percent of hospitals, autonomous organizational arrangements have emerged in the last 25 years in the form of private support foundations, public enterprises, and health social organizations (*organizações sociais de saúde*, OSSs). The discussion of the private sector is focused on nonprofit hospitals, which rely heavily on public financing from the SUS.

These arrangements are examined to determine to what extent they foster the conditions (e.g., decision-making authority) that allow managers to manage and make managers accountable for performance, and how greater autonomy and accountability contribute to efficiency, cost containment, and quality. To this end, findings from four analyses are presented: (1) a comparison of the relative efficiency of hospitals under different organizational arrangements in the public and private sectors; (2) a comparative analysis of a sample of "alternative" and "traditional" hospitals; (3) a review of efficiency and quality indicators for a sample of OSS hospitals in São Paulo state with a matched sample of the state's direct administration hospitals; and (4) a study of governance arrangements in nonprofit hospitals.

The evidence shows that organizational arrangements make a difference to hospital performance. For-profit facilities are the most efficient, followed by autonomous public hospitals. Public hospitals under flexible organizational arrangements that grant managers decision-making autonomy are the best-performing public facilities, as measured by production, efficiency, and quality. Public hospitals under the direct administration organizational arrangement are the poorest performers across the board. Autonomous public hospitals appear to achieve greater gains in efficiency and quality over time than their nonautonomous counterparts achieve.

The most promising arrangement is that of the OSS-managed public hospitals in São Paulo state. These hospitals rival private for-profit hospitals in efficiency, and their quality of care is superior to that of comparable public hospitals under traditional organizational arrangements. The OSS experience shows that hospitals with the independence and flexibility to manage inputs, set case mix, adjust capacity, reallocate resources, and perform other managerial functions are better performers than their counterparts without such independence.

Although independence is a necessary ingredient for improving performance, it may not be sufficient. As is seen in the study of OSS hospitals, accountability mechanisms such as performance-based contracting and financing, combined with vigorous contract management and enforcement, contribute to performance.

Finally, although private nonprofit hospitals demonstrate an intermediate level of efficiency, because of lack of information no definitive statement can be made about the relation between the various organizational arrangements found among nonprofits and their performance. Overlapping governance and management functions, together with informal decision-making arrangements, may, however, compromise nonprofits' performance.

Chapter 6. Inside the Black Box: Linking Organizational Arrangements, Managerial Behaviors, and Performance in Public and Private Hospitals

Chapter 6 builds on the findings reported in the previous chapter establishing a linkage between organizational arrangements and performance. The central question addressed in this chapter is, how are managerial behaviors related to organizational arrangements, and how do they influence performance? This question is answered by examining management practices related to human resource management, procurement of materials, financial management, and contracting. A comparison of public hospitals under "traditional" and "alternative" organizational arrangements establishes that managerial behaviors differ with a hospital's organizational structure.

Because many managerial functions are performed outside public facilities, the chapter reports on the findings of an expenditure-tracking survey based on a sample of state and municipal health secretariats, hospitals, and ambulatory units. The results highlight shortcomings related to public sector administration and health management.

Although autonomy appears to improve managerial practices and performance in public hospitals, it seems to work less well in private nonprofit hospitals. Management practices in nonprofit facilities are far from optimal, especially in small facilities. Many small and medium-size hospitals appear to be unmanaged or informally managed, suggesting inefficiency and low quality. In the absence of contract requirements or competition, there is little pressure to perform.

The chapter examines why OSSs perform better than direct administration facilities. OSS managers respond to the incentive environment inherent in the social organization arrangement by applying private law to human resource management, developing and implementing effective procurement processes, displaying accountability through compliance with contractual conditions, and managing and reallocating resources to meet production and quality targets. Of equal importance, the São Paulo state government shows a willingness to enforce contractual terms by reducing or denying payments or canceling contracts. In contrast, the direct administration organizational arrangement fails to create an enabling environment for effective management and performance.

Two case studies from Brazil highlight the opportunities and obstacles related to conversion of public hospitals to autonomous organizational arrangements. International experience with public hospital conversion is also examined. Drawing on the successful OSS experience, the chapter recommends a strategy for public hospital reform that consists of five elements: autonomy, flexible human resource management, strategic purchasing, contract enforcement, and a robust information environment.

Chapter 7. Quality of Care: Still the Forgotten Component?

Chapter 7 assesses the current state of quality in Brazilian hospitals. Although quality improvement has been mentioned in nearly all government health policy statements over the last 15 years, few strategies and actions have systematically addressed quality issues in publicly funded hospitals. The situation is similar in the private sector: few private purchasers monitor the quality of care delivered by contracted providers.

Two quality gaps are discussed. The first is between medical research and medical practice in Brazil. For example, evidence shows that although cutting-edge cancer research is being performed in Brazil, the quality of care for most of the country's cancer patients is lagging. The second gap is between the quality of care provided at a few world-class centers of excellence and that in the vast majority of hospitals. While many of the centers of excellence apply international quality standards, most other hospitals struggle to maintain basic standards of infrastructure, staffing, and services.

The chapter examines hospital quality on the basis of a framework proposed by Donabedian (1980) and consisting of three components: structure, process, and results. Drawing on small sample surveys and microstudies, the evidence suggests serious shortcomings in each of these components in Brazilian hospitals. Many hospitals are unsafe, as evidenced by their failure to meet licensure standards for infrastructure, equipment, and human resources, or to comply with regulations for controlling hospital infections. Clinical processes are deficient, resulting in an array of errors, adverse events, and suboptimal practices, which in turn contribute to poor outcomes.

The quality of professional practice is also examined. Mandatory physician recertification is just getting under way, and Brazil lacks a system for certifying the competence of medical school graduates. The evidence presented suggests that some medical schools do not adequately prepare their students for practice. Disciplinary mechanisms to protect patients from physician malpractice appear ineffective. Of the few malpractice cases brought before medical boards, disciplinary actions are taken in fewer than 10 percent.

Perhaps the most worrisome finding is that the quality of care in most hospitals is unknown. Despite widespread recognition that data on quality are essential for assessing and improving hospital care, the surveys and literature reviewed in the chapter suggest that measurement and comparison of quality are not priority policy concerns.

Chapter 8. Quality Assessment and Improvement

Chapter 8 examines national, local, and facility-based systems and programs for improving quality. Among the most important of these are a government-sponsored accreditation system, a certification program and benchmarking system established by a state medical society, a quality-based purchasing scheme developed by a private purchaser, and a small number of government-led national and state programs. Although these initiatives are important advances, most of them are isolated, stand-alone efforts. Broader implementation by hospitals and purchasers has been limited. Some of these efforts have been short lived, and none has been evaluated.

Brazil leads Latin America in the development of hospital accreditation systems. Yet despite the range of accreditation and certification systems in operation, uptake has been disappointingly meager. In 2003 only 55 of more than 6,500 hospitals were accredited. Facilities have few incentives to participate in and complete the accreditation requirements. An analysis of hospitals with and without accreditation found that accredited facilities demonstrate superior efficiency and quality. Unfortunately, expansion of accreditation is not on the policy agenda of the SUS, despite past support from the Ministry of Health, nor is accreditation a key consideration of private purchasers.

Accreditation forces hospitals to examine their competencies by assessing and comparing the care they provide against standards. The experiences of a number of leading hospitals in Brazil show that successful adoption of accreditation is achieved through the implementation of quality improvement programs, which in turn are facilitated by the application of one or more quality management tools. The chapter reports on the results of a survey of hospitals that applied management tools to gain accreditation.

An undetermined number of Brazilian hospitals have launched quality improvement programs, but very few evaluate impact with the use of measurable before-and-after results. A case study of one hospital that did so documents the institutionwide managerial change processes and quality management tools, implemented over a 10-year period, that resulted in significant quality improvement.

The future trajectory of the Brazilian health system is away from acute hospital care and toward coordination or integration of service provision across a range of providers and practice settings. In Brazil, despite the outwardly integrated nature of government (municipal) — operated systems, many facilities operate as islands with only limited referral linkages with primary care, ambulatory, and diagnostic services. Many specialists in these facilities act as "independent craftsmen" rather than as members of a care team and of an organization that integrates and supports care delivery. The lack of a policy framework also works against network creation. A few states and municipalities, among them Minas Gerais state and Curitiba city, are experimenting with network arrangements.

Isolated efforts to improve quality abound in Brazil, but they have yet to coalesce into a national movement for quality improvement. National leadership is sorely needed to establish the policies and institutional arrangements to support quality improvement systemwide, but particularly in hospitals. Improving and maintaining quality requires a combination of actions in three categories: system support, external controls and accountability mechanisms, and organizational development.

Chapter 9. Conclusions and Recommendations

Chapter 9 synthesizes the conclusions of this study and presents recommendations for improving hospital performance in the near and medium term. It describes a subset of best practices and promising innovations, based on Brazilian experience and highlighted in the book, that can serve as building blocks for change. The chapter concludes with insights into priority actions for fostering implementation of the recommendations.

Sources and Caveats

Readers should note that analysis or evaluation of hospitals, especially public hospitals, is very difficult. The literature gives little guidance on appropriate methodologies. What studies do exist usually come from the United States and a handful of European countries, and the findings may not be applicable to low- and middle-income countries with fewer health resources.

The findings and recommendations in this volume are based mainly on available evidence in Brazil, drawn from a mix of sources. Limitations related to the availability and quality of data and the use of small sample sizes restricted the breadth and depth of some of the analyses reported. Where possible, international experiences were consulted to fill this gap.

This volume is based on an eclectic mix of research and evaluative studies. Some of the quantitative analyses (e.g., on efficiency) use large national samples of facilities. Others, such as those on organizational arrangements and quality, are based on small, local samples. Case studies and qualitative analysis have been applied to enhance the quantitative research. Again, the research was limited by the availability of information, the quality of national databases, and the cost of securing primary data. Consequently, the mix of analyses and methods applied varies by chapter.

The report draws heavily on a number of studies commissioned for this task.[7] The studies selected share the following features: they built on the recommendations of previous sector reports, particularly by the World Bank (1994, 2002); they expanded on results and made use of databases derived from recently concluded analyses that employed robust methodologies; they applied quantitative research and evaluation methods; they filled recognized analytical and information gaps as identified by in-depth literature reviews; and they were viable and affordable with respect to scope, samples, data collection, and analysis. The volume also makes use of other studies that applied rigorous evaluative and research methods. A number of these, however, are based on small samples, making inference difficult. These limitations are noted in the text.

This study is not meant to be a broad assessment of the state of Brazilian hospitals. Instead, a more focused approach is taken to address specific information and analytical gaps related to each of the six policy areas outlined above. As noted, the scope was limited by the availability of information and by budgetary constraints. Many of the problems facing Brazilian hospitals are recognized informally but have not been analyzed systematically, or have been analyzed with methodologies that were less than rigorous. As described throughout the report, potential solutions to the problems of the country's health system can be found within Brazil. Innovative programs and interventions can serve as beacons to shed light on solutions to issues and problems in each policy area. The overall approach has been to find out what works in Brazil itself, and why; international experience is cited in cases appropriate to the Brazilian context. The intent is to provide information about and proof of effective change strategies that together can drive a hospital reform strategy and a long-term development program.

Notes

1. For example, in October 2002 the Brazilian Federation of Hospitals (Federação Brasileira de Hospitais, FBH), a trade organization representing mainly nonprofit hospitals contracted by the Unified Health System (Sistema Único de Saúde, SUS), sent an open letter (Carta de Brasilia) to the incoming administration highlighting the tenuous financial situation of member hospitals. The letter claimed that the undervalued SUS reimbursement system was driving the subsector into bankruptcy.
2. The analyses referred to include McKee and Healy (2002); Saltman and Figueras (1997); Preker and Harding (2003); Eriksson, Diwan, and Karlberg (2001).
3. There is some overlap between the external and organizational environments. Both exert considerable influence on hospital behaviors and, ultimately, on performance.
4. The assessment was based on conclusions from workshops held in 2003.
5. Priority areas include senior health, cancer control and prevention, maternal and infant health, communicable disease control, health promotion, and primary care.
6. The Basic Care Directorate of the MS has already proposed such a performance-based financing arrangement.
7. The commissioned papers are included in the Bibliography.

2

The Brazilian Hospital Sector: Structure, Financing, Spending, and Outcomes

Brazil's hospital sector is large, with more than 7,400 facilities and nearly one-half million beds. It is also complex, encompassing a multitude of funding arrangements, ownership types, and organizational arrangements. Understanding the links among the parts is a daunting task, even for Brazilian systems analysts.

The health sector is shaped by the overall configuration of the decentralized and publicly funded Unified Health System (Sistema Único de Saúde, SUS) and by a vigorous private insurance industry. Federal, state, and municipal governments own and operate many health facilities. The private sector owns and operates most hospitals, many of them under contract to the SUS. Health spending is high in Brazil compared with other middle-income countries, and hospital spending is a major component of national health expenditure.

The SUS is the main single source of financing for hospital care, yet until recently no one knew exactly how much the SUS was spending on hospitals. Information gaps compromise estimates of SUS spending on hospital care (see annex 2A). The rapid pace of the epidemiological transition and the onslaught of chronic diseases may soon cause spending to escalate.

This chapter surveys Brazil's health system and the major characteristics of the hospital sector. The questions addressed include, How is the hospital system configured within the health sector? How much does the SUS spend on hospital care? What are the main sources of funding? On what types of care are these funds spent? How do Brazilian hospitals allocate resources among the different inputs used? How much is spent, by category and by type of hospital?

The Brazilian Health Sector

The Brazilian health sector encompasses two main systems: the publicly financed and managed SUS, which was originally designed as a social security system, and a large privately financed system consisting mainly of private insurers and prepayment plans.

The Health Reform and the Creation of the SUS

In the mid-1980s Brazil embarked on ambitious reforms that changed the structure, organization, and financing of the health sector, resulting in the creation of the SUS. The first wave of reform (1984–89) focused on institutional restructuring, decentralization to the state level, and establishment of mechanisms for social participation, with a universal right to health care as the emerging system's core value. The second wave (1990–95) emphasized consolidation of the unified system, "municipalization" of service delivery, and implementation of financial mechanisms for allocating federal funds. The third wave, beginning in 1996, attempted to reorient the health care model for basic care, separate institutional roles, enact legal and regulatory changes, and introduce alternative resource allocation mechanisms to support basic care. Recent regulations suggest the inception of a fourth wave (described below) oriented toward sharpening the focus on results in federal-subnational relations.

The establishment of the SUS in 1988 was the outcome of a nearly decade-long reform process. The Constitution defined the SUS as the main provider of health services to Brazilians and limited the (privately funded) private sector to a marginal but ill-defined "supplementary" role. Access to SUS services is universal and free by constitutional mandate, and Brazilians are entitled to all the care they need. In practice, fewer than 60 percent of the population, mainly low-income Brazilians, use SUS-financed services as their regular source of care, according to household surveys (IBGE 2000b). Many middle- and high-income Brazilians covered by private insurance do, however, use the SUS occasionally, particularly for high-complexity services or for services not covered by private insurers.

The SUS can be characterized by the following features: decentralization of service organization and delivery to municipal governments and, to a lesser extent, state governments; public financing of health services delivered by public and private providers; use of federal grant transfers to cofinance care provision at subnational levels; and formalized social participation mechanisms.[1]

The health reform that took place during most of the 1980s and into the 1990s was an incremental process that redefined the responsibilities and roles of the different levels of government and public institutions in the health system. According to the SUS basic legislation,[2] these responsibilities are

- *System coordination and policy formulation.* This responsibility rests mostly with the Ministry of Health (Ministério da Saúde, MS), although state and municipal health secretariats have a role in detailing and adapting federally mandated policies. Overlap of responsibilities is a constant source of stress in the SUS. Although intergovernmental coordination with respect to planning, financing, capital investment, and service delivery is a main feature of the SUS, it is still a work in progress in terms of implementation.

- *Regulation.* As in the case of policy, regulation is primarily the responsibility of the federal government through the MS, but states and municipalities complement and adapt federal regulations and may issue local regulations. Federal legislation, however, always takes precedence over state and municipal laws. Independent federal regulatory bodies were established in the late 1990s: the National Agency for Sanitary Surveillance (Agência Nacional de Vigilância Sanitária, ANVISA), which regulates the pharmaceutical industry and health and food services, and the National Agency for Health Insurance (Agência Nacional de Saúde Suplementar, ANS), which regulates private health plans and health insurance companies. Private organizations—for example, professional, hospital, and health plan associations—have traditionally played a role in self-regulating their areas of interest (e.g., medical and nursing practice), but government authorities seldom recognize the regulating role of the private sector.[3] The overlay of federal and subnational legislation has resulted in a convoluted legal and regulatory framework in which any new initiative can legally be both supported and challenged.

- *Financing.* The public financing function is split between several government bodies. The Ministry of Finance (Ministério da Fazenda, MF) collects federal taxes and social insurance contributions, and the MS allocates and distributes federal funds. The MS is also responsible for collecting reimbursement from private health insurance and prepayment plans for patients treated in SUS facilities.[4] State and municipal governments collect their own tax revenues and allocate them to health care through their respective health secretariats. They also receive federal grant transfers. In accordance with the SUS legislation, most of the financing derived from all government levels is pooled in a general health fund created and managed by each government entity (federal, state, and municipal). For example, municipalities place all federal and state government transfers, as well as nonpersonnel financing from their own revenues, in their municipal health funds.
- *Provision of health services.* Responsibility for service provision is split among states and municipalities, usually according to the level of complexity. As a general rule, primary and secondary care is the responsibility of municipal governments, while the state assumes tertiary and referral responsibilities. The Ministries of Health and Education operate a few (mostly referral and university) hospitals. The importance of state vis-à-vis municipal roles in the delivery of hospital care—as well as subnational capacity to operate and manage these facilities—varies considerably. In short, reality is much more diverse than what is outlined in the health legislation.[5]

Decentralization has been the defining feature of the SUS reform. Significant autonomy for subnational levels was a by-product of the democratization process that emerged from (and reacted to) 20 years of a centralized military regime. At least one observer has described decentralization as a "system shock" (Akhavan 2001), in part because the subnational level was ill prepared to accept responsibility for health care provision. In the 1990s the MS established (and revised) qualifying criteria that, to the extent they were fulfilled, essentially certified the decentralized status of subnational governments, allowing them to receive recently enacted federal grant transfers for health.[6] Access to the grants created a strong financial incentive for subnational levels to seek certification.

Certification is based on subnational capacity to plan, organize, and manage specific levels of care. For example, in the case of basic care management (*gestão plena da atenção básica*), a municipality is responsible for delivering basic care services and for managing and allocating federal transfers directed to these services, but not for providing higher-level services. In full system management (*gestão plena do sistema*), a municipality (or state) assumes responsibility for the management and oversight of all publicly financed services, activities, and programs within its geographic boundaries and manages all financial resources, from its own budget or in the form of transfers from higher government levels. By mid-2006, 682 municipalities (12 percent of the total) qualified for full system management, and nearly all the remainder qualified for basic care management.

Certification is mainly a bureaucratic process and has little to do with real capacity to oversee, manage, or provide health care. For example, although nearly all municipalities have been certified for basic care management, an undetermined number have yet to structure a primary care system or provide their populations with significant coverage. Because of the diversity of local conditions and the differing capacities for planning, analysis, management, and monitoring, implementation of decentralization has been uneven. For example, some financial resources are managed federally and others by states and municipalities, depending on the level of certification and capacity. In general, larger municipalities have been certified for full system management and more or less perform these functions. Although most municipalities perform functions related to basic care, leaving higher-level services to the states, large urban municipalities generally offer a broad range of medium- and high-complexity care.

In the past the MS has used its regulatory power and financial clout to encourage subnational health authorities to adopt federal policies and programs. For example, the qualifying criteria for decentralization certification tended to impose a one-size-fits-all delivery system based on a supply-side planning approach. Although most subnational governments abide by federal regulatory mandates, they are not legally bound to do so. Once they are certified for decentralization by the MS, state and municipal health authorities have significant autonomy to determine the organization and delivery of care within their borders, including the mix of providers. In other words, in the SUS one level of government has little direct influence on another, either vertically (e.g., federal to municipal or state to municipal) or horizontally (municipal to municipal). Nor do higher levels of government make full use of financial instruments (e.g., grant transfers) to influence behaviors at lower levels. For example, the Health Care Operational Norms (Normas Operacionais de Assistência à Saúde, NOAS), which were approved in 2001 and 2002, mandated the regionalization of medium- and high-complexity care and defined the role of the state health secretariat within a regionalized delivery system. Implementation has been lax, however, partly because the incentives inherent in SUS structures and financial incentives grant subnational governments significant autonomy.

Recent regulation has attempted to remedy municipalities' excessive autonomy—coupled with limited capacity and lack of coordination—in planning and managing their local health systems. The NOAS have put forward a strategy for regionalizing certain services across defined groups of municipalities. Regulations adopted in 2006 have gone a step farther, strengthening the regionalization strategy and defining the role of states while increasing their responsibilities in a to-be-developed regional system. A 2006 federal regulation revised the legislation on municipal consortiums and provided further incentive for municipalities to consolidate certain services between them. Still, although some experiments are under way, regionalized and coordinated services have yet to take hold in Brazil (see chapter 8 for a discussion of service coordination).

The SUS established a complex web of participatory consensus-building mechanisms to complement MS regulatory and policy-making authority and to serve as a system of checks and balances. These mechanisms consist of health councils at the state and municipal levels and joint commissions with participants from two or more levels of government. The councils, which are composed of representatives of government, health care providers, health professionals, and health service users, review and approve all health plans and policies. In theory, the purpose of the councils is to ensure democracy in decision-making processes.[7] The joint health commissions are the main forums for policy negotiation, approval, or rejection, at both the state and national levels. At the state level the "bipartite" commission consists of state and municipal health authorities. At the national level the "tripartite" commission seats federal, state, and municipal health officials.

The combination of subnational autonomy with mandated participatory mechanisms has resulted in an intricate system of shared responsibilities and negotiated decision making. The system functions through a mixed bottom-up, top-down decision process, implying constant and successive rounds of negotiation at multiple levels (see World Bank 2007 for an analysis). Although the MS is responsible for defining national health policies and priorities, state and municipal governments are autonomous and are not legally bound by federal policies as long as their actions do not directly infringe on federal legislation. Consistency and implementation of national health policies and priorities are ensured mainly through the participatory councils and commissions and, to a lesser extent, through financial incentives embedded in federal transfers to states and municipalities for specific programs.[8]

As suggested above, decentralization focused on empowerment of local governments, not facility or program managers. In most cases decision-making authority was centralized in subnational health secretariats or elsewhere in the public administrative apparatus. The way most public hospitals were governed and managed, or publicly financed private hospitals were contracted or monitored, changed little with the reform.[9] With the exception of periodic adjustments of hospital payment mechanisms, until very recently hospitals received little systematic attention from policy makers. In short, the reforms introduced few changes in the organization and delivery of hospital services.

Finally, both the negotiation and financing features of the SUS were strengthened in early 2006 through the approval of a policy collectively known as the National Covenants for Health and the Strengthening of the SUS (pacto pela saúde 2006—Consolidação do SUS).[10] This fourth wave of reforms represents the first step in an important shift in federal-subnational relations in the health sector. Unlike previous regulations that normatively specified a one-size-fits-all delivery structure, the *pactos* aim to provide subnational entities with the flexibility to design and organize their delivery systems to fit the local context. The pactos specify performance targets for each level of government and stipulate practical steps for regionalization and intergovernmental coordination. Although still a work in progress, the pactos establish the foundation for a stronger role for the federal government in using its financial leverage to strengthen subnational performance. The policy is innovative in that it promotes change in three ways: by directing resources to priority areas; by streamlining SUS management and financing; and by introducing contracting into the relationship between public entities. Furthermore, it introduces the possibility of performance-based payment mechanisms—a key feature for promoting change. Achievement of compliance with performance targets, however, will require development of instruments to enable federal monitoring of municipal and state performance, as well as strengthening of state and municipal capacity for planning, budgeting, management, and monitoring of service provision. Moreover, the reforms sidestep the difficult issue of subnational autonomy.

Despite these limitations, implementation of the SUS has restructured the public health system in Brazil and has been successful in several respects. It has implemented a national health system, rationalized the roles of the different government levels, improved coordination between them, and decentralized health care provision to the municipal level. It has expanded coverage to the whole population (even though a quarter of Brazilians choose not to use the SUS as their main source of care) and has reduced inequalities in access to care. Finally, it has moved from a vertically structured, disease-focused approach to an integrated health care model and has ensured participation of civil society in health care planning and evaluation.

The Challenge of Epidemiological Transition

The health reform, which, as noted above, was implemented in overlapping waves, was incremental but nonlinear. Measuring impact is difficult because changes occurred systemwide and no baseline data were collected, but time series data suggest significant improvements in health status over the past 25 years (table 2.1). Infant mortality has decreased sharply: mortality rates from vaccine-preventable diseases in children are negligible and diarrheal diseases cause less than 7 percent of all deaths among children under five years of age. The number of new cases of HIV/AIDS has leveled off, in part thanks to an aggressive prevention, promotion, and treatment system. For lack of comparable data, it is nearly impossible to attribute these achievements to SUS reforms, but specific programs developed and implemented through the SUS (e.g., Family Health, Disease Surveillance, and HIV/AIDS) have contributed to improved health outcomes, especially in life expectancy and infant mortality (MS 2005, 2006a; Macinko, Guanais, and de Souza 2006).

Neonatal and maternal mortality rates, which are closely related to the quality and effectiveness of hospital care, show much slower progress, considering that in Brazil over 90 percent of deliveries take place in a hospital. Maternal mortality reported for 2004 was 53.9 per 100,000 live births, down from 67.0 in 1980 (see table 2.1). These figures, however, are greatly underreported, and the adjusted MS figure for 2004 (not shown in table 2.1) was 75.4 per 100,000 live births. Establishing a trend over the long run is difficult because of the absence of precise data. Nevertheless, available data suggest a slow decrease over the past 20 years, little change in the last decade, and a worsening in 2004. The unadjusted figures have been stagnant since 1996, the first year of systematic reporting, when the maternal mortality rate was 51.6 (MS/Datasus 2007; IBGE 2004b).

During the last two decades, Brazil has experienced a demographic transition, with its population growth rate decreasing from nearly 2.3 percent to 1.4 percent (table 2.1). This, together with a concurrent epidemiological transition, has led to a shift in the burden of disease from infectious to noncommunicable diseases (NCDs). The latter now account for nearly two-thirds of the burden of disease (measured in disability-adjusted life years, DALYs).

TABLE 2.1
Demographic and Health Trends

Indicator	1980	1990	2004
Population growth (%)	2.3	1.7	1.43
Dependency ratio <15	66.2	59.5	42.8
Dependency ratio 65+	6.9	7.1	9.1
Fertility rate	4.1	2.8	2.3
Life expectancy at birth (years)	62.6	66.6	71.6
Infant mortality (per 1,000 live births)	69.1	47.0	26.6
Maternal mortality (per 100,000 live births)	67.0	51.6	53.9
Neonatal mortality (per 1,000 live births)	26.7	17.8	16.5

Source: IBGE 2004b; MS/Datasus 2007; Siqueira et al. 1984.

Note: The dependency ratio is the proportion of the population in the specific age group to the population in the working-age group (age 15–64).

The main causes of mortality include circulatory diseases (33 percent of all deaths), injuries (16 percent), and cancer (14 percent).[11]

The rapid pace of the demographic and epidemiological transitions will increase the demand for health care and the pressure on financial resources. The incidence of NCDs is likely to rise as the Brazilian population ages. The health system currently faces a dual challenge: to continue addressing the burden of communicable diseases and maternal and child health, while restructuring health care and directing resources to meet the growing challenge of NCDs.

Treatment of NCDs already consumes nearly one-half of hospital spending (World Bank 2005a). Continuation of the status quo will add US$34 billion to Brazil's health care expenditures over the next five years and will also result in economic costs of US$38 billion in lost productivity (table 2.2). In 2003 the financial and economic costs together represented about 10 percent of Brazil's gross domestic product (GDP). "Status quo" here refers to underprovision of health promotion and prevention interventions, weakness of referral systems, failure to disseminate and use cost-effective treatments, and the absence of functional networks to facilitate the application of case-management protocols across all levels of care (see chapter 8).

Health Spending and Value for Money

Health spending is a controversial subject in Brazil. Authorities at all levels of government generally claim that the insufficiency of (public) resources for health is the main driver of system deficiencies, particularly for the SUS.[12] For its income level, however, Brazil is already a big health spender—but only an average performer. Brazilian national health expenditure in 2004 amounted to R$147 billion (US$50 billion), about 8.3 percent of GDP.[13] That proportion is higher than in most middle-income countries and is close to the average for Organisation for Economic Co-operation and Development (OECD) countries. Even in per capita terms, the country's spending as a whole is commensurate with that of other middle-income countries (table 2.3). Nevertheless, public spending is probably insufficient given the universal nature of the SUS. By constitutional mandate, the SUS offers free of charge to all

TABLE 2.2
Financial and Economic Costs Related to the NCD Burden of Disease, 2005–9

(US$ billions)

Disease	Financial costs	Economic and financial costs
Ischemic heart disease	26.3	39.3
Cerebrovascular disease	3.5	19.7
Diabetes mellitus	1.2	3.9
Chronic obstructive pulmonary disease	3.2	6.8
Cancer	0.2	1.8
Total	34.4	71.5

Source: World Bank 2005a.

Note: Assumes status quo will continue. Financial costs are for the treatment of patients with NCDs. Economic costs correspond to productivity losses due to NCDs.

TABLE 2.3
International Comparison of Health Expenditure, 2002

Health expenditure indicator	Brazil	LAC	MIC	Low OECD	OECD
Percentage of GDP	7.9	7.0	6.0	7.2	8.6
Per capita (current US$)	206	217	109	1,743	2,283
Per capita (PPP US$)	566	486	569	1,755	2,341
Public share of total spending (%)	45.9	47.8	49.4	69.7	73.3

Source: World Bank 2005b; OECD 2005; WHO 2005.

Note: LAC, Latin America and the Caribbean; MIC, middle-income countries; PPP, purchasing power parity. Country group averages are not weighted.

Brazilians a comprehensive set of services that is compatible with service packages offered in high-income countries—yet its financial capacity is commensurate with health spending in middle-income rather than in high-income countries.[14] It is also worth noting that the public share of total spending in Brazil is lower than in most middle- and high-income countries (table 2.3).

Inefficiencies in resource allocation and use contribute to the relatively poor outcomes observed in relation to Brazil's current level of spending and in comparison with similar countries (see chapter 3). Although Brazil's health indexes have improved across the board over the last 25 years, given its spending Brazil is an average performer in terms of health outcomes (see table 2.4). Comparison of spending and health indicators such as infant and maternal mortality places Brazil at an average performance level in Latin America and among middle-income countries.[15] Many other countries spend less but achieve equal or superior health outcomes for their populations.

Health spending alone is not a good predictor of health outcomes across countries. Other factors, such as access to water and sanitation, education of girls, and the distribution of resources, can influence comparisons between spending and outcomes (Médici 2005; World Bank 2004c). Yet even controlling for these factors, some countries perform better than others at similar levels of spending and economic development (World Bank 2004c). This suggests that additional factors may modulate the effectiveness of public spending on health. Policies that direct spending toward addressing the health needs of the poor and

TABLE 2.4
International Comparison of Health Spending and Outcomes, 2002

Country or group	Health expenditure per capita (PPP US$) (1)	Health expenditure as % of GDP	Immunization rate (%)	Life expectancy at birth (years) (2)	Infant mortality/1,000	Ratio (1)/(2)
Brazil	566	7.9	94.5	69	25	8.4
LAC	486	7.0	89.5	71	28	6.7
Upper MIC	611	6.4	92.0	73	19	8.3
Lower MIC	307	5.8	81.0	69	32	4.5

Source: MS/Datasus 2005a; WHO 2005.

that seek to improve the quality of spending can help enhance health outcomes, whereas increased spending on, for example, high-complexity hospital care may have little impact on overall health outcomes.

The epidemiological transition, together with the demand for modern technology and the dissemination of medical innovations and new treatments, will exert pressure to increase spending. According to Ferraz (2006), at current levels of health system inefficiency, by 2025 total health spending as a percentage of GDP will increase from 8 to 12 percent, while household spending on health as a percentage of income will rise from 5 to 11 percent.[16] Ferraz expressed the dilemma facing Brazil as "how to meet the demand for 21st century standards of health care and technology with funds that, as a percentage of . . . GDP, remain lower than what developed nations were investing in health in the 1980s." Major additional resources are not likely to be forthcoming from government coffers. Financial authorities are increasingly concerned about the mounting costs of health care, which already represent 11 percent of public expenditures. As discussed in this volume, this relatively low value for money is in part attributable to a delivery model that overemphasizes acute care provided in inefficiently run and low-quality hospitals.

Financial Sources and Flows in the Brazilian Health Sector

The Brazilian health sector is financed by several different sources and through many types of intermediary arrangements. Figure 2.1 presents a simplified schematic of the main actors and resource flows. Following a national health account framework but with a focus on hospitals,

FIGURE 2.1
Main Players and Fund Flows in the Brazilian Hospital Sector

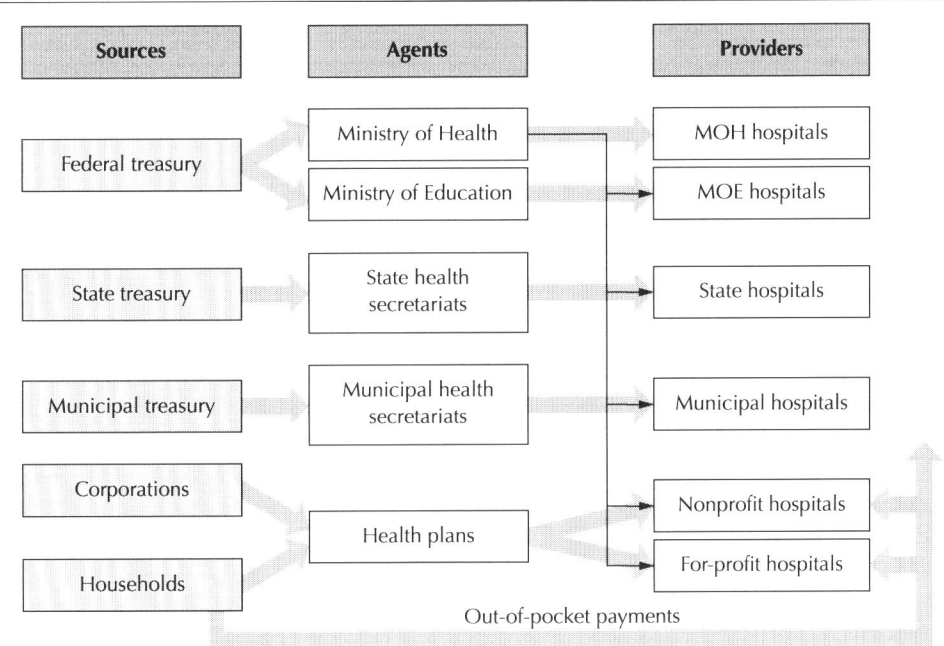

Source: Authors' elaboration.

Note: Arrows signify financial flows. Broad gray arrows are for direct flows/payments. Narrow black arrows are for transfers from MoH to public and private hosp itals.

the figure illustrates flows from financing sources to financial agents to providers (public and private hospitals). The major public financing sources are federal, state, and municipal treasuries, while firms and households constitute the main private sources. Resources are channeled to hospitals through a number of financing agents and payment mechanisms. For example, the federal treasury allocates funds to the MS, which transfers the funds to state and municipal health secretariats and directly to some hospitals, including MS-operated facilities and private facilities under contract to the SUS.[17] Not shown in the figure, hospitals then allocate resources to buy inputs such as labor, supplies, and equipment to produce health care services (e.g., patient stays, outpatient and emergency consultations, and diagnostic tests).

About 45 percent of national health expenditure originates from public sources (SUS), consisting of the three levels of government; the remainder comes from private sources.[18] Private financing overall is distributed almost equally between various private insurers[19] and household out-of-pocket spending, but household spending, mainly for drugs, medical supplies, and health services such as dental care and eye care, is the largest single source of private financing. Figure 2.2 shows the distribution of financing by source, including the four major categories of private insurance: group medicine and medical cooperatives (prepaid schemes), self-insurance, and indemnity insurance. More than 80 percent of federal financing is transferred to states and municipalities, which are responsible for the organization and delivery of health care.

The federal share of total public financing for health has decreased steadily since the onset of decentralization, from 72 percent in 1985 to 48 percent in 2004 (figure 2.3). Municipalities and, to a lesser extent, states have picked up the slack. State funding increased sharply after 2000 because of the earmarking mandate stipulated in Constitutional Amendment 29 (EC 29).[20]

FIGURE 2.2
Distribution of National Health Expenditure, by Source, 2004
(percentage)

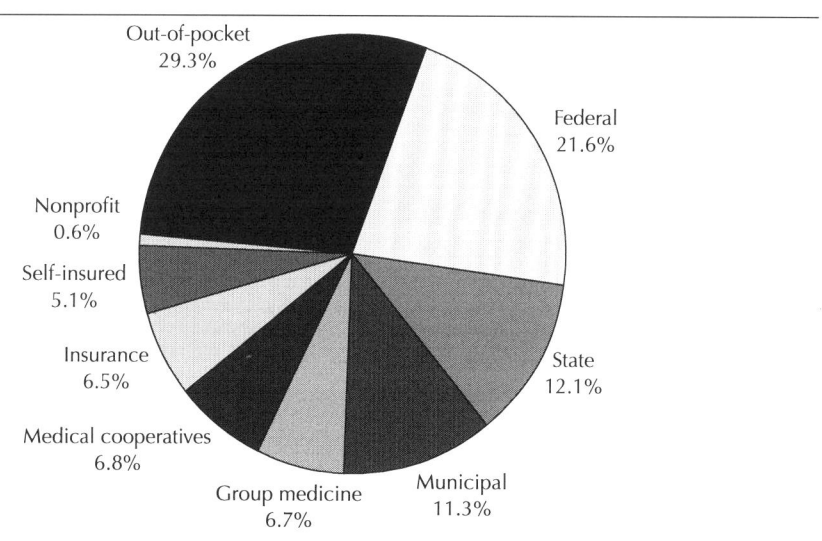

Source: Authors' elaboration based on IBGE (2003) and MS/SIOPS database.

FIGURE 2.3
Trends in SUS Financing, by Source, 1985–2004

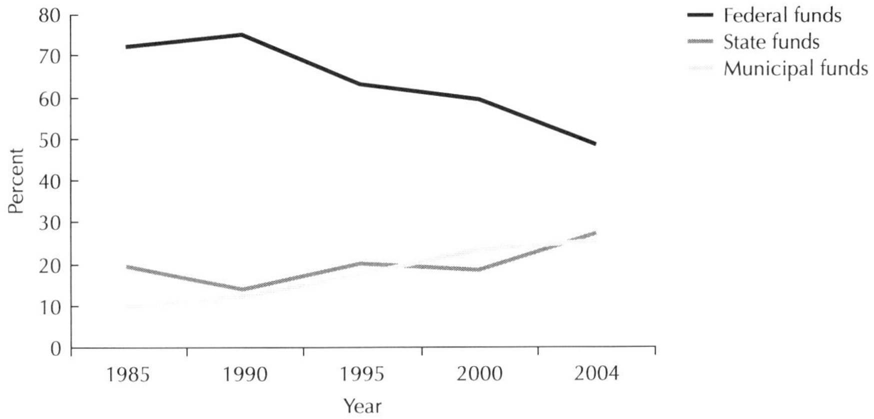

Source: Authors' elaboration based on MS/SIOPS database.

Although federal health authorities cite municipal buy-in as one of the major achievements of decentralization, the limits of municipal health financing are becoming increasingly apparent. Since a federal takeover of municipal hospitals in Rio de Janeiro city in 2005, a constant stream of press reports on sordid conditions in municipal hospitals has called into question municipal capacity to finance and manage these facilities. Some politicians and journalists have called for refederalization of hospitals that had been turned over to municipalities as part of the decentralization reform.[21]

SUS Resource Transfer and Hospital Payment Mechanisms

SUS financing is based on a complex system of fund transfers and payment mechanisms designed to channel funding to hospitals:

- The Authorization for Hospitalization System/Hospital Information System (Autorização de Internação Hospitalar, AIH; Sistema de Informação Hospitalar, SIH), consisting of federal payments from the MS for inpatient care.[22]
- The Ambulatory Care Information System (Sistema de Informação Ambulatorial, SIA) consisting of federal payments for outpatient and emergency services.[23]
- Federal transfers or block grants to state and municipal health secretariats relating to hospital care. These payments, generally bundled into a single grant transfer for "medium- and high-complexity care," are allocated to state or municipal health funds or accounts rather than being paid to individual hospitals. The funds are typically channeled to hospitals through subnational budgets.[24]
- Additional federal payments for university and high-complexity facilities (Fator de Incentivo ao Desenvolvimento Ensino e Pesquisa em Saúde, FIDEPS) and for facilities providing specialized care (e.g., cardiac surgery and transplants) and emergency care. For public hospitals, these payments are increasingly consolidated in hospital-related transfers to states and municipalities.

- Budgeted funds from general or earmarked tax revenues, from federal, state, or municipal governments. These are directed to public hospitals directly managed by government.
- Other sources, including sale of services to private health plans and out-of-pocket payments from private patients.

Whether an SUS-financed hospital is paid through budgets or production-based direct payments (e.g., AIH/SIH, SIA) depends on the management status of the states and municipalities where a facility is located, and on the public or private status of the facility. Where the municipality has full responsibility for the SUS network in its territory (full system management), private hospitals are paid by the municipal health secretariat using funds received from the MS. In municipalities not under this status, private hospitals are paid by the state health secretariat or directly by the federal government. Federal funds are increasingly transferred to state and municipal health secretariats rather than directly to individual hospitals (including private ones). In fact, as of 2005 AIH and SIA are no longer used as payment mechanisms by the federal government and serve only as the basis for computing the amount of federal transfers for middle- and high-complexity care. States and municipalities still use AIH and SIA as a basis for paying private hospitals under contract with the SUS.

Private financing agents such as insurers and prepayment plans are responsible for most private funds paid to non-SUS hospitals, usually through a fee-for-service payment mechanism. Self-insured private corporations and some large public enterprises may also pay providers directly when they manage their own provider networks. Individuals may pay out of pocket for some hospital care, usually deliveries and plastic surgery. Both types of private payment mechanisms are a big source of funding for most private hospitals and for a few large public facilities.

The principal SUS transfers and payments systems for hospitals are illustrated in figure 2.4. As mentioned above, the most important source of revenue for public hospitals is usually the public budget of the respective level of government. For private hospitals under contract with the SUS, the AIH and SIA systems, which used to be the main payment conduits, are increasingly consolidated in federal transfers to states and municipalities. As described in this volume, the variety and complexity of flows and payment mechanisms, together with the limitations of existing information systems, prevent consolidation of public expenditure by type of facility or level of care. Worse, a number of municipalities have yet to establish a health fund and register the funding from different sources in a single account (e.g., for hospital services). This situation complicates any attempt to estimate hospital spending by the SUS.[25]

The Brazilian Hospital Sector

The Brazilian hospital sector consists of 7,400 hospitals with 471,000 beds.[26] Table 2.5 presents a breakdown of all health facilities by type and ownership.

Supply Characteristics

The hospital sector consists of three main subsectors:

- *Public hospitals owned and managed by federal, state, or municipal health authorities.* Nearly all are publicly financed and managed. Most (71 percent) are municipal hospitals, and most

FIGURE 2.4
Payment and Transfer Flows for SUS Hospitals

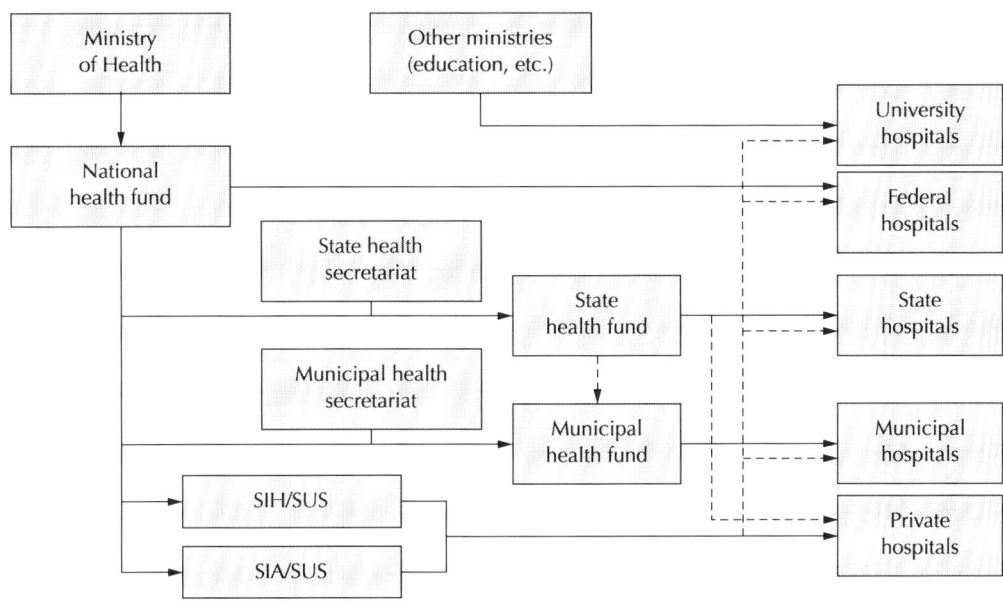

Source: Authors' elaboration.

of the rest are state facilities. The federal government operates a relatively small number of hospitals through the MS and the Ministry of Education.

- *Private hospitals under contract to the SUS.* About 70 percent of private facilities receive public funding. These include most nonprofit facilities (*filantrópicos* and *beneficientes*) and about half of the for-profit hospitals (*lucrativos*). SUS-contracted nonprofit facilities operate under an arrangement known as *convênio* and are required to offer at least 60

TABLE 2.5
Hospital Ownership, 2002

Ownership	Number of hospitals	% of total
Public		
Federal	147	2.0
State	610	8.2
Municipal	1,831	24.8
Subtotal	2,588	35.0
Private		
SUS financed	3,357	45.4
Non–SUS financed	1,452	19.6
Subtotal	4,809	65.0
Total	7,397	100.0

Source: IBGE 2003.

percent of their beds to SUS patients. Most private hospitals receiving SUS financing to a greater or lesser degree also derive funds from private sources.

- *For-profit and some nonprofit private hospitals not financed by the SUS.* These privately financed and managed hospitals constitute about 20 percent of all facilities but 30 percent of all private hospitals.

In sum, the private sector, with 65 percent of the hospitals and nearly 70 percent of the beds, is the main provider of hospital services in Brazil. Most public hospitals are municipally owned and operated. The federal government is responsible for only 147 hospitals, including many large teaching facilities.

Hospital Size

Most Brazilian hospitals are small: more than 60 percent have fewer than 50 beds, and 64 beds is the average size. (The median is 38.) Figure 2.5 displays hospital size by ownership. Municipal hospitals are the smallest, with a mean size of 36 beds, followed by for-profits (mean: 53 beds). The largest, on average, are federal facilities (118 beds), followed by state and nonprofit facilities, with averages of 103 and 88 beds, respectively. The small size of most of the country's hospitals has important implications for quality and for scale efficiency and is out of line with international standards.[27]

Since the mid-1970s the total number of hospitals has grown by 40 percent, but most of this growth has been concentrated in the public sector. Bed growth has been much more modest. Figure 2.6 shows a steady increase in the number of public hospital beds since the mid-1980s and a decrease in the number of private hospital beds. Most of the new beds were in small municipal facilities. For example, between 1976 and 2002 the public sector added 1,620 hospitals (a 170 percent increase) but only about 27,000 beds (a 23 percent increase). The average size of these new facilities was 17 beds.[28]

FIGURE 2.5
Hospitals, by Size and Ownership, 2002

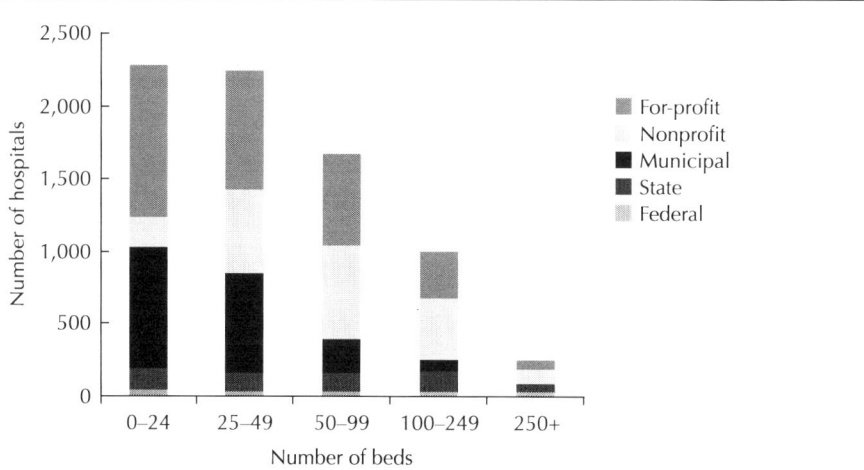

Source: IBGE 2003.

FIGURE 2.6
Long-Term Trends in Bed Supply, 1976–2002

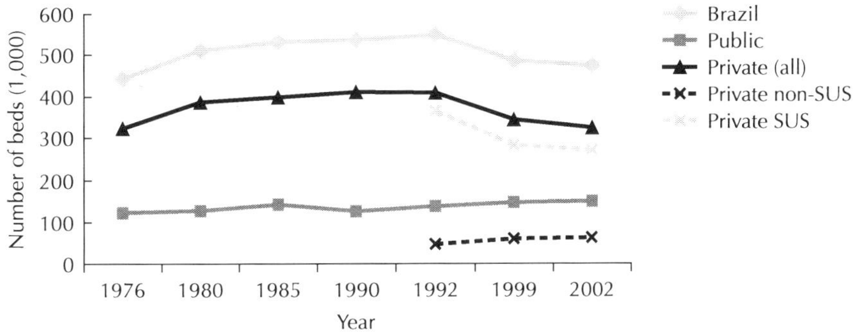

Source: IBGE 2003.

This trend is a response to reform-linked policies aimed at prioritizing and expand-ing the public network while containing AIH/SIH reimbursement rates.[29] The latter policy, directed mainly at private hospitals, financially crippled a number of them, especially non-profits fully dependent on the SUS.[30] Box 2.1 describes the historical circumstances that led to this not-so-implicit policy, as well as the challenges facing private hospitals in the SUS.

In addition to SUS investment policies for expanding the public hospital network to improve hospital access, during the last two decades decentralization has been a driver of growth, particularly for small facilities. As Brazil enthusiastically embraced democracy, campaign promises by newly elected mayors, combined with the political benefits of hospi-tal inaugurations, resulted in the construction of many small "me-too" municipal facilities throughout the country. Municipal governments became the main benefactors of public largesse extended to support the SUS and expand the delivery system. Financial support was often secured through political contacts in the federal Congress. A common mecha-nism for financing these capital investments, still used today, was through amendments or riders attached to congressional laws. These capital investments were allocated haphaz-ardly, often through "pork barrel"–like handouts from the Congress. The introduction of the grant-based financing system gave rise to another incentive: many mayors mistakenly believed that federal transfers would cover the cost of operating a hospital, once built. The resulting construction spree left small municipalities with relatively high bed densities (average: 3.2 per 1,000 inhabitants), comparable to those in medium-size and large munic-ipalities, with averages of 3.0 and 3.4, respectively.[31] Most of these facilities are severely underutilized, at occupancy rates of less than 30 percent (see chapter 3 for a discussion of occupancy and efficiency issues).

Regional Disparities
Although hospital infrastructure has been expanded and access to hospital care has improved considerably in the last two decades, more disaggregated analysis shows that inequalities remain in the spatial distribution of hospital resources, particularly for high-technology ser-vices. As indicated in annex tables 2B.1 and 2B.2, the density of both beds and diagnostic

Box 2.1
A Brief History of Hospitals in Brazil

The Santa Casa de Misericórdia in Santos, established in 1565 by Jesuit priests, was the first Brazilian hospital. The model of religious hospitals, which assumed that caring for the sick was a religious rather than medical responsibility, was inspired by the experience of several European countries, especially Portugal and Spain, and was fully adopted in Brazil, to the point that nearly every medium-size Brazilian city has a hospital founded by a religious organization. Over time, the religious character of the hospitals waned, and management was gradually taken over by physicians and, in some cases, health authorities, although formal governance by a religious order survives in many hospitals.

During the 20th century, until the 1980s, medicalization of patients' treatment gave rise to university (mostly public) hospitals and social security hospitals. These were operated initially by pension and sickness funds and, following the consolidation of social security in the 1970s, by the Social Security Medical Institute (Instituto Nacional de Assistência Médica da Previdência Social, INAMPS). Forty-two such hospitals existed in the mid-1980s. The MS, dealing as it did mostly with national preventive activities and vertical disease programs, targeted its hospitals on the care and treatment of specific diseases such as mental illness, cancer, and tuberculosis, and on rehabilitation. State and municipal hospitals focused primarily on emergency care. The consolidation of the 1970 social security reforms, combined with a policy of the military regime in the 1970s and early 1980s of improving the health system to support rapid economic growth, led to the expansion of the hospital network. This was mainly realized through subsidized interest rates for the construction of for-profit private hospitals. As a result, the bulk of INAMPS hospital payments in the early 1980s paid for care at private, for-profit facilities (see table).

Federal Payments to Hospitals, by Facility Ownership, 1981–2002

(% of total payments)

Hospital type	1981	1988	1995	2002
Federal	20.2	17.9	1.6	0.2
University	2.5	0.4	17.2	22.3
State and municipal	5.6	52.6	30.4	27.5
Nonprofit and union	6.4	0.7	21.5	33.8
For-profit	64.0	28.4	29.2	16.2

Source: INAMPS; World Bank 1994.

Note: Columns may not sum to 100 because of rounding.

(continued)

equipment is relatively high and balanced across regions and across different sizes of municipality. At the microregional and municipality levels, however, wide disparities are evident.

The density of high-complexity diagnostic and treatment technologies, as measured by an indicator of equipment complexity, reflects a distorted distribution.[32] It is excessively high in some municipalities, both large and small,[33] but is almost nonexistent in large parts of the country. Unexpectedly, most of the 189 municipalities exhibiting high equipment density are small; most have fewer than 20,000 inhabitants. Although an undetermined number of these facilities may function as referral centers for neighboring municipalities, the

Box 2.1 *(continued)*

This model, deemed by many as tantamount to privatization, was strongly criticized by the designers of the SUS reforms of the 1980s, which reversed this pattern. Investment funds were directed toward expanding public facilities, SUS payments to private hospitals (through the AIH and SIA systems) failed to keep pace with inflation, and public facilities were favored with additional budgetary resources.

The private hospital sector represents 69 percent of the country's beds, 70 percent of hospital admissions, 59 percent of emergency procedures, and 54 percent of hospital outpatient consultations. It accounts for 68 percent of national hospital spending and 56 percent of spending by the SUS. Despite the importance of private facilities in the SUS, the sector has faced severe constraints in recent years. SUS policies favor the public sector and, to a lesser extent, the private nonprofit subsector, which is perceived as a quasi-public sector. [a] As a direct result of the health reform, the proportion of public funding going to private facilities was reduced, and public facilities began to receive an increasing proportion of federal transfers. At the same time, AIH/SIA payment levels deteriorated; they currently represent less than half the real cost of care for most hospital procedures (see chapter 4). As a strategy for survival, an undetermined number of for-profits have dropped out of the SUS system but may continue to treat SUS patients for high-complexity care that is well compensated by the SUS. A number of nonprofit hospitals, most of them heavily dependent on SUS patients and funding, have opted to establish their own private prepayment plans to capture a fixed clientele of private patients. Others have closed or have been rescued by government bailouts or "public donations." Some bailouts have been sizeable, but they have been mostly ad hoc and unpredictable (see chapter 4).

Source: Castelar, Mordelet, and Grabois 1995; MS/Datasus 2007.

a. Both the 1988 Constitution (Article 199) and Law 8080 state that participation in the SUS is open to private providers in an ill-defined "complementary" role.

analysis suggests an irrational and inefficient distribution of hospital technology resources. This inefficient pattern relates to political factors (every mayor and local politician wants hospital beds and technology for his own constituency—whether they are needed or not);[34] the organizational and financial structure of the SUS, which grants full autonomy to municipalities; the absence of national or state policies guiding technological assessment and distribution; and economic incentives. For example, higher-than-cost reimbursements by the SUS for some complex procedures and diagnoses give a strong incentive for specializing in those procedures and downplaying less-well-reimbursed treatments.

A striking example of these distortions is the density of computerized tomography (CT) and magnetic resonance imaging (MRI) scanners. Nationally, the density rate is 9.3 per million population for CT and 2.5 per million for MRI. These are comparable to density rates in the lowest (density) quartile of OECD countries, including such countries as France and Canada. The density of this equipment in several Brazilian cities and metropolitan areas is, however, much higher. Metropolitan Rio de Janeiro has 75 percent more CT and MRI scanners than metropolitan Paris, with a similar population (IBGE 2000a, 2003; OECD 2005).

Service Production and Utilization Characteristics

Brazilian hospitals are responsible for 20 million inpatient admissions annually, a rate of 115 admissions per 1,000 population. This rate compares favorably with international benchmarks; the mean for OECD countries is 165 admissions, and for the lower quartile of these countries it is 112 (OECD 2005). In addition to inpatient care, hospitals administer nearly three-fourths of all emergency care within the Brazilian health system (70 percent, 240 million procedures) and a significant amount of outpatient care (27 percent, 162 million medical consultations).

The SUS provides the lion's share of hospital services, accounting for 68 percent of admissions, 73 percent of emergency care, and 67 percent of outpatient care in hospitals. As shown in figures 2.7 and 2.8, despite the above-mentioned policy orientation toward expanding public hospitals, most SUS-financed inpatient care is still delivered in private facilities. This is especially the case for the nonprofits that cater more to the SUS than to private or privately insured patients. Public hospitals account for less than half of admissions (43 percent). As expected, private (or non–SUS financed) inpatient care is concentrated in private facilities, particularly in the for-profits.

The average rates of medical consultations (2.6 per person per year) and hospital admissions (11.5 per 100 persons per year) are within international ranges, at or above the levels in middle-income countries, and in the lowest quartile of OECD countries. These utilization ratios are above the benchmarks set by the MS (2.5 medical consultations per person per year and 9.0 hospitalizations per 100 persons per year).

Based on the founding principles of universal and equitable access to health services, the SUS has aimed to reduce inequalities, at least in terms of access.[35] Expansion of the SUS-financed facility network has helped expand access to health care. Average outpatient utilization rates are comparable to international averages, suggesting adequate overall supply. Household health surveys show that only 5 percent of respondents experiencing a sickness episode fail to obtain care because of physical or financial access barriers; the proportion increases to 6 percent for low-income groups nationally (IBGE 2000a). The figures compare favorably with results from household demand surveys in middle-income countries (WHO 2000f).[36]

FIGURE 2.7
Privately Financed and SUS-Financed Patients, 2002

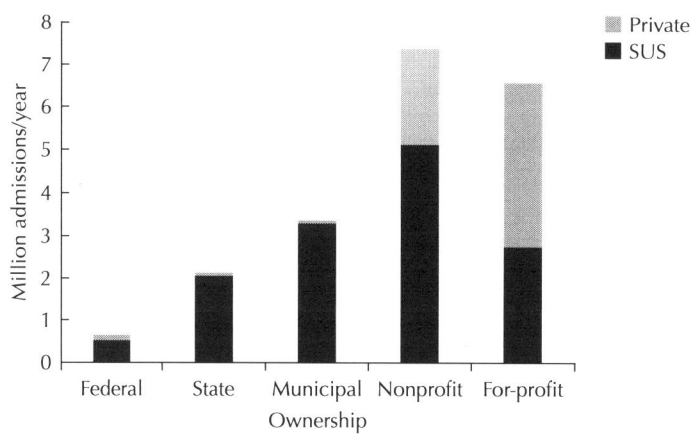

Source: Authors' elaboration based on IBGE (2003).

These national averages, however, hide important differences and distortions. A recent MS study paints a more precise picture, indicating the existence of important inequalities in specific types of care (Vianna 2005). The study found that access to health care becomes increasingly inequitable as complexity and costs increase. For example, blacks and mixed-race (*mestiço*) persons represent 27 percent of the population in São Paulo state but account for only 9.6 percent of cardiac surgeries in a large public hospital. Among private patients, the proportion drops to 2.4 percent.

According to the 1998 National Household Survey (Pesquisa Nacional por Amostra de Domicílios, PNAD), 7 percent of the general population was hospitalized in the 12 months prior to the survey (IBGE 2000b). The proportion was larger among low-income households: 7.3 percent for the poorest income group, compared with 6.5 percent for the highest. Regional and urban-rural variations were not significant. In all income groups, individuals covered by a private health plan were hospitalized at a rate 30 to 50 percent higher than those without insurance coverage. People with little or no education and the elderly registered significantly higher utilization rates. Their employment situation had no significant effect except for the economically inactive, who had a much higher rate of hospitalization. Self-reported low health status was a major factor in hospitalization across all income groups.

The survey also showed that the SUS finances the preponderance of hospital care for the poor (90 percent in the lowest quintile and 82 percent in the next lowest), while the well-off tend to draw on insurance and out-of-pocket payments. The SUS, however, finances a significant number of hospitalizations (21 percent) demanded by high-income households.

The 1998 PNAD also reported service utilization by type of provider. Whereas 72 percent of those demanding health care did so at an ambulatory facility, about 20 percent sought care in a hospital as their primary source. Emergency care centers received 5 percent of demand. Low-income populations sought care in hospitals much more frequently than their high-income counterparts. The main reason for seeking care in hospitals was for a medical visit (71 percent).

FIGURE 2.8
Inpatient Care, by Clientele and Hospital Ownership, 2000–3

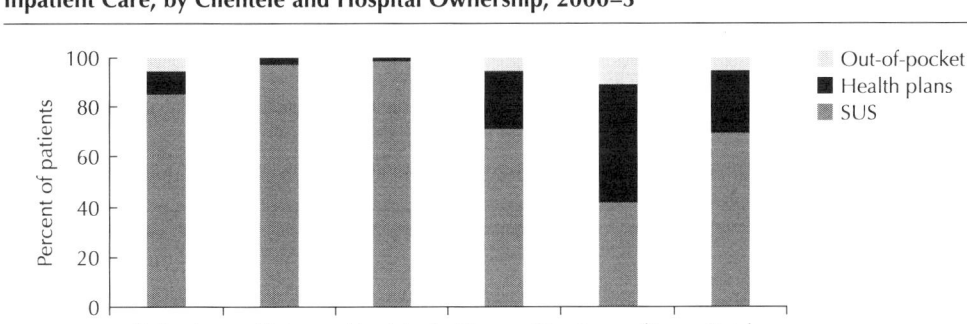

Source: Authors' elaboration based on IBGE (2003).

TABLE 2.6
Disparities in Health Indicators in the Municipality of São Paulo, 2002–3

Indicator	Mean	Best	Worse
Neonatal mortality/1,000	9.6	3.2	24.2
Infant mortality/1,000	15.1	4.3	30.0
NCD mortality, <60 years[a]	25.4	10.4	46.9

Source: PMSP/Secretaria Municipal da Saúde/CeInfo 2002.
a. Due to hypertension, cerebrovascular disease, and diabetes.

Finally, outcome indicators such as infant and maternal mortality show wide regional and social differences. For example, infant mortality per 1,000 live births varies from 22 to 58 percent across regions (see table 2B.3 in annex 2B) and from 10 to nearly 100 across municipalities. As shown in table 2.6, even within a well-served municipality like São Paulo, where nearly the entire population resides within one hour's travel of a public referral facility, neonatal mortality varies from 3 to 24 per 1,000.[37] Other health indicators show similar variations. Such disparities are to some extent associated with general socioeconomic disparities rather than with supply of health services.

Hospital Finance and Spending

Total spending on hospital care was estimated at R$47.3 billion (US$16.1 billion) in 2002.[38] In the same year, hospital spending represented 67 percent of total health expenditures (R$70.4 billion). Figure 2.9 shows that the SUS is the major source of hospital finance, contributing 58 percent (R$27.5 billion, US$9.4 billion) of hospital spending, while private insurance and out-of-pocket financing account for 33 and 8.5 percent, respectively.[39] The federal government is the source of nearly a third of all public funding and 29 percent of total hospital finance.

FIGURE 2.9
Sources of Hospital Care Financing, 2002

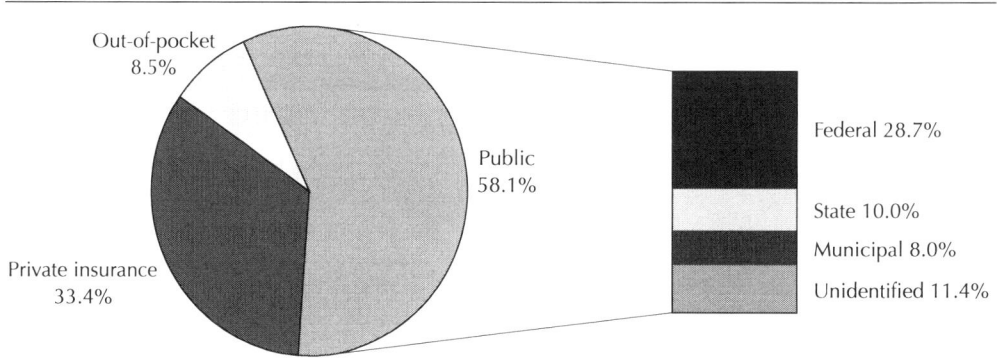

Source: Authors' estimates, using the approach described in annex 2A and government budgets.
a. "Unidentified" refers to ad hoc transfers with specific source not identifiable in budget documents.

The second largest public source is classified as "unidentified." This generally consists of ad hoc bailouts, sometimes referred to as "public donations," to private hospitals by municipal and state governments. These transfers are directed to facilities in financial crisis or with political ties to subnational governments.[40] None of these subsidies are recorded systematically in subnational budgets.[41] Combining state, municipal, and "unidentifiable" sources, subnational levels together pay half of the public hospital bill.

Spending by Hospital Ownership

Reflecting the pluralistic nature of the Brazilian hospital sector, nearly 67 percent of total hospital expenditure is allocated to private facilities.[42] Nonprofits take up 38 percent of spending and for-profits, 29 percent; public facilities account for 33 percent of the total. Private facilities absorb 56 percent of SUS outlays on hospitals, and public hospitals the remainder (see annex table 2B.6). As shown in figure 2.10, nearly all private hospital spending goes to private facilities, and for-profit facilities receive about 60 percent of that. About 8 percent of private spending occurs in public hospitals, mostly large referral hospitals operated by the federal and state governments. Though still limited, revenue from selling services to private patients has increased as public hospitals seek to expand and diversify their funding sources. Many federal hospitals have set up nonprofit organizations—"support foundations"—that function in part as organizational conduits for tapping private revenues (see chapter 5).

Spending by Line Item

Figure 2.11 displays spending by expense category. Fifty-two percent of all hospital sector spending goes for staff.[43] When personnel spending for outsourced contractors (e.g., cleaning, laundry, security, dietary) and payments to contracted physicians and other medical personnel are included, labor costs reach 64 percent. Personnel costs as a percentage of total spending are higher among municipal hospitals (78 percent) than among private hospitals

FIGURE 2.10
Hospital Spending, by Facility Ownership, 2002

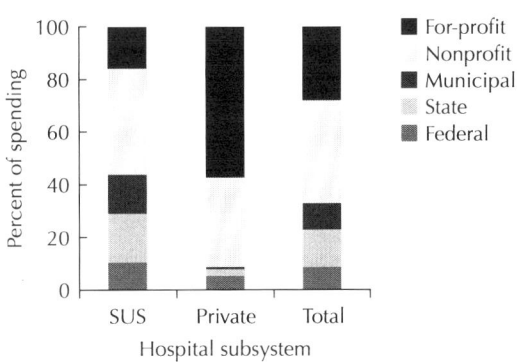

Source: Authors' elaboration.

FIGURE 2.11
Hospital Spending, by Line Item, 2002

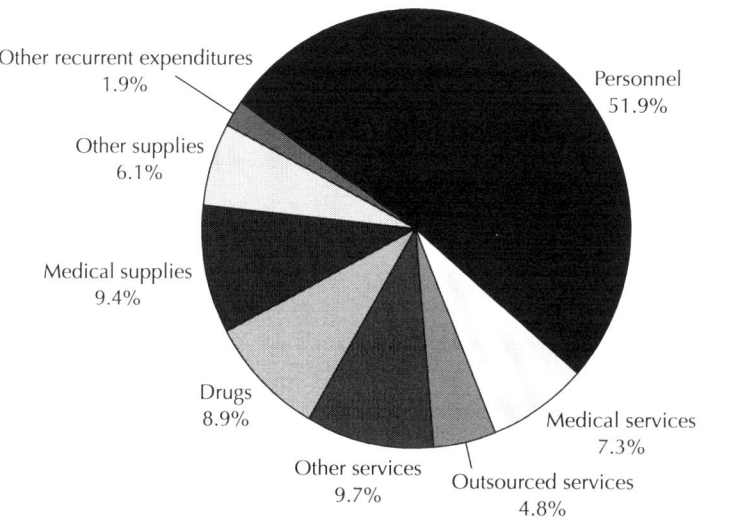

Source: Authors' elaboration based on World Bank (2007) and De Matos (2002).

(60 percent). Little difference was found in the proportions of labor costs in private hospitals under SUS contracts and in facilities catering entirely to private patients. State and municipal hospitals usually have larger staffs, but their salaries are generally lower than at private facilities. Supplies, chiefly medical supplies and drugs, constitute the second largest expenditure category (24 percent). Other services, such as utilities and transportation, and other recurrent expenditures add up to 12 percent.[44]

This pattern is in line with international practice except for labor costs, which in Brazil consume a higher share of spending than in most other countries. In the United States, for instance, wages and benefits, including professional fees (5 percent), account for 62 percent of total hospital spending, and drugs and supplies represent 18 percent (annex figure 2B.1).

Spending by Type of Service

The distribution of SUS hospital expenditure by type of service is displayed in figure 2.12. The bulk of SUS hospital expenditure (64 percent) goes for inpatient care. Ambulatory and emergency care account for 8 and 11 percent, respectively, and spending on "external" outpatient diagnostic services, for 4 percent.[45] Administration represents 13 percent of the total.[46] The data for public hospitals only (not shown in figure 2.12) are slightly different, with larger proportions of spending allocated to outpatient care (12 percent), emergency care (12 percent), and administration (15 percent). In contrast, private hospitals concentrate spending on inpatient care (70 percent) and spend a lower proportion on administration (9 percent).

Since these distributions are based on estimates, spending in a small subset of public hospitals that have standardized cost accounting systems was analyzed for comparison.[47] The data from these hospitals allow for a more robust estimate of expenditure composition.

FIGURE 2.12
SUS Hospital Spending, by Type of Care, 2002

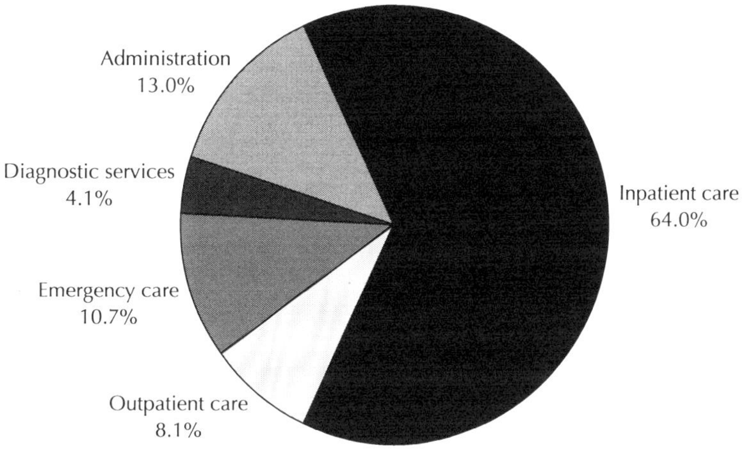

Source: Authors' elaboration using approach described in annex 2A.

The results compare well with the spending estimates presented in figure 2.12. The hospitals in the subset direct 68, 16, and 10 percent of total expenditure to inpatient, emergency, and outpatient care, respectively.

Compared with high-income countries such as Canada, Brazil's hospitals spend proportionately more on emergency care and administration and less on inpatient care and diagnostics. For instance, Canadian hospitals spend 5 percent of their total expenditure on emergency care and 8 percent on administration (CIHI 2005), and in the United States the proportion of central-level administrative costs is 6.3 percent (CMS 2002). Factors contributing to these differences include the use of Brazilian emergency rooms for nonurgent care, partly because of low primary care coverage or effectiveness; inadequate governance and organizational arrangements combined with poor management practices that contribute to inefficiencies (see chapters 5 and 6 for a discussion of these topics); and low quality of care, particularly in terms of clinical management.

Spending by Care Level and Specialty

The MS classifies health services according to three care levels: (1) basic or low-complexity care—mostly outpatient primary care; (2) high-complexity care, often defined by its unit cost and the technology involved rather than by its complexity—for example, cardiac care and surgery, organ transplants, oncology, neurosurgery, diagnostic tests such as magnetic resonance imaging and computerized tomography, and expensive drugs; and (3) medium-complexity care, an amorphous classification that includes whatever is excluded from the other two groups.

In principle, allocation of spending by care level should reflect a country's epidemiological profile and stated health priorities. Analysis of volume and spending by care level provides insight into how well the actual pattern reflects policy priorities and how efficiently

TABLE 2.7
SUS Hospital Expenditure, by Care Level, 2002

(percent)

| Care level | Inpatient care | | Outpatient care | | Emergency care | | % of total spending |
	Volume	Spending	Volume	Spending	Volume	Spending	
Basic/low complexity	41.5	24.3	61.1	50.0	42.6	28.7	25.9
Medium complexity/ specialized	51.5	48.3	38.9	50.0	57.4	71.3	50.9
High complexity	7.0	27.4	N/A	N/A	N/A	N/A	23.2[a]
Total	—	73.3	—	8.5	—	13.5	4.8

Source: MS/Datasus AIH databank; De Matos 2002; SES-SP 2004.
N/A, data not reported or not available.
Note: Following the categories generally used within the SUS, basic or low-complexity care includes primary care or ambulatory care in the four main medical specialties: general medicine, general surgery, gynecology and obstetrics, and pediatrics. Medium-complexity or specialized care includes services in the other medical specialties. High-complexity care was identified only for inpatient care, from the MS/Datasus AIH database. The amounts shown are based on mean costs obtained from the cost studies cited: the De Matos (2002) study for hospitalizations, and health social organization (*organização social de saúde,* OSS) data from São Paulo state for ambulatory and emergency care. An MS study (Vianna 2005) arrived at slightly different figures for spending than those presented in this table: high-complexity ambulatory and hospital services accounted for R$5.2 billion (US$1.7 billion) in 2003, or 19.2 percent of MS spending on health services, an increase from 13 percent in 1995. Per capita spending on high-complexity care increased 21 percent in real terms during 1995–2003.
a. Includes high-complexity diagnostic tests for external patients.

resources are allocated. Table 2.7 shows the distribution of spending at the three care levels, as defined in the table. Specialized or medium-complexity care represents 51 percent of total hospital spending and about half the admissions (52 percent) and inpatient expenditures (48 percent). High-complexity procedures represent only 7 percent of inpatient volume but 27 percent of inpatient expenditure and 23 percent of hospital spending.

Low-complexity care accounts for 42 percent of admissions, 61 percent of ambulatory medical consultations, and 43 percent of emergencies. The relatively large volume of procedures, and the corresponding spending, at this level suggest an inefficiently high utilization of hospital services for conditions that could be treated at lower cost outside the hospital, in ambulatory care. In addition, many emergency procedures are performed on nonurgent cases because patients bypass the primary care facilities.[48] Although the MS has prioritized the extension of primary care coverage since the mid-1990s, considerably more needs to be done to improve coverage and effectiveness at this level of care.

Summary Assessment

The overview of the Brazilian hospital sector presented in this chapter has focused on financing, supply, utilization, and spending characteristics. Several of the themes touched on here are taken up in greater detail in subsequent chapters. As is typical of most large middle-income countries, the hospital sector in Brazil is large, with more than 7,000 facilities. Atypical features are the pluralistic mix of federal, state, municipal, and private non-profit and for-profit hospitals and the predominance of publicly financed private facilities. Also unusual is the complex and sometimes overlapping web of financial flows and payment mechanisms.

Hospitals are the main engines of the service delivery system. In addition to delivering all inpatient care, they provide a very large share of outpatient care, and they employ 56 percent of all health facility personnel. They consume 67 percent of total health expenditures and 70 percent of public spending.

Brazil has made great strides in improving access to hospitals and to health care in general. Yet compared with other middle-income countries, Brazil is only an average performer relative to its level of spending. Considering the large amounts of resources directed to hospitals, finding ways to contain hospital spending is a pressing policy objective. The data presented in this chapter suggest that resource allocation to and within the hospital sector differs from international patterns.

Brazil's health system and hospital sectors have several defining characteristics:

- Access to hospital care is broadly satisfactory for most Brazilians, and financial protection against the cost of illness is considerable. Universal access to the public system is constitutionally guaranteed, and private insurance coverage is high among middle-income groups.
- Brazil spends more on health care, in both absolute and relative terms, than comparable middle-income countries, but it obtains less value for the money.
- Hospitals consume about two-thirds of total health spending. Approximately 70 percent of hospital spending is publicly funded (under the SUS), but most care is delivered by private providers, especially nonprofit hospitals. More than 60 percent of Brazilian hospitals have fewer than 50 beds. Most hospitals are severely underutilized.
- Health care delivery in Brazil can best be described as "hospital-centric." The supply of hospitals (e.g., bed density) and the use of hospital care are similar to levels found in higher-income countries and are well above those in most middle-income countries. Brazil, however, has a much younger population and a disease burden composition that does not require intense use of hospitals. Hospital emergency rooms appear to be the gateway to the delivery system. In 2002 SUS hospitals provided more than 121 million emergency medical consultations, or 25.8 percent of all medical consultations supplied by the SUS. There is growing evidence that not all this demand requires hospital-based emergency care.
- Hospital resources are not rationally distributed, either geographically or by type and level of care. The density of expensive, high-technology hospital and diagnostic services in many Brazilian cities is higher than in OECD countries. An increasing number of Brazilian hospitals excel in organ transplants, cardiac surgery, and other high-complexity procedures. A hospital payment system that favors—and may overpay for—these procedures contributes to this distortion. Oversupply of high-technology equipment in some cities coexists with lack of access to referral services in large parts of the country.
- Brazil is ill prepared for the rising incidence of NCDs. The health care system is organized to provide expensive hospital-based care for acute illnesses that are resolved quickly. The number of Brazilians with chronic disease has, however, risen dramatically. These patients

require care that is coordinated across a number of medical care providers, as discussed in chapter 8.

Although Brazil has a much younger population and a lower NCD disease burden than the average OECD country, its supply and use of hospital care are at similar levels, suggesting over-reliance on hospital services and inpatient care (see table 2.8). The widespread use of inpatient care, especially emergency rooms, is related to the low effectiveness and quality of the primary care network. A significant proportion of low-complexity hospital and inpatient care in Brazil could be administered more effectively—for less—at ambulatory facilities. Because hospital care is usually more expensive than ambulatory care, the current pattern is likely to significantly and unnecessarily sap financial resources for health. In the next chapter, costs and efficiency are examined in detail.

TABLE 2.8

Brazilian and International Patterns of Hospital Resource Allocation, 2000–2

Indicator	Brazil	OECD
Percentage of population over age 60	8.1	20.1
Percentage of disease burden from NCDs	55.0	85.3
Percentage of disease burden from injuries	20.8	8.9
Percentage of disease burden from communicable, maternal, and prenatal conditions	24.2	5.7
Bed density (per 1,000)	2.7	3.1
Hospitalizations (per 1,000)	11.5	11.2
Hospitals as percentage of health personnel	56.5	64.7
Hospitals as percentage of health expenditure	67.0	N/A
Inpatient care as percentage of health expenditure	43.0	41.6
Outpatient care as percentage of health expenditure	31.8	32.5
Prescription drugs as percentage of health expenditure	17.0	15.9

Source: IBGE; MS/Datasus; public budgets; OECD 2005; authors' estimates based on annex 2A and annex table 2B.4.
N/A, data not reported or unavailable.

Annex 2A

An Indirect Method for Estimating Hospital Spending

Hospital spending in Brazil is difficult to ascertain or estimate because of the diverse structure of the hospital sector and the gaps in available data. Three main approaches were used in this volume to estimate sector funding and allocation.

The first builds on existing public budget information and other partial expenditure information. This approach requires some extrapolation because of information gaps. The second approach uses information on facility personnel and wages to estimate facility-level expenditure, as described below. Though indirect, this approach allows complete coverage of the facility network by ownership. The third approach attempts to estimate expenditure by care type and uses available information on service production and costs. Despite their limitations, these three approaches yield similar estimates for aggregate hospital spending, although disaggregated estimates show some significant differences.

The indirect estimation method used in this chapter is based on the number of hospital personnel by category (e.g., medical, nursing) and by type of employer (ownership) and on the mean salary paid to each group. Personnel expenditure thus estimated can be used to estimate total hospital expenditure. Two major assumptions are needed for this strategy: (1) the proportion of personnel expenditure relative to total hospital expenditure is relatively constant across types of hospital, or the proportion extracted from partial studies is valid for all hospitals; and (2) aggregate personnel expenditure can be reasonably estimated from data on the number of personnel working in hospitals and on mean wages.

Personnel expenditure is estimated in three steps: (1) the number and skill levels of personnel located in hospitals and other types of health facilities are extracted from the National Health Facility Survey (Assistência Médico-Sanitária, AMS), reported in IBGE (2003); (2) the mean wage earned by each category of personnel, by state and type of provider, is extracted from the National Household Survey (Pesquisa Nacional por Amostra de Domicílios, PNAD), reported in IBGE (2004c); and (3) the number of personnel is multiplied by the mean annual wage and adjusted for nonwage payroll charges (27 percent for public hospitals and 72.7 percent for private hospitals). Finally, hospital expenditure is estimated from personnel expenditure by assuming, on the basis of available information, that personnel expenditure, on average, corresponds to 65 percent of total hospital expenditure.

This approach does not control for differences in case mix, and it implicitly assumes that wage differences across ownership groups constitute the only cost driver explaining cost differences. Despite these limitations, the method proved to provide reasonable estimates, especially at the aggregate level.

Annex 2B
Supplementary Data

TABLE 2B.1
Health Facilities, by Region

Indicator	All Brazil	North	Northeast	Southeast	South	Central-West
Hospitals	7,397	642	2,328	2,376	1,206	845
Public	2,588	345	1,211	499	258	275
Private SUS	3,357	149	841	1,169	803	395
Non-SUS	1,452	148	276	708	145	175
Hospital beds	471,171	27,653	122,164	205,099	79,379	36,876
Public	146,319	13,582	51,736	54,434	15,301	11,266
Private SUS	269,028	10,471	62,726	117,000	57,732	21,099
Non-SUS	55,824	3,600	7,702	33,665	6,346	4,511
Ambulatory facilities	46,428	3,959	14,764	16,647	7,826	3,232
Public	35,086	3,586	11,848	11,298	6,019	2,335
Private SUS	1,619	97	650	516	276	80
Non-SUS	9,723	276	2,266	4,833	1,531	817
Diagnostic facilities	11,518	536	1,820	5,389	2,725	1,048
Public	673	64	139	324	80	66
Private SUS	3,699	190	625	1,312	1,238	334
Non-SUS	7,146	282	1,056	3,753	1,407	648
Total	65,343	5,137	18,912	24,412	11,757	5,125

Source: IBGE 2003.
Note: SUS, Sistema Único de Saúde (Unified Health System). The number of SUS beds varies between the National Health Facility Survey (Assistência Médico-Sanitária, AMS), reported in IBGE (2003), and the Ministério da Saúde (MS)/Datasus figures because hospitals tend to inflate their official offer of SUS beds while effectively using fewer of them.

TABLE 2B.2
Geographic Distribution of Hospital Infrastructure

Group	Population	Beds	Beds/1,000	Equipment points	Equipment points/1,000
Brazil	174,632,960	471,157	2.70	292,510	1.67
State capitals	41,583,935	143,029	3.78	125,764	2.72
Metro areas	69,497,490	186,228	1.74	155,125	0.86
Large municipalities[a]	29,542,522	98,977	3.41	65,331	2.10
Medium-size municipalities[b]	17,082,060	50,986	3.00	24,779	1.41
Small municipalities[c]	46,440,482	134,966	3.31	47,275	1.12
Municipalities without a hospital[c]	12,070,378	0	0.00	0	0.00

Source: IBGE 2003.
a. More than 100,000 inhabitants.
b. 50,000–100,000 inhabitants.
c. Fewer than 50,000 inhabitants and not lying within a metropolitan area.

TABLE 2B.3
Regional Variation in Socioeconomic Indicators, 1998–2002

Indicator	North	Northeast	Southeast	South	Central-West
Population	11,850	45,925	69,174	24,223	11,048
GDP per capita (US$)	4,932	2,136	6,824	5,168	5,018
Infant mortality (%)	35.2	57.9	24.8	22.4	25.1
Life expectancy (years)	67.4	64.4	68.8	70.2	68.5
Human Development Index	0.727	0.608	0.857	0.860	0.848
Illiteracy rate (%)	20.8	28.7	8.7	8.9	11.6
People with <4 years education (%)	37.1	53.4	26.5	25.7	31.7
Urban access to potable water (%)	69.9	88.4	96.1	95.0	85.3
Urban access to sanitation (%)	52.9	50.9	89.9	77.4	46.7
Urban access to garbage collection (%)	79.5	82.3	96.9	97.5	9

Source: IBGE 2004c; IPEA/PNUD 2000; MS/RIPSA 2000; MS/Datasus 2005a.

TABLE 2B.4
Hospital Financing, by Source, 2002

(R$ billions)

Source	SUS	Public non-SUS[a]	Private	Total expenditure
Federal	13.1	0.5	0.0	13.6
State	4.6	0.2	0.0	4.7
Municipal	3.8	0.2	0.0	3.8
Unidentified[b]	5.4	0.0	0.0	5.4
Total public	26.8	0.7	—	27.5
Private insurance	N/A	0.0	15.8	15.8
Out-of-pocket	N/A	0.0	4.0	4.0
Total	27.5	0.7	19.8	47.3

Source: Authors' estimates using the approach described in annex 2A and government budgets.
Note: US$1.00 = R$2.92. N/A, not available.
a. Expenditure for civil servants and the armed forces.
b. Ad hoc transfers with specific source not identifiable in budget documents.

TABLE 2B.5
Hospital Expenditure, by Financing Source, 2002
(R$ thousands)

Hospitals by ownership	Federal budget	MS transfers	State health sector	Municipal health sector	Total SUS funding	Health plans	Out-of-pocket	Total funding
Public budget, all health care[a]	26,415,511	—	10,260,107	12,073,360	48,748,968	N/A	0	48,748,968
Hospitals								
Federal MS	1,017,885	33,698	N/A	N/A	1,051,583	238,754	157,038	1,664,481
Federal Ministry of Education	1,562,384	593,475	N/A	N/A	2,155,859	50,544	12,452	2,551,683
State	0	1,745,244	3,940,098	274,567	5,685,342	248,402	124,709	6,967,221
Municipal	0	990,042	204,825	3,289,663	4,279,705	121,060	69,091	5,140,334
Nonprofit	0	3,384,870	629,972	3,233,103	3,384,870	6,166,733	1,542,499	11,648,807
For-profit	0	1,969,082	907,328	2,296,512	1,969,082	11,341,380	2,702,428	16,813,535
Total SUS	2,580,269	8,716,410	3,940,098	3,289,663	18,526,440	0	0	21,305,406
Share of total SUS (%)	13.9	47.0	21.3	17.8	100.0			*
Public non-SUS	501,143	0	159,223	16,254	676,620	658,760	363,290	1,953,470
Total public and central	3,543,624	10,023,872	4,714,219	3,801,805	22,083,519	757,574	417,783	23,258,877
All hospitals[b]	3,543,624	10,023,872	4,714,219	3,801,805	22,083,519	18,265,688	4,662,710	45,011,917
Share of total (%)	7.9	22.3	10.5	8.5	49.1	40.6	10.4	100.0

Source: Authors' calculations.
Note: SUS expenditure given here is lower than that in table 2B.4 because of financial transfers not identifiable in budget data. (The data in table 2B.4 are estimated.) Amounts in italics are payments by state and municipal secretariats to private providers. When identifiable; they were not added to the totals because of likely double counting with federal transfers.
a. Does not include expenditure on non-SUS facilities.
b. Total funding by source (line) and hospital ownership (last column) includes expenditure on support services to hospitals executed at the central level.

TABLE 2B.6
SUS Expenditure, by Facility Ownership, 2002

(R$ thousands)

Ownership	Hospitals	Percentage of total	Ambulatory	Diagnostic	All facilities
Federal	2,914,750	10.13	189,111	7,330	3,111,191
State	5,523,114	19.20	839,330	86,076	6,448,520
Municipal	4,201,448	14.60	9,556,696	79,276	13,837,420
Nonprofit	11,535,189	40.09	583,091	362,734	12,481,014
For-profit	4,597,585	15.98	804,389	80,474	5,482,448
SUS facilities	28,772,086	100.00	11,972,617	615,890	41,360,593
SUS total[a]	33,087,898	—	13,768,509	708,274	47,564,682

Source: Authors' estimates using the approach described in annex 2A.
a. Includes allocated expenditure at the central level.

FIGURE 2B.1
Total Hospital Costs, United States, by Type of Expense, Fiscal 2003

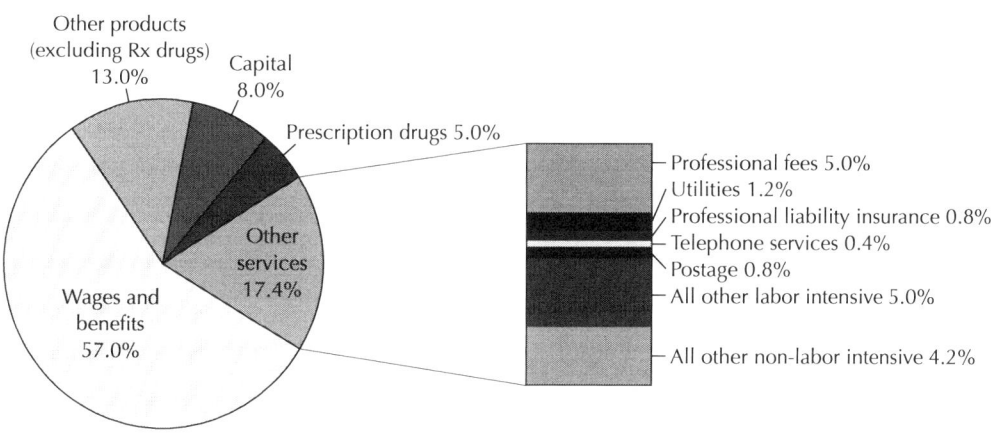

Source: CMS 2002.

Notes

1. These participation mechanisms include health councils and commissions at each level of government, as described later in this section.
2. The SUS basic legislation includes the 1988 Constitution, which established citizens' right to health care and created the SUS; the health organic laws (Laws 8.080/90 and 8.142/90), which defined the system's basic rules and policies; the Basic Operational Directives (Normas Operacionais Básicas, NOB) published in 1991, 1993, and 1996; and the Health Care Operational Norms (Normas Operacionais de Assistência à Saúde, NOAS) of 2000 and 2001. The NOB and NOAS defined and regulated specific aspects of the system and set forth action plans.
3. For example, despite private initiatives to accredit hospitals, the MS established its own accrediting agency (see chapter 8). MS initiatives tend to duplicate existing private initiatives instead of building on them.

4. This policy has failed to meet expectations. Reimbursements are meager, and the policy has been challenged in court by private insurers (see chapter 4).

5. Smaller municipalities and a number of large urban municipalities struggle to manage basic care. Out of 5,560 municipalities, 4,375 (78.7 percent) have fewer than 10,000 inhabitants; these entities represent 23.4 percent of the population.

6. Provided in the 1996 MS regulations (NOB 01/96) and revised in 2001 and 2002 (NOAS 2001/2002).

7. Anecdotal evidence suggests that, in practice, most councils have little power and are mere rubber stamps for government health authorities.

8. The Family Health Program is arguably the best example of a performance-linked financial system: levels of finance are partially linked to population coverage levels.

9. The exception was autonomous public hospitals under "indirect administration," which were essentially converted to directly managed facilities (see chapter 5).

10. Published in Portaria MS/GM 399, February 22, 2006, and Portaria MS/GM 699, April 3, 2006.

11. Infectious and childhood diseases, representing 24 percent of the disease burden, are concentrated in the North and Northeast regions of Brazil.

12. In response to calls for additional financing, Constitutional Amendment 29, passed in 2000, required each government level to earmark a defined percentage of revenues for health (12 percent for the states and 15 percent for the municipalities). There are no generally accepted definitions of health expenditure or hospital expenditure in Brazil and no accepted criteria for such a definition. This leads to lack of precision, significant discrepancies in estimates, and great difficulties in comparing estimates across time and regional entities. The main definitions used are the "institutional" definition, which takes into account all expenditure incurred by a health department or agency, even if not health-related; the "budget" concept of health function (*função saúde*); the definition of "public (financed) health services and activities" used by the Information System for Public Budgets in Health (Sistema de Informações sobre Orçamentos Públicos em Saúde, SIOPS); "expenditure on budget subfunctions," especially "hospital and ambulatory care," which includes most hospital expenditure except personnel costs; and "hospital expenditure," defined as all spending incurred in hospitals regardless of budget classification.

13. Expenditure figures are authors' estimates based on IBGE (2003, 2004a) and a compilation from various sources. The mean exchange rate was R$2.92 per US$1.00 for both 2002 (to which most figures refer) and 2004.

14. A common argument states that Brazil spends too little in comparison with the level of spending of richer countries. This argument can be misleading because, as shown in table 2.3, achieving the levels of per capita health spending of the lower quartile of OECD countries would imply multiplying national health spending threefold, which would mean committing nearly 25 percent of the country's GDP (in PPP dollars) to health. This level is significantly higher than that of the big spenders among OECD countries, and it is an unrealistic and unsustainable goal.

15. A WHO report on the performance of national health systems ranked Brazil 125th among 191 countries worldwide and 28th among 33 countries in the Latin America and the Caribbean region. Despite the methodological and data issues, the results are indicative of the low performance of the Brazilian health system when outcomes are related to expenditure (WHO 2000a).

16. Other study variables included population increase, GDP growth, average income, general inflation, health inflation, and health system efficiency. Various scenarios were simulated, but the data presented here reflect the most "optimistic" scenario, with household income rising 1 percent annually (Ferraz 2006).

17. The federal treasury also directs funds to the Ministry of Education, which operates most teaching hospitals.

18. Authors' estimation based on IBGE (2004a); MF 2005; MF/SIAFI information system; and ANS (2006a).

19. Insurance schemes covering public servants are considered private insurance.

20. Constitutional Amendment 29, passed in 2000, was intended to secure stable and increased funding for the SUS. It is being elaborated in complementary legislation by Congress.

21. *Jornal do Brasil*, March 20, 2005, p. A16; *O Estado de São Paulo*, April 5, 2005, p. A10.

22. The AIH/SIH (discussed in chapter 4) is an information system that authorizes and records SUS hospital admissions. The AIH/SIH functions as a billing system for reimbursement purposes when the hospital is paid directly, as is usually the case for private hospitals under contract with the SUS. It is also a prospective payment system based on general hospital procedures or treatments rather than individual services.

23. The SIA records all ambulatory services provided by the SUS, including emergency care, and serves as the mechanism for reimbursing providers (see chapter 4).

24. These transfers constitute an increasing proportion of federal funding as more states and municipalities qualify for full system management (a requisite for such transfers).

25. Even estimating spending for a single hospital is difficult because most public facilities do not possess a separate budget and have little or no information on the use of financial resources (World Bank 2007).

26. The Brazilian Census Bureau (Instituto Brasileiro de Geografia e Estatística, IBGE) defines a hospital as a health facility with beds. Only facilities that were operational at the time of the annual national survey of health facilities (IBGE 2003) are considered in this volume.

27. It is generally accepted that to attain efficiencies of scale and scope, a hospital should have between 150 and 250 beds (Posnett 2002). The implications are explored in chapter 3.

28. In contrast, the number of private hospital beds decreased, while the number of private hospitals increased by 10 percent (personal communication, Pedro Barbosa, April 10, 2005).

29. See for example Law 8080 (Título III, Capítulo II); World Bank (1994). For the Social Security Medical Institute (Instituto Nacional de Assistência Médica da Previdência Social, INAMPS), the proportion of spending on public hospitals to total expenditure increased from 26.5 percent in 1984 to 55.0 percent in 1987.

30. Public facilities rely heavily on public budgets. The creators of the SUS had a strong public sector bias. Some policy makers and public health professionals still frown on public financing of private facilities, asserting that the SUS should finance only public facilities. In line with this thinking, SUS advocates maintain that the system should follow the constitutional mandate of financing private providers on a supplementary basis only in areas, or for care, not publicly covered (see box 2.1).

31. The average bed density was 2.7 per 1,000 population in 2002, down from over 4 in the early 1980s. This rate is commensurate with international averages (see table 2.8) but is still higher than elsewhere in Latin America. It is also higher than the reference benchmark of 2.18 per 1,000 set by the MS. The decrease in bed density is consistent with international trends. Bed density varies from over 4 in Goiás, Maranhão, and Rio de Janeiro states to less than 2 in Amazonas, Amapá, and Pará. Bed density is decreasing because the increase in public beds has not kept pace with the decrease in private beds, while the population is growing.

32. The equipment complexity indicator was constructed as the weighted sum of different types and complexities of diagnostic and treatment equipment (especially imaging equipment), with weights assigned according to complexity. Though biased toward imaging services, the indicator proved a reasonable proxy for the overall level of hospital technological complexity.

33. In these municipalities the level is comparable to or higher than in high-income countries.

34. The implementation completion report (ICR) on the SUS Reform Project (REFORSUS), cofinanced by the World Bank and the Inter-American Development Bank, mentioned the political pressure exerted by the Brazilian Congress to distribute equipment that is unnecessary often to a wide array of hospitals (World Bank 2004a).

35. Brazil is one of the most unequal societies in the world, with a Gini coefficient of 0.59 in 2001 (World Bank 2006c).

36. For example, in Guatemala, Paraguay, and South Africa only about 50 to 60 percent of those in the lowest-income quintile seeking care are actually seen by a physician.

37. Neonatal mortality is strongly influenced by access to care and by quality of care.

38. Annex 2A describes estimation methods, and annex table 2B.4 presents detailed breakdowns of hospital expenditures by funding source. These estimates are based on available data and on the

indirect estimation method. No precise information is available regarding hospital funding by level of government, given the complexity of SUS financial mechanisms and the limited detail in budget documents.

39. The figure for SUS financing may overestimate the actual proportion because it assumes (according to the methodology used, as described in annex 2A) similar costs in public and private facilities. In contrast, the lower figure reported in annex table 2B.5 (49 percent) is underestimated because it does not account for ad hoc government transfers to private facilities. These transfers are difficult to identify in subnational budget ledgers.

40. The low level of SUS reimbursement to private hospitals is a major driver of the financial predicament facing private facilities, mostly charitable nonprofits, under contract with the SUS. The financial crisis of nonprofit hospitals is discussed in chapter 4.

41. Another practice with spending implications is the seconding of civil servants to private hospitals. Unless the cost of this staff is registered in a specific public hospital or as hospital personnel in public budgets, it is difficult to account for such spending.

42. Estimates based on AMS 2002 data (IBGE 2003).

43. Hospital expenditure by category (line item) was estimated from two samples of public and private hospitals (World Bank 2007; de Matos 2002).

44. Capital expenditure was not analyzed because its variability results in distorted allocation patterns.

45. The "external" category consists of patients who receive diagnostic tests at the hospital without receiving an outpatient or emergency consultation or being admitted for inpatient care. Spending on diagnostic services for inpatient, outpatient, and emergency care is included in the respective expenditure categories.

46. Administration refers to managerial and support services provided at the central level and not attributable to particular types of health and medical services; it does not include in-hospital administration costs.

47. These include 14 hospitals in São Paulo state that apply an organizational form known as health social organizations (organizações sociais em saúde), as discussed in chapters 5 and 6.

48. The lack of clarity in both the AMS survey and the Datasus classification of emergency services precluded more definitive estimates.

3

Comparative Analysis of Costs and Efficiency

Brazil's spending on health care and hospitals is not being fully reflected in outcomes. Policy makers have begun to realize that they are not getting their money's worth. Either more money will be needed—but money is tight—or systemic efficiency will have to be improved. Unfortunately, there is little empirical evidence to show where resources are being wasted. Sparse knowledge about the efficiency and costs of hospital service delivery contributes to fragmented, short-term, and discontinuous policies intended to improve hospital performance.

This chapter attempts to inform policy makers and to provoke debate by examining the evidence and issues related to hospital efficiency in the context of production, productivity, and costs. Using the data available, it seeks answers to these questions: Do Brazilian hospitals use resources in ways that minimize production costs (for a given level of quality)? Do hospitals maximize health outcomes by providing appropriate mixes or types of treatment within budgetary limits? What are the determinants of hospital costs? How does efficiency vary by hospital type and size? What policies can improve the efficiency of resource use and contain escalating costs? The tools of cost and efficiency analysis applied in this chapter can assist in addressing these questions.

As a main driver behind the establishment of the Unified Health System (Sistema Único de Saúde, SUS), the federal government has for nearly two decades played a major role in forging a health policy framework. This framework has focused on promoting wider access, decentralization, and financial equity. Cost and efficiency issues have been conspicuously absent from the policy agenda until very recently.

Recent macroeconomic factors have hastened recognition that cost and efficiency must be addressed in order to stretch tight budgets and obtain full value for money. In 2005 public debt accounted for 46 percent and public sector expenditure for 41 percent of gross domestic product (GDP), and the tax burden amounted to nearly 34 percent. These indicators—among the world's highest—imply that Brazil has little room for increasing public spending. In this uncertain fiscal situation, government financial authorities are preoccupied with public expenditures on health. Because hospitals absorb the lion's share of SUS spending and the SUS is the main source of hospital financing, the emerging policy debate will focus on cost containment and efficiency gains in the delivery of hospital care. Cost and efficiency arguments will be countered by calls to increase financing, protect gains made by the SUS, and improve access to free hospital care for the poor.

High spending on health care—unlike in other areas of the economy—is usually seen as a bad thing, as a diversion of scarce resources from more productive sectors. In addition, findings from international studies suggest that more spending does not necessarily mean better health outcomes. How resources are allocated and used appears to be the key to understanding the lack of correspondence between spending and end results in health. Technically, this notion can best be expressed in terms of efficiency (see box 3.1).

Because hospitals receive the largest share of Brazilian health spending, any improvements in efficiency and cost control could yield significant benefits for the entire health sector by freeing up resources in order to expand other services or improve the quality of care. Systematic information on hospital costs and efficiency helps identify the main sources of inefficiency and waste and thus contributes to the design of policies and actions to make better use of available resources, yet little is known about the real cost of hospital services or how efficiently these resources are being employed. Information is scattered, incomplete, and disparate and is therefore difficult or impossible to analyze and compare. The few analyses of efficiency in Brazilian hospitals that have been undertaken do not point to clear conclusions because of their limited sample size and scope.

Hospitals are complex, multidimensional institutions that produce a variety of services or products: patient care (inpatient, ambulatory, emergency, and diagnostic), research and training, hotel services (from food to laundry), social work, and community outreach for health promotion and prevention. Any analysis of hospital costs and productivity requires the correct definition and measurement of these outputs. Depending on the type of analysis, the "product" of a hospital can be defined in terms of patients, treatment of illness episodes, procedures, end results, and health outcomes, or in terms of composite units that aggregate measures of different outputs. Costs can be measured only for specific outputs or sets of outputs. Drawing on available studies and datasets, this chapter employs several methodologies that define and analyze the efficiency and costs of different hospital outputs.

Box 3.1
Types of Efficiency

Efficiency is generally defined as a ratio between the quantity of output produced and the quantity of inputs used in the production process. It is closely associated with productivity and costs in the sense that an efficient producer will exhibit higher productivity (an index of output per input used) and incur lower production costs. Efficiency can be classified into different types according to the main factors determining it.

Technical efficiency is a characteristic of the production process itself and best corresponds to the general definition given above. The more product is generated with a given quantity and combination of inputs, or the fewer inputs are used to turn out a given quantity of product, the more efficient is the process in the technical sense.

As explained in detail in annex 3D, technical efficiency can be broken down into two main components: *pure,* or *internal, technical efficiency,* associated with internal factors such as management and control of the production process; and *scale efficiency,* determined by operational size or scale. Small hospitals are usually inefficient because small scale results in higher unit costs. Increasing production volume would raise efficiency and reduce unit costs.

In contrast to technical efficiency, which takes the combination of inputs used (labor, medical supplies, technology, and so on) as given, *allocative efficiency* focuses on how inputs are combined. A production process using the optimal combination of inputs—the one leading to lower production costs—is said to be allocatively efficient.

In a context of limited resources and growing demand, cost containment has become a goal of health care reform in many countries, and the issue is also relevant to Brazil.[1] Cost containment is closely linked both to health care costs and to the efficiency with which resources are utilized. These are the two major themes of this chapter.

Hospital Costs: Measurement Challenges and Findings

Information on the cost of hospital procedures is fundamental for realistically pricing products and services, evaluating efficiency, and designing policies that will promote rational use of resources. The cost information available in Brazil, however, suffers from limitations that compromise its effective use. Furthermore, most existing cost information presents average costs by cost center rather than by specific procedures and treatments. An exception is a recent study that estimated the cost of 107 inpatient procedures (De Matos 2002). A complementary study by Dias, Couttolenc, and De Matos (2004), commissioned for this volume, adjusted the original data by case mix and provided comparisons across hospital types.

Challenges to Cost Measurement in Brazilian Hospitals

Cost information available from Brazilian hospitals suffers from a number of limitations.[2] These include overall poor quality, multiple and unstandardized cost accounting systems (where they exist), and managerial failure to apply available data to operations. Because many cost information systems are poorly designed and implemented, they reduce the reliability of the existing data and its usefulness for evaluation and decision making. Deficient medical information and record keeping prevent meaningful analysis of medical practices and frustrate efforts to track costs and link them to specific cases or treatments. These shortcomings are discussed in detail next.

Cost Accounting Systems
No one knows precisely how many Brazilian hospitals have cost accounting systems, but it is generally accepted that fewer than 5 percent do; most of these are large private facilities.

Traditionally, three costing methodologies have been applied to Brazilian hospitals. *Classical absorption costing*, which allocates all costs and expenses to final cost centers, is used in most hospitals that have a cost accounting system. *Direct costing*, which considers only the direct costs of production, is most often used ad hoc to meet a specific need. *Activity-based costing*, with its demanding needs for information, is used by very few hospitals. These approaches are applied for different purposes and are not mutually exclusive. Few, if any, facilities have installed a permanent system for estimating procedure, case, or treatment costs.[3] This absence of comprehensive and systematic cost information constitutes an important obstacle to reforming hospital payment mechanisms or introducing case-based hospital payments such as those based on diagnostic groups (discussed in chapter 4).

System Design
Although most of the Brazilian hospitals that have a costing system have chosen the absorption costing general methodology, the particular methods and approaches used and the way they

are applied are not standardized in terms of definition and measurement of cost centers, outputs, and appropriation criteria.[4] Moreover, published cost data seldom specify the methodology used, which makes comparisons difficult or arbitrary. Most systems have been designed from an accounting perspective and do not lend themselves to cost analysis and decision making, nor do they allow direct estimation of costs of treatments or of hospital procedures.

The final objective of hospital costing often goes beyond estimating the mean cost of the product or service of a cost center. In many cases the issue of interest is the cost of individual patients or groups of patients according to the type of procedure performed or the particular diagnosis or treatment.

Nevertheless, nearly all existing costing systems estimate mean costs by the unit cost of a patient-day, a medical visit, or other service. These data require considerable manipulation to yield case-based cost estimates.

System Implementation

Most cost accounting systems in Brazilian hospitals were introduced from the top down, following a decision at the central level or under the leadership of a charismatic and inspired hospital manager. Seldom has the technical staff in charge of the system been involved in the design and implementation strategy. Managers and decision makers at the hospital level or at the central level receive little or no training in cost analysis and interpretation and usually do not know what to do with information generated by cost accounting systems. Cost data—where they exist—are usually considered confidential, and researchers encounter difficulty in obtaining them from hospitals for analysis or comparison. Because of this approach to implementation, many costing system applications have been quickly abandoned, usually after a change in leadership or in the technical team responsible for implementation and management.

Information Management and Use

Most public hospitals in Brazil, especially small and medium-size facilities, do not manage their budgets and therefore have little financial information.[5] Even when hospitals do have financial information, it is often of questionable quality and reliability and, in the case of public hospitals, is oriented toward financial control and budget monitoring and is thus not directly suitable for cost estimation. Financial management is weak in nearly all public facilities and most small private hospitals. As a result of these limitations, the partial cost information on hospital services that is available is often difficult to use for comparison purposes, requiring careful scrutiny of methods and data and adjustment for methodological differences. The available data often do not lend themselves to generalization because of limited sample size.

The limited use of cost accounting systems, the lack of uniformity in these systems, and the nonstandard organization of medical and statistical information complicate the processing, analysis, and comparison of cost data, resulting in important unexplained variations. In the De Matos (2002) sample, only 11 hospitals out of 25 had implemented a cost accounting system; 6 had some basic cost information (usually simple spreadsheets), and 8 had no cost information. In most hospitals patient statistical information, especially regarding morbidity (by diagnosis or treatment), is disorganized or unreliable, making it difficult to collect and analyze data for a given procedure or treatment. Different kinds of data—on patients, costs, and hospitals—often refer to different time periods, requiring adjustments to make them comparable.

Medical Records

Collecting and using patient information by reviewing medical records is cumbersome and time consuming, even under ideal conditions. In most Brazilian hospitals medical records are incomplete and poorly maintained. Records are disorganized, physician or nursing annotations are absent or illegible, and order forms for diagnostic tests or medical reports are often missing. In general, medical records present little or no information on inputs and their volume. Expense or consumption sheets completed in nursing units or operating rooms are hard to find and, when present, are not part of patient records. Finally, diagnostic test prescriptions and orders for special medical supplies either are not kept with medical records or disappear. Measures of utilization and resource consumption (e.g., activities and inputs) that are recorded in patient charts are not standardized across patients.

Treatment Protocols

Patients undergoing the same procedure can receive quite different treatments requiring different sets and quantities of inputs, both within a given hospital and across institutions. Often, no difference in severity is evident to explain the observed variation in treatment. In the absence of standardization, and given the limited information in medical records, it is almost impossible to control or adjust for differences in case severity at the patient level or for the presence of comorbidities and complications. There is little standard description and coding of diagnostic tests, medical supplies, and drugs. This absence of standardization within and between hospitals leads to significant variations in data collected for similar procedures or patients and precludes meaningful comparisons.

Billing Information

The SUS billing information system, the Authorization for Hospitalization (Autorização de Internação Hospitalar, AIH), contains detailed claim forms for recording a patient's treatment and thus could be used to complement or validate information collected from medical records.[6] In many cases, however, there are important discrepancies between medical records and AIH forms. Patient bills are usually not attached to the corresponding medical records because they pertain to a different information system and serve a different purpose. Diagnostic tests and other ancillary procedures registered on medical records often do not appear on AIH claim forms. Lengths of stay (LOSs) are often inconsistent between the two sources of information. In a number of cases, reasonable medical practice would result in a lower LOS than defined in the AIH schedule, and in lower costs. To receive payment, however, hospitals have to submit data aligned with the AIH payment schedule and rules, even when these are based on outdated practices or result in higher costs. In addition, incompatibility between the resource groups defined in the AIH schedule and the hospitals' accounting structures creates a major difficulty in obtaining a "homogeneous procedure," as established in the AIH schedule.

Hospital Procedure Costs: Results of In-Depth Costing Research

The hospital costing analysis performed by De Matos (2002) is the most comprehensive study of hospital procedure costs to date.[7] The estimated cost of 107 inpatient procedures is based on a sample of 16,500 cases randomly selected from 25 publicly (SUS) financed public and private hospitals. Although the hospital sample was biased toward larger teaching hospitals, the procedures represented 62 percent of volume and 61 percent of the inpatient care payments made by the federal government.[8] They can thus be considered representative of inpatient care provided by the SUS.[9] Annex 3A presents a detailed description of the costing methodology applied by De Matos (2002).

Cases of a particular disease or treatment are expected to have, on average, similar costs. Variations in (average) cost can stem from several factors: differences in individual case severity; differences in hospital characteristics such as the mean severity or complexity of cases treated or the nature of the hospital's work as a teaching facility; differences in efficiency and use of resources, as well as in input prices; differences in medical practice regarding treatment; and differences in quality. The mean severity or complexity of the cases treated is often measured by a case-mix index (CMI) that is used to adjust the cost of particular procedures or treatments.[10] Measuring the importance and pattern of cost variations and identifying their sources can help in diagnosing sources of inefficiencies and waste and in identifying reasons for poor quality of care.

Dias, Couttolenc, and De Matos (2004) found wide variations in mean costs, even after adjusting for case-mix differences. Such variations for the same procedure were found both across cases within a given hospital and across hospitals.

Average Costs and Cost Variations

The mean cost of the 107 procedures in the sample was R$2,606 (US$1,055 at 2002 exchange rates), varying between R$513 for conservative treatment of cranial trauma to R$48,436 for a lung transplant. (See annex 3C for a complete listing of procedures and mean costs.) Nearly two-thirds of the procedures, including most of the clinical procedures, had a mean cost less than the sample mean. The remaining one-third, with a mean cost above the sample mean, consisted mostly of surgical interventions.

Average costs varied widely for a given procedure across cases and hospitals. The coefficient of variation (CV) in the sample ranged from 20 percent (intracranial vascular microsurgery) to 221 percent (kidney receptor transplant, live donor), with a mean of 55 percent.[11] In order to identify the main factors contributing to cost variation, the CV was computed along three dimensions: (1) all cases pooled, which resulted in the largest variation (CV equal to 86.4 percent) because the pool included all the possible factors affecting cost variation; (2) interhospital cases, in which the average cost variation was 61.0 percent, which may reflect differences in case mix, efficiency, quality, input prices, and other hospital characteristics; and (3) intrahospital cases—cases treated within the same hospital—for which the average variation was 41.1 percent, reflecting mostly differences in resource use within the hospital and variation in treatment practices. The main factors contributing to cost variation were differences in case mix, hospital characteristics, length of stay, clinical practice, and type of procedure. The remainder of this section examines each factor.

Case Mix

Differences in case mix can be a major source of variation in hospital costs because case mix reflects the complexity of care and the severity of illness.[12] To estimate the importance of case mix, a case-mix index was computed, drawing on cost data in the sample and based on the relative cost for a given procedure across hospitals (annex 3A). Figure 3.1 shows that most cases in the sample were within the lower ranges of the CMI, indicating low complexity and

FIGURE 3.1
Distribution of Cases and Costs, by Case-Mix Index Range, 2001
(*N* = 16,493 cases)

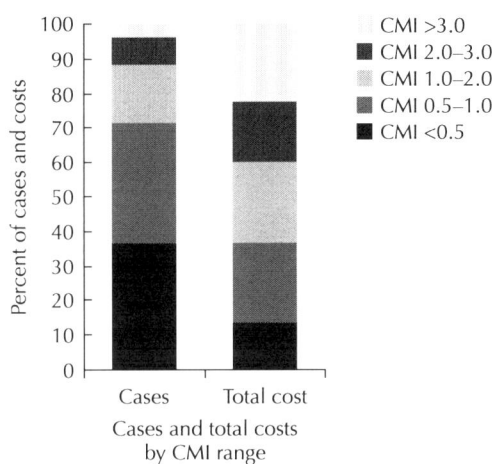

Source: Dias, Couttolenc, and De Matos 2004; De Matos 2002.

cost. For example, 32 low-complexity procedures (those with CMI less than 0.5) accounted for 37 percent of volume (number of cases) but for 13.4 percent of the total cost incurred by the 107 procedures in the sample. In contrast, 23 high-complexity procedures (CMI greater than 2) represented 11.5 percent of volume but nearly 40 percent of total cost. Procedures with an intermediate level of complexity represented around 51.5 percent of volume and 46.7 percent of total cost.

Because differences in severity inflate cost variations, the case-mix adjustment reduced the variations in procedure cost, with little change in the mean cost itself. It also shifted the distribution toward higher-cost categories, with more procedures falling in the cost intervals above R$2,000 (figure 3.2). However, important variations remained even after the case-mix adjustment, indicating that other factors were at work, such as hospital characteristics and clinical practice patterns.

Hospital Characteristics
Mean costs differed significantly across types of hospital. Teaching hospitals had a higher mean cost (23.2 percent) than nonteaching hospitals (figure 3.3). Consistent with international experience, higher costs among teaching hospitals were expected because of the additional cost of teaching and research activities, greater use of high-complexity equipment, and treatment of more complex—and thus more costly—cases. The CMI was indeed higher among university, especially public, hospitals than among general hospitals (CMI = 1.5, against the mean of 1). In fact, it explained most of the observed differences between teaching and nonteaching hospitals, and nearly all of these differences disappeared after adjusting for case mix (figure 3.3).

Public hospitals showed a higher mean procedure cost than private hospitals and had the highest costs for more procedures. Again, much of the difference in average cost was attributable

FIGURE 3.2
Distribution of Procedures, by Cost Intervals, 2001
(N = 107 procedures)

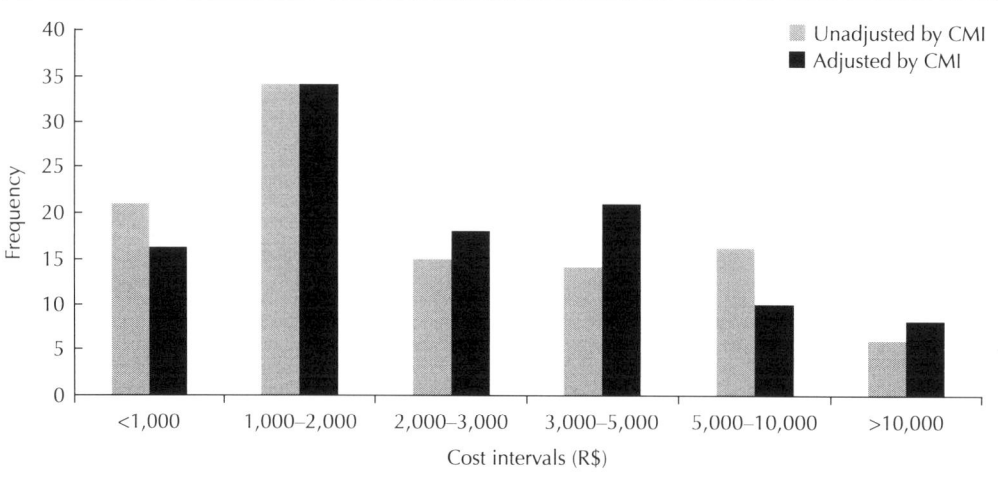

Source: Dias, Couttolenc, and De Matos 2004; De Matos 2002.

FIGURE 3.3
Costs by Hospital Type, Unadjusted and Adjusted for Case Mix, 2001
(N = 107 procedures)

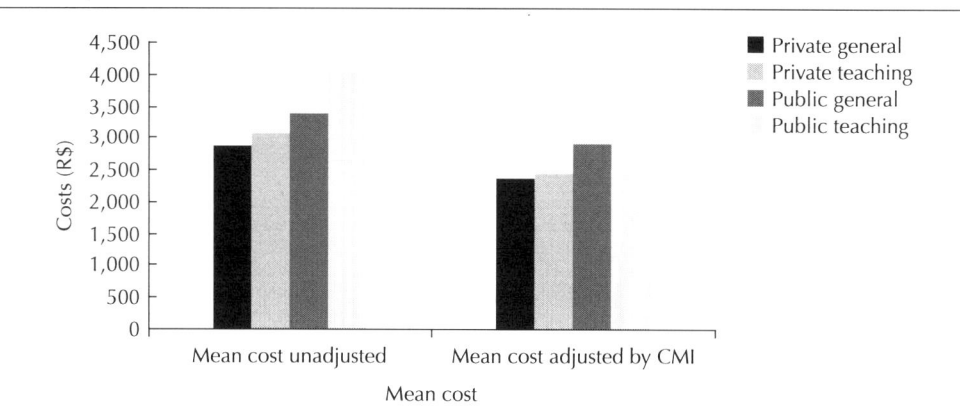

Source: Dias, Couttolenc, and De Matos 2004; De Matos 2002.

to differences in facility case mix. In other words, public hospitals usually handle a more severe case load than their private counterparts.[13] But other factors may contribute to higher costs in public facilities. First, public hospitals are, on average, less efficient than private ones, as is discussed below. Second, public hospitals receive more SUS funding for treating SUS patients than do comparable private hospitals under an SUS contract. The reduced levels of financing place a severe constraint on these private facilities, reflecting distortions in the SUS purchasing systems.[14] This difference in funding levels and the corresponding absence of fair competition directly impair hospital and systemic efficiency because they encourage providers to select (higher-paying) cases or to cut costs indiscriminately.

Length of Stay

Another important source of cost variation was patients' length of stay. To isolate the effect of differences in LOS, the CV was computed for the cost per patient-day for each procedure and compared with the CVs of the procedures themselves. As reported in figure 3.4, the CVs for patient-days were systematically smaller than for the procedures, for both the case-mix-adjusted and the unadjusted costs. After controlling for average length of stay (ALOS), the CV fell by about 20 percent, demonstrating the strong effect of ALOS on hospital costs. This is illustrated in figure 3.4 by the difference between the procedures (PROC) and patient-day (P-D) bars for each group of cases—all cases, interhospital cases, and intrahospital cases.

Figure 3.4 also illustrates the effect and size of case-mix adjustment and other hospital characteristics. After adjustment for CMI, the CVs for procedures and patient-days were significantly lower, by 11–18 percent and 5–10 percent, respectively, than the unadjusted CVs, whether for all cases pooled or across hospitals (the "interhospital" bars). The average difference was 10–15 percent. Finally, facility characteristics, including efficiency, teaching status, governance, and other characteristics, drive the observed differences between CVs (for both procedures and patient-days) in the interhospital category.[15]

Clinical Practice

Even after adjusting for case mix and ALOS, significant cost variation remains. This appears in the variance within hospitals (figure 3.4, intrahospital bars). Because for a given procedure different cases in a particular hospital are expected to face identical facility characteristics, case mix, and input prices, the large observed variation within hospitals is likely to be

FIGURE 3.4
Main Sources of Variation in Hospital Costs, 2001
(N = 16,493 cases/25 hospitals)

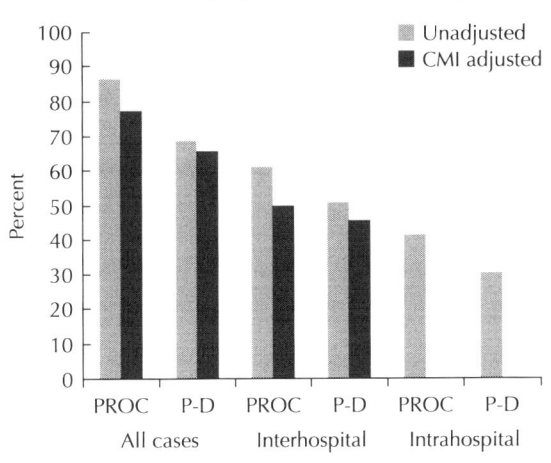

Source: Dias, Couttolenc, and De Matos 2004; De Matos 2002.
Note: PROC, procedures; P-D, patient-day.

associated either with differences in individual case severity or with lack of standardization in medical procedures and related input use.[16] Although input use could not be measured directly, the review of medical records used to extract data for the study indicated that lack of standardization was indeed a major problem. This was evidenced by incomplete or incorrect recording of medical information in patient charts, the near-absence of treatment protocols in the sampled facilities, and large variations in medical practice. Patients with the same diagnosis and procedure and with no notation in the medical records of significant variations in severity or health status received different treatments, most often implying different combinations and quantities of inputs (e.g., duration of surgery, length of stay, diagnostic tests).

Procedure Type

The procedure type was also shown to affect cost variation. Figure 3.5 compares the CVs for clinical cases, surgical cases, and all cases in the sample. Clinical cases had markedly higher CVs, on average, than surgical cases (65 and 43 percent, respectively). This may reflect greater standardization of surgical procedures or greater variation in patient severity among clinical cases. There is some evidence of the latter effect; adjusting for case mix changed the pattern slightly, reducing the mean CV among clinical procedures to 61 percent, with little change among surgical procedures. Further analysis, however, suggests that much of the cost variation between clinical and surgical cases is associated with differences in average length of stay. As shown in figure 3.5, correcting for ALOS greatly reduced the CV among clinical procedures, to 47 percent, while increasing it among surgical procedures, to 53 percent. In short, length of stay is the main factor in cost variation among clinical procedures, probably because of the low use of standard treatment protocols in clinical cases, as well as wider variation in case severity.

Examination of variations among specific procedures provides a more focused notion of the scope of cost variations. Table 3.1 compares the range of variation for the eight procedures with lowest and highest CVs (unadjusted for case mix) for all cases and for intrahospital

FIGURE 3.5
Coefficient of Variation for Surgical and Clinical Cases, 2001
(*N* = 107 procedures/16,493 cases)

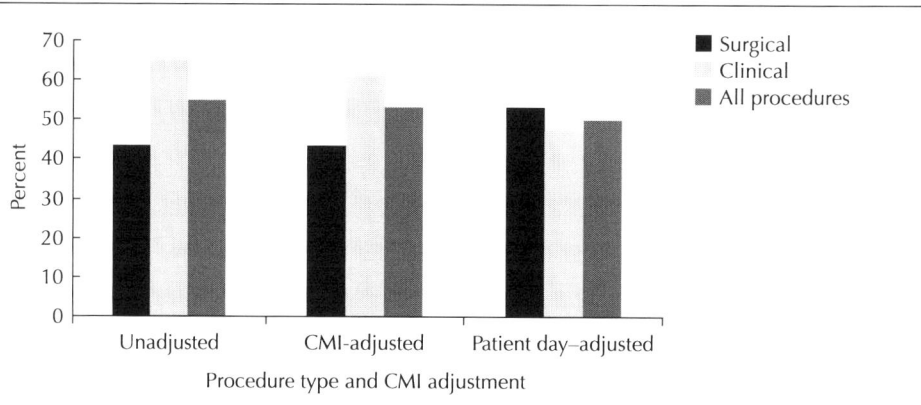

Source: Dias, Couttolenc, and De Matos 2004; De Matos 2002.

TABLE 3.1
Total and Intrahospital Cost Variation and Ranges for Procedures
with Low and High CVs, Unadjusted for CMI, 2001

(*N* = 107 procedures, 16,493 cases)

Procedure	All cases, mean CV (%)	All cases, range (R$)	Intrahospital CV, procedure (%)	Intrahospital CV, patient-day (%)	Intrahospital, range (R$)
Low CV					
Cesarean section	41.1	304–3,865	19.9	19.2	304–1,402
Normal delivery	45.8	141–1,844	24.5	27.0	289–1,746
Appendectomy	48.7	236–6,259	30.9	30.9	772–6,259
Endoscopic prostate resection	49.4	462–6,924	25.5	23.8	1,219–6,924
High CV					
Lung tuberculosis	114.4	357–14,641	60.5	32.2	487–10,402
Digestive hemorrhage	123.1	87–13,473	67.4	38.2	87–3,540
Acute lung edema	123.4	226–26,326	69.5	45.4	471–26,326
Pediatric septicemia	125.3	208–67,791	69.5	46.1	997–37,132

Source: De Matos 2002; Dias, Couttolenc, and De Matos 2004.

cases. Cost ranges across all cases vary from approximately 15:1 in low-variation procedures to over 300:1 among high-variation procedures.[17] Intrahospital variations are lower than variations among all cases pooled (by around 50 percent) but are still large, as shown in the last column of the table, with average ratios of 6:1 for low-variation procedures and 39:1 for high-variation procedures.

Cost Structure

The cost structure of procedures can show how efficiently resources are being allocated among inputs. For example, a hospital spending too much on labor may have few resources left for other essential inputs such as drugs and medical supplies. An inefficient mix of inputs (resulting, for example, in a shortage of essential medical supplies) can compromise the quality of care.

Cost composition varies widely among procedures and across hospitals, according to the AIH billing and payment system.[18] This is not surprising because different procedures require different input mixes. On average, hospital services account for nearly two-thirds of a procedure's total cost; professional services account for about 11 percent, as do drugs and medical supplies (figure 3.6). Surgical procedures requiring use of prostheses or expensive drugs will show a very high proportion of costs going to those categories.

FIGURE 3.6
Composition of Procedure Costs, by AIH Category, 2001
(*N* = 16,493 cases)

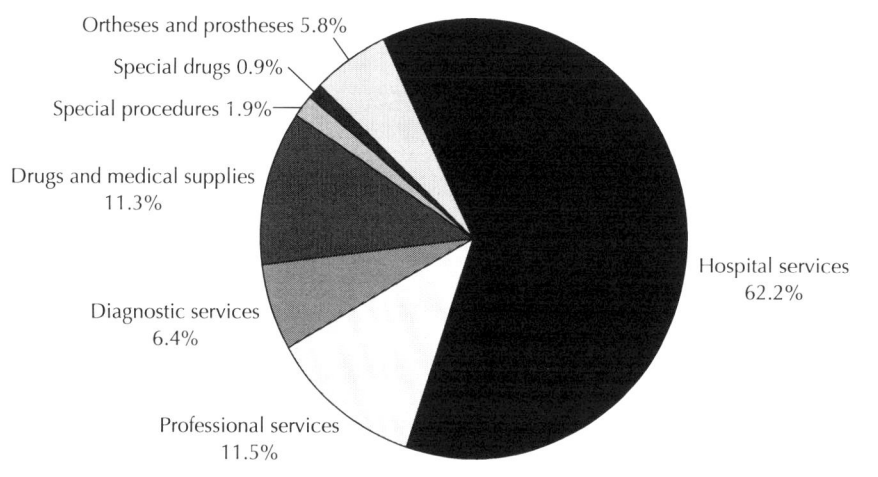

Source: Dias, Couttolenc, and De Matos 2004; De Matos 2002.

The AIH structure has more to do with how and to whom payments are made than with categories of inputs and is thus not appropriate for the analysis of resource allocation. A more useful breakdown is by input type (shown in table 3.2 by hospital ownership) or by type of hospital services (box 3.2).

Personnel costs account for 61 percent of total hospital costs; inclusion of nonmedical outsourced manpower increases labor costs to 65 percent of the total. Supplies make up another 28 percent, mostly for drugs (9.4 percent of total cost) and medical supplies. Other costs, including nonphysician outsourced labor and general expenses such as maintenance,

TABLE 3.2
Composition of Hospital Costs, by Ownership and Line Item, 2002

(Percent)

Cost	Private nonprofit	Private for-profit	OSS	Average
Personnel	59.8	57.2	68.2	61.3
Salaried	46.9	40.8	57.0	47.7
Outsourced physician	12.9	16.4	11.2	13.6
Supplies	28.8	31.9	22.8	28.2
Drugs	10.5	10.5	6.4	9.4
Other medical supplies	13.3	17.1	10.1	13.7
General and other	11.4	10.9	9.0	10.5
Outsourced other	3.0	2.1	2.7	2.6

Source: Data supplied by PLANISA.
Note: N = 22 hospitals. OSS (Health Social Organizations) are public facilities managed by private organizations under a management contract (see chapters 5 and 6 for a discussion of this organizational arrangement).

Box 3.2
Hospital Cost Structures in Brazil and Canada

The structure of hospital costs is somewhat different in Brazil than in other countries. Compared with Canadian hospitals, for instance, Brazilian hospitals, as shown in the table, spend a much lower proportion on diagnostic services, ambulatory care, and support services such as cleaning, surveillance, and maintenance. Conversely, they spend a higher proportion on emergency care, operating room, and administrative costs. Three factors enter into the cost differences: differences in the product mix, associated with greater use of hospital services and emergency care compared with primary care and ambulatory facilities; the relative cost of the inputs used (hence the relatively small proportion of support service costs in Brazil); and differences in the environment in which hospitals operate, especially regulatory and payment mechanisms, which can put a big burden on Brazilian hospital administration. The relatively high administrative costs in Brazil can, however, also be interpreted as an indication of inefficient management.

Distribution of Costs by Component

(Percent)

Cost component	Brazil	Canada
Inpatient care	44	N/A
Nursing	N/A	30
Diagnostic services	4	20
Ambulatory care	8	8
Emergency care	10	5
Operating room	10	5
Support services	10	16
Administration	13	8
Other	0	6

Source: For Brazil, figure 2.12, this volume, and *organizações sociais em saúde* (OSSs) cost data; for Canada, CIHI (2005).
Note: N/A, not available.

utilities, depreciation, marketing, and equipment leasing, account for the remainder. Public hospitals spend, on average, a higher proportion of their costs on personnel than do private facilities (68 percent against 58 percent) and a significantly lower proportion on supplies. This suggests problems related to allocative efficiency because a high proportion of spending on personnel can shortchange resources for drugs, maintenance, and other critical inputs. Public managers often view hiring more personnel as the solution to their problems and do not consider the allocative implications of this action. Brazilian hospitals in general, and public hospitals in particular, are overstaffed, as discussed below.

The Fiscal Responsibility Law of May 4, 2000 (Lei Complementar 101), set caps on personnel expenditures of government organizations, including public hospitals. For federal hospitals the ceiling is 50 percent of recurrent revenue, and for state and municipal hospitals it is 60 percent. To circumvent this legislation, many public hospitals which used to spend well above those limits have been outsourcing nonclinical services such as food, security, and laundry. Staff costs are within the limits, but overall labor costs, including outsourcing, are not (table 3.2). Overall, cost composition varies widely across hospitals as a result of facility-based policies (e.g., outsourcing versus in-house production of support services), other facility characteristics, and patient mix.

Costs in the Private Sector

Information is scarce regarding costs in private hospitals, especially those not affiliated with the SUS. An undetermined number of private hospitals have installed cost accounting systems, but the resulting cost information is considered proprietary and is thus unavailable to outsiders. The National Agency for Health Insurance (Agência Nacional de Saúde Suplementar, ANS) and the National Association of Self-Insured Health Plans (União Nacional das Instituições de Autogestão em Saúde, UNIDAS) have published data on payments by private health insurance carriers (*operadoras*) to providers of hospital and ambulatory services.[19] This information can be considered a proxy for costs in privately funded hospitals. São Paulo state has installed cost accounting systems in 16 public hospitals known as health social organizations (*organizações sociais de saúde*, OSSs), which are privately managed.

Table 3.3 compares cost data from these sources with those from the De Matos (2002) study, which included public hospitals as well as private hospitals under contract with the SUS. Inpatient costs are higher for UNIDAS, perhaps because of the more generous coverage under self-administered plans than under other health insurance plans and a hhigher than average proportion of reitred (and therefore elderly) in their covered population. It is important to keep in mind that the values shown for ANS and UNIDAS are payments to providers, not providers' costs as estimated by De Matos (2002) or as generated for the OSSs. Nonetheless, these values are on the same order of magnitude as the mean cost estimated by the De Matos study for the 107 procedures (R$2,607), considering that the estimates from that study are biased upward because of the larger proportion of complex procedures and university hospitals in the sample.[20] Costs for medical consultations and diagnostic tests are almost identical for the four sources because they are much more standardized and less subject to variation associated with case severity.

Cost Containment Strategies

The government has applied cost containment measures for many years, and the track record has been mixed. Because of their fragmentation and inadequacy, the measures have been

TABLE 3.3

Mean Costs in the Private Sector, 2002–4

(R$)

Service	ANS (2004)	UNIDAS (2003–4)	De Matos (2002)	OSS (2003)
Hospitalization	2,063	2,855	2,607	1,861
Medical consultation	26	25	N/A	24
Diagnostic tests	19	18	N/A	189

Source: ANS 2005; UNIDAS 2005; De Matos 2002; for OSS, SES-SP 2004.
Note: US$1 = R$3.08 (2003). N/A, not available.

only partially successful in limiting growth of expenditures; between 1990 and 2004 real SUS spending increased by about 50 percent. Some measures compromise efficiency and lead to lower quality. A 1994 World Bank report highlighted the problems of the cost control policies and strategies applied by the SUS (World Bank 1994).

The SUS has addressed cost containment through three main approaches. The first—although not an explicit policy—consists of systematically adjusting hospital reimbursement rates at below-inflation rates. This practice has kept an informal cap on expenditures but has severed reimbursement rates from actual costs. Below-cost adjustments have generated a wide gap between costs and payments, threatening the sustainability of private providers. Caps on reimbursement rates have not necessarily improved efficiency in service delivery, for two reasons. First, severe underpayment for simpler (and high-volume) procedures has induced hospitals to specialize in complex, expensive procedures. Second, low payment levels drive private hospitals to lobby subnational governments for ad hoc bailout payments to make ends meet (see the discussion in chapter 4).

The second strategy consists of setting volume or financial ceilings on the number of admissions or procedures paid by the SUS for each state or municipality. For instance, the number of admissions authorized by the SUS as a whole was reduced from 11.7 million in 2000 to 11.4 million in 2005, or 7 and 6.2 admissions per 100.[21] These caps help contain expenditure, but they are based mostly on historical supply trends, not actual population needs, and therefore create imbalances across geographic areas and socioeconomic groups. Lobbying by interest and political groups also influences the determination of the ceilings.

The third approach consists of controls on the use of expensive procedures and inputs through prior registration of suppliers, definition of authorized ceilings by states, improved information systems that include verification of the validity of treatment (with respect to diagnosis or procedure), and auditing.[22] The Information System for High-Complexity Procedures (Sistema de Informações para Procedimentos de Alta Complexidade, SIPAC) was the main system for that purpose, but it is gradually being merged into the Hospital Information System (Sistema de Informação Hospitalar, SIH) and the Medium and High-Complexity (Media e Alta Complexidade) federal transfer (see chapter 4). These latter systems now generate automatic checks on consistency between diagnostic and treatment parameters and the procedures that are actually provided. Although they simplify payment mechanisms, they do not necessarily help control costs.

More recent initiatives that contribute to better cost control and containment include an online price database (Banco de Preços em Saúde) sponsored by the Ministry of Health (Ministério da Saúde, MS), which records recent prices paid to suppliers for many medical inputs, and an online bidding system (Pregão Eletrônico) that allows suppliers to bid on purchases to be made by public agencies. Although these tools have great potential to contain costs, they are still insufficiently or irregularly used in most municipalities and smaller states (World Bank 2007).

A third initiative worth mentioning is aimed at the private insurance sector. The ANS (the public agency regulating private health insurance) has introduced limits on yearly increases in insurance premiums for family/individual plans by requiring health insurers to demonstrate that their input costs have increased. None of these initiatives has been rigorously evaluated in terms of impact on spending.

Efficiency Analysis

The relative efficiency of Brazilian hospitals was assessed by applying two methodologies: data envelopment analysis (DEA) and benchmarking. Benchmarking is an important complement to DEA because it contributes to the explanation and interpretation of DEA results. Whereas DEA presents a global view of hospital efficiency by working simultaneously with several inputs and outputs and summarizing efficiency in a single score, benchmarking examines one indicator or dimension at a time. Both DEA and benchmarking are evaluation techniques for measuring the relative performance of different organizations. They can indicate best performers and thus serve as a guide for others to improve their own performance.

Methodological Background and Literature Review

In its production process, a hospital combines manpower, drugs, supplies, equipment, and other inputs to produce multiple outputs such as inpatient discharges, patient-days, outpatient consultations, and diagnostic tests. The relation between the quantity of outputs produced and the quantity of inputs used indicates the efficiency of the production process.

DEA is a method for estimating technical efficiency—the ratio of outputs to inputs used. It involves the use of linear programming to rank organizations producing goods or services according to their relative efficiency scores. DEA is based on the idea that production units seek to maximize their output per unit of input (output orientation) or, alternatively, minimize the quantity of inputs per unit of output (input orientation). Box 3.3 summarizes the advantages and limitations of DEA, and annex 3D explains its basic methodology. DEA relies on the construction of an efficiency frontier that joins all the possible points for a fully efficient organization to produce a given output. Organizations with a lower ratio of inputs to outputs relative to

---

Box 3.3
Advantages and Limitations of Data Envelopment Analysis

Advantages
- Allows for multiple inputs and products—an important plus in the analysis of hospitals.
- Ranks productive units in order of efficiency.
- Allows estimation of various types of efficiency—pure, or internal, efficiency; scale efficiency; total technical efficiency; or allocative efficiency—using different models.
- Indicates differences in input allocation between efficient and inefficient units.
- Does not require a particular functional form relating inputs to outputs.
- Allows measurement of inputs and outputs in different units.

Limitations
- Results are sample specific and are sensitive to data problems such as measurement error.
- Estimates gauge relative efficiency rather than absolute efficiency; that is, the same hospital will be ranked differently depending on the sample.
- Statistical hypothesis testing is difficult because DEA does not require a functional form relating inputs and outputs.

Source: Bowlin et al. 1985; Jacobs 2001.

other firms are said to be efficient, are located on the frontier, and receive a score of 1. Inefficient organizations are below the frontier and receive a score between 0 and 1.

DEA permits a breakdown of technical efficiency (referred to as total technical efficiency, TTE) into its two main components: pure technical efficiency (pure TE) and scale efficiency. In this study, the more intuitive term internal technical efficiency (ITE) is used to denote the former because it is associated with factors internal to the organization, such as management practices, organizational structure, and the production process. Scale efficiency relates mostly to external or environmental factors such as demand and sector policies, which often determine facility size. Total technical efficiency is the product of internal and scale efficiency.

Review of Hospital Research on DEA and Benchmarking

This section briefly examines international and Brazilian literature on DEA and benchmarking. It focuses on objectives, findings, and issues involving these techniques.

International Studies Applying DEA

The extensive international literature on hospital efficiency shows that DEA has been used for different purposes. Many studies have used DEA in microanalysis to rank individual production units, identify the most efficient units as role models for inefficient facilities, and define strategies for improving efficiency. For example, Ersoy et al. (1997) used DEA to analyze the technical efficiency of 573 general acute hospitals in Turkey. The results showed that inefficient hospitals had more beds, used more physicians, performed fewer surgeries, and delivered fewer inpatient and outpatient services than efficient institutions.

Other researchers have used DEA to examine the effect of structural or institutional variables on efficiency by comparing mean scores of provider groups or types. These studies have looked at the effect of hospital ownership, for-profit status, governance, or teaching status. Since these institutional characteristics are subject to policies, such analyses are useful for policy making.

The research results are mixed. Several studies found no significant effects of hospital institutional variables, especially ownership (Webster, Kennedy, and Johnson 1998; Register and Bruning 1987; Gruca and Nath 2001; Puig-Junoy 1999). Others found a significant difference in efficiency associated with public-private ownership, often favoring public hospitals (Grosskopf and Valdmanis 1987; Valdmanis 1992; Ozcan, Luke, and Haksever 1992; Ozcan and Luke 1993; Grosskopf, Margaritis, and Valdmanis 2001).[23] Several studies found that teaching hospitals were less efficient than nonteaching ones (Grosskopf, Margaritis, and Valdmanis 2001); the difference was attributed to the use of medical residents and greater use of other inputs. Burgess and Wilson (1996) found that ownership had different effects on technical efficiency, scale efficiency, and input use, which may explain some of the contradictory findings in the literature. Market structure and policy were also found to affect hospital efficiency; facilities operating in more competitive markets tend to be more efficient (Dalmau-Matarrodona and Puig-Junoy 1996).

An important topic in the DEA literature is the relation between size and efficiency. Again, the results are inconclusive. Some authors found a positive relation between size and efficiency (McKillop et al. 1999), while others found the opposite, that smaller hospitals were more efficient (Zere 2000; Ersoy et al. 1997; Marinho and Façanha 2001). An issue often related to size is the relation between efficiency and hospital bed occupancy, but few studies estimated the cost of low occupancy.

The possibility of a trade-off between quality and efficiency is a key and recurrent question in efficiency analysis and its policy implications. Finkler and Wirtschafter (1993) estimated a cost-efficient frontier using DEA and found a trade-off between quantity and quality, based on a sample of nine obstetric hospitals. Tambour and Zethraeus (1998) assessed efficiency in the treatment and rehabilitation of hip fracture patients in Sweden and argued that costs could be reduced by 11 percent without any change in quality and quantity. Maniadakis, Hollingsworth, and Thanassoulis (1999) studied the impact of the U.K. National Health Service reform on acute care hospitals and found that the productivity gains were accompanied by diminishing service quality. Efficiency-quality analysis, however, encounters difficulties in properly assessing quality.

International Research on Benchmarking

Benchmarking has been defined as

> a continuous systematic process for evaluating products, services and work practices of organizations that are recognized as representing best practice for the purpose of organizational improvement. The benchmarking focus may be internal, external or functional, comparing performance to a particular function or process with the best performance regardless of the industry. (Higgins 1997: 61)

Benchmarking can be used to increase performance by identifying organizations with best practices as partners or models, by measuring and comparing a selected work process against partners, by conducting interviews with the benchmark organizations, and by adopting or adapting their best practices (Gohlke 1997).

Benchmarking in health care has a rich history of accumulated experience. As applied to hospitals, benchmarking has contributed to policies and initiatives to redeploy and reallocate staff, reduce length of stay, manage pediatric pain, reduce postsurgical extubation, and decrease operating room hours, among other improvements.[24] Benchmarking can be a valuable marketing tool and an instrument for increasing consumer information by helping consumers and insurers identify the best providers in a specific geographic area. By identifying both high and low performers, it can motivate change and improvement.

The use of benchmarking as a management and evaluation tool is gaining acceptance as part of a larger movement to measure specific aspects of health services functioning, quality, and effectiveness (see chapter 8 for a discussion of quality benchmarking). Under increasing pressure to evaluate and improve performance in health systems, several countries have designed and implemented systems for performance evaluation, quality assessment, and management. International organizations such as the World Health Organization (WHO) and the Organisation for Economic Co-operation and Development (OECD) have proposed methodologies for comparing health system performance. Evaluation of hospital performance through benchmarking is more widespread. Several countries, including Australia, Canada, the United Kingdom, and the United States, have developed and used benchmarking to assess their national health systems or hospital services (box 3.4).

Box 3.4
International Experience in Health System Evaluation and Benchmarking

Benchmarking is increasingly used as a policy tool, and international experience can show how it is applied in different contexts to foster performance and quality in health care.

Australia. Three national databases have been used for benchmarking: the National Hospital Morbidity Database, the National Public Hospital Establishments Database, and the Health Expenditure Database.

United States. The Joint Commission on Accreditation of Healthcare Organizations (JCAHO) has a department entirely dedicated to measuring performance in health and hospital care. Periodically, it produces a detailed severity-adjusted report analyzing the performance of hospitals in each U.S. state. Key statistics are compared with their expected values (that is, the severity-adjusted averages for each hospital's Metropolitan Statistical Area, state, or region) for the top 50 diagnosis-related groups (DRGs), ranked by volume.

A customizable Internet subscription service (http://www.hospitalbenchmarks.com), developed by the U.S. company Ingenix, provides health care executives with immediate access to decision-critical information via one of the most comprehensive health care databases in the United States. The database offers detailed statistics on more than 6,000 U.S. hospitals and publishes benchmarked indicators in the areas of finance, patient care, consumer satisfaction, key departments, multispecialty practices, and advanced markets.

An interesting benchmarking program in the hospital sector is HCIA-Sachs' "100 Top Hospitals: Benchmarks for Success." The program, in existence since 1993, uses Medicare cost reports on more than 6,000 hospitals and other sources to rank hospitals on seven measures of clinical quality practices, operations, and financial management: risk-adjusted mortality index; risk-adjusted complications index; severity-adjusted average length of stay; expense per discharge, adjusted for case mix and for wage cost; profitability (cash flow margin); proportion of outpatient revenue; and productivity (total asset turnover ratio).

Source: Hurst and Jee-Hughes 2001; CMS data (http://www.cms.hhs.gov); JCAHO 1990; Solucient 2004; WHO 2003b.

Brazilian Research Involving DEA and Benchmarking

Empirical studies on the estimation of hospital efficiency in Brazil are few. Most studies have focused on productivity ratios such as output per bed or per staff member. Only nine studies were found that used DEA or similar statistical analyses to estimate efficiency; their main features—their methods, variables, and results—are summarized in annex 3E. A common finding is that the average Brazilian hospital operates with a staff surplus and produces below its output potential. For example, Marinho (2001a) reported that the average hospital uses 39 percent more personnel (excluding doctors) than more efficient facilities. In his study of municipalities in Rio de Janeiro state, Marinho (2001b) found that many municipalities had an excess supply of hospitals and ambulatory units. Efficiency was often inversely associated with average length of stay (Marinho 2001c; Prefeitura da Cidade do Rio de Janeiro 2002).

Calvo (2002) compared the productive efficiency of public and SUS-financed private hospitals in Mato Grosso state. The analysis of input rates for the efficient hospitals suggested that public hospitals saved on financial resources, while private ones saved on the number of doctors. Overall, the author found no significant difference in efficiency between public and private hospitals. The author concluded that ownership (public or private) did not affect productive efficiency in hospitals providing services to the SUS.

The effect of size on hospital efficiency is controversial in Brazil. Marinho and Façanha (2001) compared Brazilian federal university hospitals and found that hospitals with fewer than 200 beds had a higher mean efficiency score (0.946) than those with 200 or more beds (0.712). Proite and Souza (2004), by contrast, encountered increasing economies of scale in most SUS surgical hospitals, probably because of the small size of those units. Other variables found to be negatively correlated with efficiency in Brazilian studies include ALOS (Proite and Souza 2004; Marinho 2001b, 2001c), municipal GDP (Holanda, Petterini, and Nogueira 2004), and a higher number of surgical and nonsurgical procedures per LOS (Proite and Souza 2004).

As is the case with broader efficiency research, Brazilian studies on hospital efficiency suffer from a number of limitations. First, most use small samples or include too many input and output variables to reach stable results.[25] Second, the frequent use of the value of hospital bills (that is, AIH payments), whether as an input or as an output variable, can distort the results because the AIH value does not reflect real use of resources or real hospital outputs.[26] Third, most of these studies have a limited focus and scope, either geographically or with respect to ownership or type of hospital.

Brazilian experience with hospital benchmarking is scarce and is limited to quality certification programs such as the Controle de Qualidade Hospitalar (CQH) and to research programs such as the Programa de Estudos Avançados em Administração Hospitalar e de Sistemas de Saúde (PROAHSA). The CQH is a hospital certification program based in São Paulo and sponsored by the Paulista Medical Association and the Medical Regional Council. It has 120 member hospitals and collects and publishes a limited set of quality indicators. PROAHSA is a joint teaching and research program in hospital management, operated by the Getúlio Vargas Foundation and the Hospital das Clínicas in São Paulo, that publishes a bimonthly standard set of performance and cost indicators. The database is, however, limited to a few indicators and is based on only 30 participating hospitals. More recent approaches to systemwide performance assessment have been proposed, but they are overambitious, given the availability and quality of data in Brazil.[27]

DEA Study Findings

This section describes the sample from the National Health Facility Survey (Assistência Médico-Sanitária, AMS) used for the DEA (IBGE 2003)[28] and presents the DEA findings based on that sample.[29] Efficiency scores across hospitals by ownership, size, and case load complexity are compared in order to identify the main factors affecting efficiency.

Descriptive Analysis of the AMS Sample

The 2002 AMS survey (conducted in 2001–2) collected data from 65,343 health facilities throughout Brazil, including 7,397 hospitals.[30] A random sample of 671 facilities was selected and was stratified by region and ownership, approximately in proportion to the number of hospitals in each category. Outliers, data errors, and hospitals offering exclusively or mostly chronic care were then excluded, reducing the sample to 588 hospitals. The sample distribution closely resembled the size and regional distribution of the Brazilian hospital network as a whole.[31]

The average hospital size of the sample was 64 beds and the median, 40 beds. As is typical of the Brazilian hospital sector, most facilities were small: nearly 60 percent had fewer than 50 beds, with 27 percent fewer than 25 beds.[32] Only 17 percent had 100 beds or more. Figure 3.7 illustrates the variation in hospital size by ownership. Federal and state hospitals are usually larger than municipal and nonprofit facilities. Most facilities have fewer than 50 beds. Nonprofit hospitals are likely to be of intermediate size: 61 percent have between 50 and 249 beds.

Figure 3.8 displays technological complexity, by ownership.[33] The average complexity was 4.4, on a scale of 1 to 10. Most Brazilian hospitals exhibit a low level of technological

FIGURE 3.7
Distribution of Sample Hospitals, by Size and Ownership, 2002
($N = 588$)

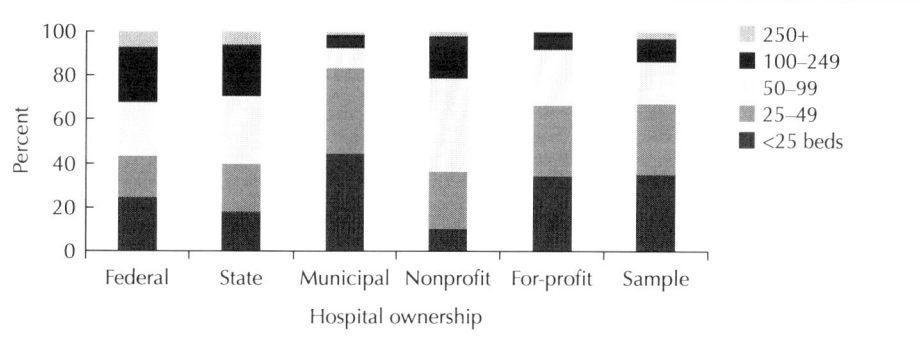

Source: IBGE 2003.

FIGURE 3.8
Technological Complexity, by Ownership, 2002
($N = 588$)

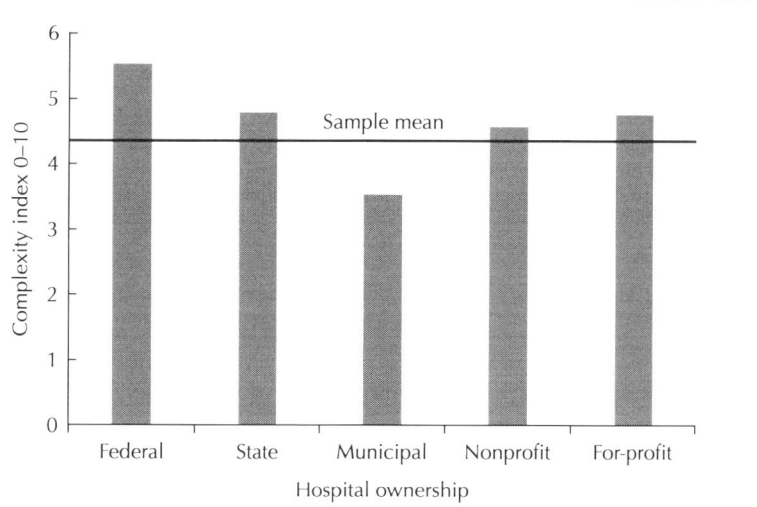

Source: Authors' elaboration based on IBGE (2003).

complexity: 63 percent were placed in the lowest categories (0 and 1). As expected, technological complexity increases with bed number, from 3.1 in hospitals with up to 24 beds to 8.3 in hospitals with 250 beds or more. The correlation coefficient between size and technology was 0.63. Complexity also varies with ownership. Because of the concentration of teaching hospitals, federal hospitals display the highest degree of complexity. State, nonprofit, and for-profit facilities are at an intermediate level, and most municipal hospitals provide low-complexity care.

Figure 3.9 shows admissions by client type: SUS, privately insured, and private out-of-pocket. SUS or public patients are the predominant clientele of state, municipal, and nonprofit hospitals. This makes sense because these facilities are nearly fully financed by the SUS and are expected to cater to public patients. Nevertheless, SUS patients account for 50 percent of the total clientele of federal hospitals. Because most federal hospitals are referral facilities, many have established arrangements to sell services to private health plans.[34] Patients covered by health insurance plans are for-profit hospitals' largest clientele group. Private patients paying out-of-pocket make up only 6 percent of total admissions and are important only for for-profit facilities.

The practice of treating (and charging) private patients—whether covered by private insurance or paying out-of-pocket—in public referral hospitals is the subject of a heated debate within the SUS. It is seen by some as a strategy for diversifying and expanding the sources of funding for public hospitals. For others, this strategy runs contrary to the SUS legislation, which stipulates universal, equal, and free coverage for all Brazilians.

General DEA Results

The general findings of the DEA analysis, presented in table 3.4, indicate high inefficiency among the sampled hospitals and wide dispersion of efficiency scores across hospitals. Of

FIGURE 3.9
Hospital Admissions, by Clientele, 2002
($N = 588$)

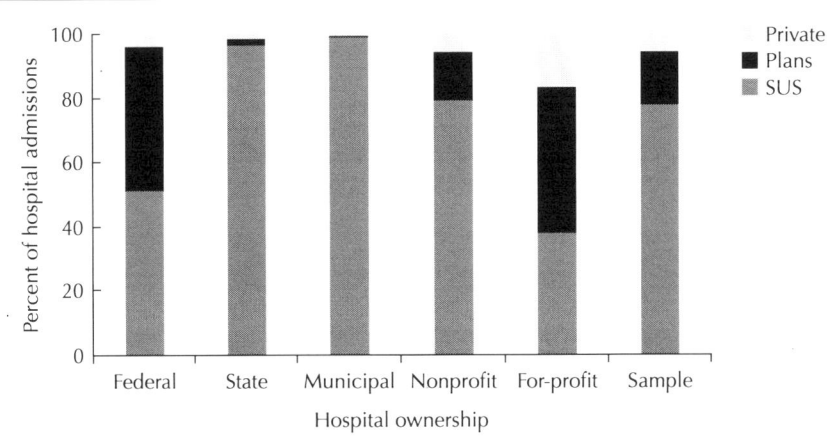

Source: IBGE 2003.

TABLE 3.4
Summary of DEA Results

($N = 428$)

Item	Total technical efficiency	Internal technical efficiency	Scale efficiency
Efficient hospitals (number)	25	63	25
Inefficient hospitals (number)	403	365	403
Mean score, efficient hospitals	1.000	1.000	1.000
Mean score, all hospitals	0.341	0.667	0.520
Mean score, inefficient hospitals	0.301	0.610	0.490
Median score, all hospitals	0.264	0.635	0.467
Standard deviation	0.249	0.225	0.291
Minimum score	0.014	0.228	0.014

Source: Couttolenc et al. 2004.

the 428 hospitals with 25 or more beds, 25 were efficient with respect to total technical efficiency (TTE), receiving a score of 1. The rest (403) placed well below the efficiency frontier, with an average score of 0.341 on a scale of 0 to 1. This score can be interpreted intuitively to mean that the average hospital produces one-third of the output produced by its efficient peers using a similar volume of inputs. Alternatively, the average hospital could produce two-thirds more output with the same input volume if it produced this output as efficiently as the 25 hospitals on the efficiency frontier. The internal technical efficiency score was 0.667, and scale efficiency scores were 0.520, on average.

Internal Technical Efficiency

Internal ("pure") technical efficiency, which is associated with factors such as management practices, control over input use and waste, and staff productivity, and the mix of services produced was, on average, 0.667. This means that the average hospital could greatly improve its efficiency by tightening resource management and stretching available resources. In fact, the average Brazilian hospital uses too much of every input relative to efficient hospitals. Excess personnel is a particular issue, especially medical personnel and administrative and support personnel. To be as efficient as the most efficient hospitals in the sample, the typical hospital would have to reduce medical personnel (physicians and interns) by 51 percent, nursing personnel by 45 percent, other personnel by 46 percent, equipment and beds by 36 percent, and consultation rooms by 46 percent (table 3.5).

Federal hospitals use more of every input than do other ownership categories, in part because of the relatively large proportion of university hospitals in that group. But federal hospitals exhibit low efficiency and high input use across the board (table 3.5). The table shows that the target changes needed for the typical hospital to be as efficient as its efficient peers varies with hospital ownership. Federal facilities need to reduce general input use in larger proportions than other hospitals, while the main issue for private hospitals is excess use of consultation rooms and medical personnel.

TABLE 3.5
Target Reduction in Resource Use, by Hospital Ownership, 2002
(Percent; *N* = 428)

Item	Beds	Consultation rooms	Technological complexity	Medical personnel	Nursing personnel	Other personnel	Inpatient discharge
Sample mean	36	46	36	51	45	46	4
Federal	54	78	56	83	67	79	11
State	45	55	44	57	64	68	6
Municipal	25	34	27	43	35	38	3
Nonprofit	38	45	37	48	42	43	2
For-profit	31	45	33	55	40	39	6

Source: Couttolenc et al. 2004.

Efficiency and Scale

Small size (measured by the number of beds) is the main single factor contributing to low total efficiency. The average scale efficiency score (associated with size) of 0.52 caused the total technical efficiency score to drop to 0.341.[35] Most hospitals, by far (91 percent), showed increasing returns to scale. In other words, these hospitals would significantly improve their efficiency and reduce unit costs by increasing their scale of operations.[36] Six percent of the hospitals exhibited decreasing returns to scale, which means they may generate inefficiencies by being too large and would therefore reduce costs by reducing their size.

Most Brazilian hospitals (61 percent) are too small, at less than 50 beds, to be efficient. The international literature suggests an optimal hospital size of between 150 and 250 beds to achieve economies of scale (Posnett 2002). As figure 3.10 shows, efficiency scores are strongly associated with hospital size, measured by the number of beds. Increased scale drives robust improvements in efficiency. Nevertheless, small hospitals exhibit higher internal technical efficiency scores (0.827 in the 25- to 49-bed category).[37] The relatively high internal efficiency achieved by small hospitals—including many municipal hospitals—can be attributed to the fact that they treat less severely ill patients, focus more intensively on simple emergency services (treating few true emergency cases), and therefore use less personnel and technology.

Efficiency by Ownership Type

Efficiency scores vary by hospital ownership (figure 3.11). Private for-profit hospitals are the most efficient group, followed by private nonprofit facilities. Public, especially federal, facilities are the least efficient. Municipal hospitals achieve the highest internal efficiency scores because, as noted above, before controlling for size, they are found to use less personnel and technology per bed, and they produce relatively large volumes of low-complexity, low-cost services. But their small size reduces their total efficiency in a higher proportion than other ownership groups. Federal hospitals are the least efficient in almost every respect, partly because many are university-based teaching facilities, which are much more resource-intensive than other groups.

FIGURE 3.10
Total Efficiency Scores, by Hospital Size, 2002
(*N* = 428)

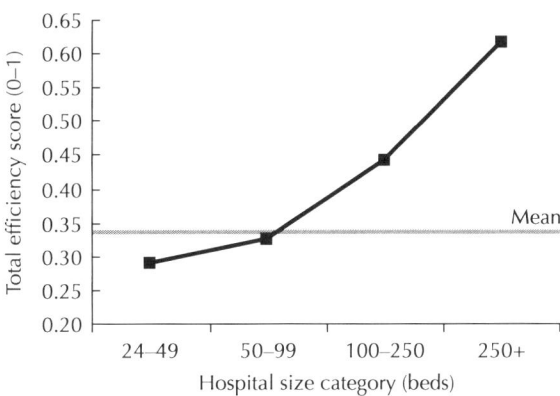

Source: Couttolenc et al. 2004.

The results by ownership hide important differences because hospitals under the same type of ownership may operate under different organizational arrangements. Some organizational arrangements in public hospitals are associated with high efficiency scores, often exceeding those registered by for-profit facilities. This is true of hospitals in São Paulo state under the OSS arrangement in which the management of state-owned hospitals is contracted to the private sector. In contrast, efficiency scores are much lower among public hospitals directly managed by government.[38]

FIGURE 3.11
Efficiency Scores, by Hospital Ownership, 2002
(*N* = 428)

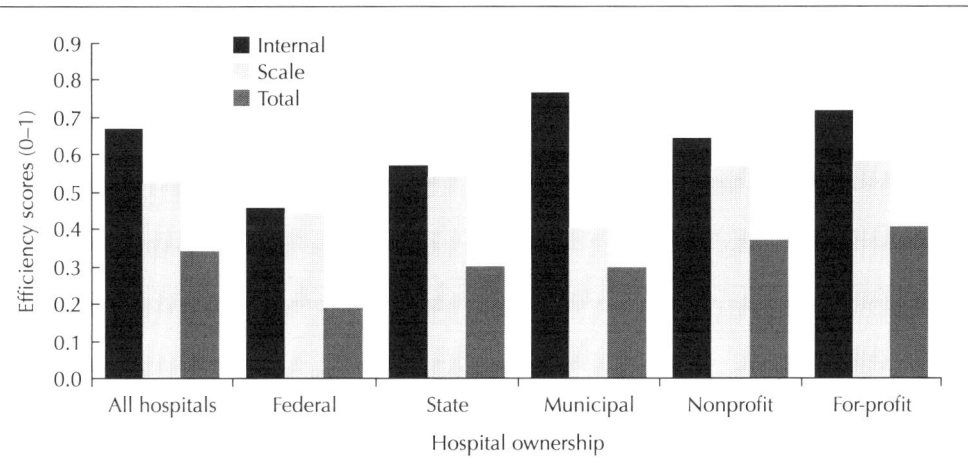

Source: Couttolenc et al. 2004.

Efficiency, Technological Complexity, and Teaching Status

Complexity and teaching status can also confound the efficiency findings. Technological complexity, measured by the availability of diagnostic equipment, was strongly and positively correlated with size, measured by the number of beds ($r = 0.62$). Increases in technological complexity were thus associated with increases in both scale and total efficiency (figure 3.12), similar to the pattern observed for facility size. Hospitals with a lower level of complexity exhibit higher internal efficiency scores, but their total efficiency is significantly lower because of their small size.

Teaching status was found to be associated with greater total efficiency (figure 3.13), but it was also correlated with both size and technological complexity. In fact, size was respon-

FIGURE 3.12
Efficiency Scores, by Technological Complexity, 2002
($N = 428$)

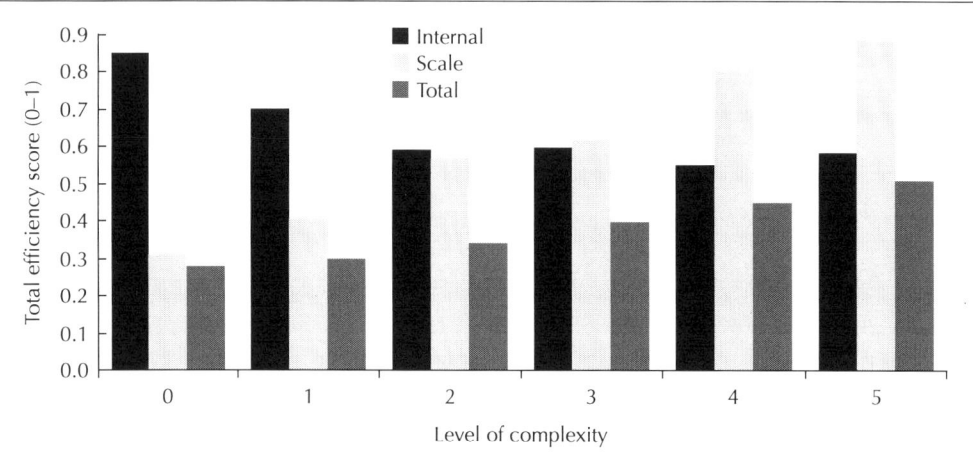

Source: Couttolenc et al. 2004.

FIGURE 3.13
Efficiency Scores, by Teaching Status, 2002
($N = 428$)

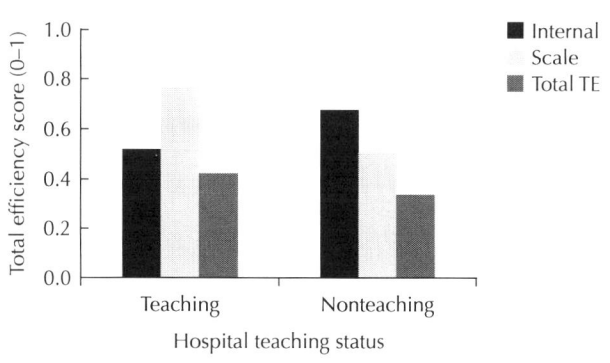

Source: Couttolenc et al. 2004.

sible for most of the observed differences between the total efficiency scores of teaching and nonteaching facilities. In other words, for a given size, teaching hospitals are actually less efficient because they use significantly more inputs to produce a given output than nonteaching hospitals. The likely reasons are the additional costs connected with a university hospital's special teaching and research mission and, perhaps, less concern about efficiency and costs among the physicians leading the hospital's teaching and research activities.

Benchmarking Analysis

To complement the DEA findings, several performance indicators were generated based on the AMS sample. Given that no single recommended standard exists for most indicators, four external reference values or benchmarks were applied for comparison purposes.[39] Even though international data are often not strictly comparable, they proved useful as references for this analysis.[40] As is typical of benchmark-based analyses of hospital performance everywhere, the findings for Brazil demonstrated considerable dispersion across hospitals for most indicators. Such dispersion, which corroborates the DEA findings, is indicative of great inefficiency in many hospitals. This section reports on findings, depending on the availability of data, for both statistical and nonstatistical measures of efficiency, including bed turnover, occupancy rates, average length of stay, personnel per bed, surgical productivity, and use of technological inputs.

Bed Turnover

The bed turnover rate (BTR), the ratio of annual patient discharges to beds, is a common indicator of hospital performance for inpatient services. It provides a measure of the efficiency of physical resource use. Figure 3.14 presents the BTR findings from the AMS sample by hospital ownership and includes benchmark values for comparison. The average for the sample was 50.4, which was higher than the OECD average (32.6) but lower than that for CQH facilities (64.7).[41] Huge dispersion was found across hospitals and, to a lesser extent, across ownership types. The BTR was highest for private for-profit hospitals (56.9), followed by municipal hospitals (53.7), state hospitals (50.0), and nonprofit hospitals (45.5). Federal hospitals registered the lowest performance (32.6), which again may be related to the large proportion in this group of university hospitals that treat more complex cases requiring longer stays. The relatively high turnover rate observed in the sample suggests that Brazilian hospitals may be efficient, but the rate is biased by a significant number of small private and municipal hospitals that hospitalize low-severity patients for short stays.[42] The average turnover rate for SUS facilities reported by the MS is a lower 28.8. Finally, bed turnover displayed the highest correlation coefficient with efficiency scores among all the variables in the analysis ($r = 0.53$) and was the single best predictor of total technical efficiency among these variables.

Bed Occupancy

The bed occupancy rate—the percentage of total bed-days in which beds are in use—is another common performance indicator because it captures the degree of utilization of existing physical resources. A bed occupancy rate between 75 and 85 percent of capacity is desirable.[43] The findings demonstrate that Brazilian hospitals suffer from low occupancy rates. The mean rate is 45 percent for all SUS hospitals and only 37 percent for acute care beds

FIGURE 3.14
Bed Turnover Rate, 2002
($N = 588$)

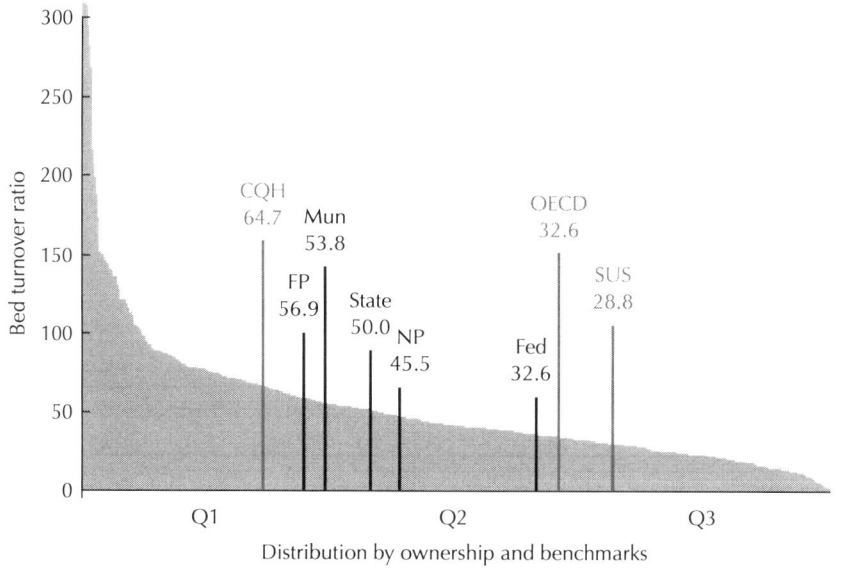

Source: Couttolenc et al. 2004.

(MS/Datasus), compared with the benchmarks of 65 percent for CQH and 71 percent for OECD hospitals.[44] Many hospitals (58 percent of the facilities in the sample) exhibit occupancy rates below 30 percent, and only 8 percent—usually, larger facilities—have rates of 80 percent or more.[45] Small hospitals register the lowest occupancy rates; facilities with fewer than 50 beds reported rates of 22 percent. Bed occupancy also varies by ownership (figure 3.15). State hospitals show the highest rates, and for-profits, the lowest.

Low occupancy rates are widespread among Brazilian hospitals, partly as a result of access extension policies initiated in the mid-1980s, after the decentralization reforms and the establishment of the SUS (see chapter 2). A case can be made that too many small hospitals were built, offering low-complexity and generally low-quality care. Many of them are poorly maintained. Patients often bypass these facilities to seek care at larger, more distant, referral facilities that offer a broader range of services. For example, occupancy rates were positively correlated with hospital size ($r = 0.38$ in the sample); they range from 21 percent in hospitals with fewer than 25 beds to 77 percent in hospitals with 250 or more beds. This is worrisome because nearly two-thirds of Brazilian hospitals are small.

Larger teaching and referral hospitals reported occupancy rates similar to those of the reference groups (figure 3.15). In general, these facilities treat a more severe case mix. High occupancy rates, however, do not necessarily reflect superior hospital performance or the efficiency of the facility. Occupancy rates are sensitive to average length of stay, which may reflect quality of care (e.g., extended stays because of hospital-acquired infections), quality of clinical management (e.g., scheduling, case management, productivity of diagnostic services), or

FIGURE 3.15
Mean Occupancy Rate for SUS Acute Care Hospitals, by Ownership, 2002
(*N* = 5,794)

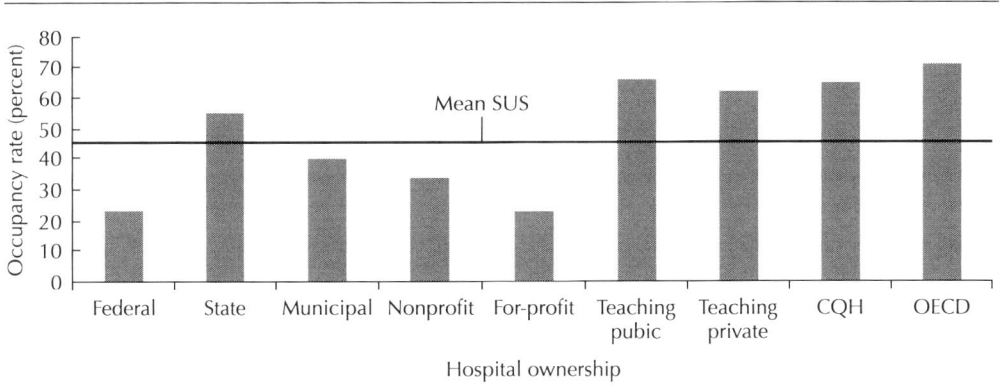

Source: Couttolenc et al. 2004.

case-mix severity. Furthermore, high occupancy rates may respond to overcrowding, which has been observed in an undetermined number of large referral facilities in Brazil.

Average Length of Stay (ALOS)
The average number of days patients occupy a bed during a hospital stay is a key indicator of efficiency of resource use. It varies with case severity, the more severe and chronic cases usually requiring longer stays.[46] Quality of care and efficiency of clinical management also affect ALOS. Technical inefficiencies in resource use and care management have been found to contribute to high ALOS (Barnum and Kutzin 1993). Longer-than-necessary stays waste hospital resources and may crowd out access to beds by patients with more severe, even life-threatening, conditions. There is no evidence that longer ALOS results in better quality of care or improves health outcomes. Finally, extended but unnecessary stays may artificially inflate bed occupancy rates.

Private facilities demonstrate the lowest ALOS and federal hospitals, the highest (figure 3.16). ALOS for the AMS sample (mean value of 2.9) is lower than both the CQH benchmark (3.4 in 2002, based mainly on private facilities in São Paulo) and the mean value for SUS hospitals reported by MS/Datasus (4.5 for the same year). The sample mean is likely to reflect the low ALOS reported by private hospitals, which account for a larger proportion of the total than in the MS/Datasus dataset. In any case, all the values reported by Brazilian hospitals are much lower than the mean value (7.8) reported by OECD hospitals for the late 1990s. The OECD hospitals, however, treat a much older population than hospitals in Brazil and are thus not strictly comparable. The low ALOS exhibited by Brazilian hospitals may indicate efficient use of resources, but if patients are sent home too early, it may lead to low-quality care.

As suggested above, case mix and hospital size influence ALOS. Larger federal and state hospitals, especially teaching and referral facilities, treat more severe cases than smaller municipal and private facilities. A separate analysis of the AMS sample showed that ALOS

FIGURE 3.16
ALOS for SUS Acute Care Hospitals, by Ownership, 2002
(N = 5,794)

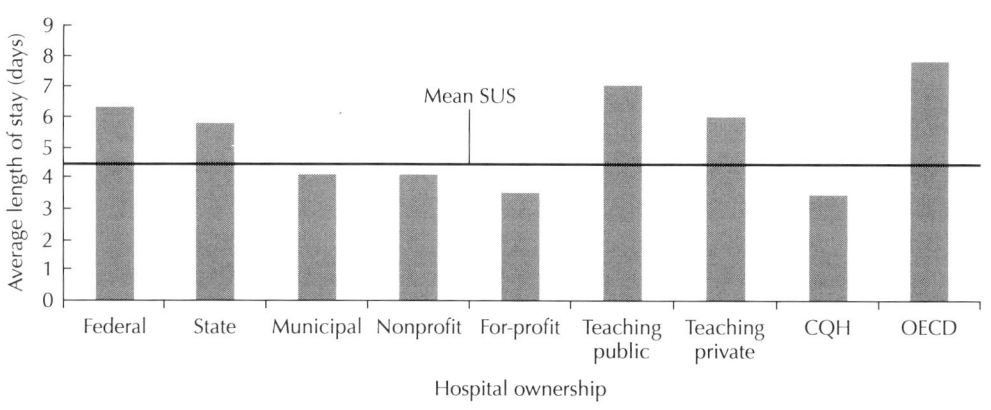

Source: Couttolenc et al. 2004.

was positively correlated with hospital size (r = 0.34). The low ALOS for private for-profit hospitals may reflect the fact that these facilities can more easily refuse to treat complex cases than their public counterparts, but it may also be true that public hospitals have few incentives to manage clinical care efficiently, resulting in needlessly high ALOS.

Personnel per Bed

Staffing per bed ratios are proxy measures of allocative efficiency because they are an indication of the use of a major input in the production of hospital care. Because staffing ratios depend on hospital size and case complexity, there are no international norms to guide the establishment of optimal or target benchmarks.[47] Comparisons among similar hospitals can, however, provide insights into potential inefficiencies.

Figure 3.17 presents staffing ratios by hospital ownership and type of personnel. The mean sample ratio is 3.0 for total personnel, but the ratio varies widely across the sample, from 5.0 to 0.1.[48] Public hospitals have the highest ratios, especially federal and state hospitals, which exhibit a ratio over 4.5. Nonprofit hospitals report the lowest staffing ratios. The average Brazilian hospital uses 50 percent more personnel (all categories) per bed than the average OECD hospital. Hospitals enrolled in the CQH program, however, use even more (figure 3.17). This confirms the DEA finding that the overuse of human resources is an important source of inefficiency in Brazilian hospitals.[49]

The ratio increases consistently with the level of technological complexity, from 2.4 among hospitals at the lower end of the complexity index to 5.7 at the higher end. The likely reason is that more technology-intensive hospitals treat more complex cases and therefore need more staff per bed. Contrary to patterns observed in other countries in which staffing ratios increase with size (Barnum and Kutzin 1993), very small facilities, with fewer than 25 beds, display higher staffing ratios (3.9) than medium-size facilities (2.5). This may be attrib-

FIGURE 3.17
Ratio and Composition of Personnel per Bed, 2002
($N = 588$)

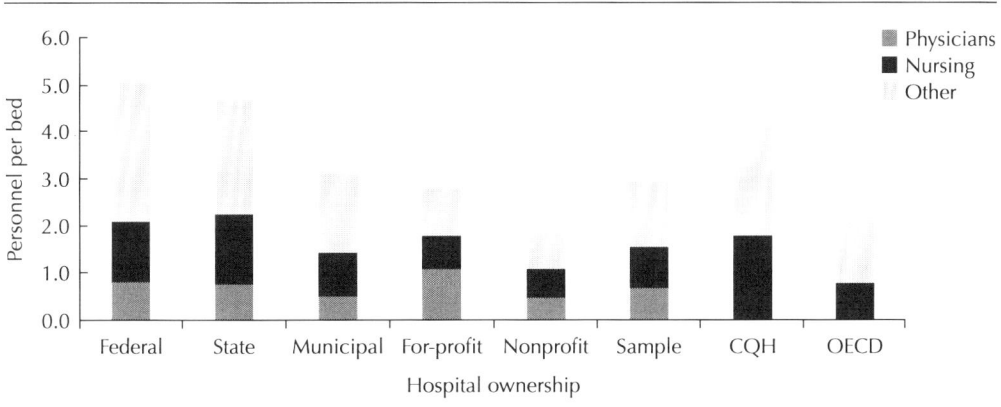

Source: Couttolenc et al. 2004.

utable to fixed labor costs or to the minimal number of personnel required for operation. In view of the low occupancy rate of small hospitals, this finding suggests scale inefficiencies related to the oversupply and underuse of personnel.

Hospital staffing by professional category varies significantly across ownership types. On average, physicians and nurses make up 22 and 30 percent, respectively, of total personnel; administrative and general support personnel account for the remainder (48 percent). The variation in the "other" personnel category, consisting of administrative and support staff, is much larger across hospital groups than for physicians or nurses (see figure 3.17). Public hospitals use almost twice as much "other" personnel (2.1 per bed) as private facilities. In sum, overstaffing in public facilities in Brazil results from high numbers of nontechnical personnel, especially administrative and nontechnical support staff (e.g., cleaning and security). This category accounts for 29 percent of hospital staff in the sample hospitals. For comparison, these personnel account for only 19 percent of hospital staff in France (IBGE 2003; DREES 2005; MSPS 2004).

Overstaffing becomes more obvious when staffing ratios per occupied bed are examined (figure 3.18). The average number of staff per occupied bed for the sample was 10.5. This compares unfavorably with reference benchmarks, CQH (6.3) and "top 100" U.S. hospitals (5.2). Public and for-profit facilities have significantly higher staffing ratios than the benchmarks. In sum, average ratios of personnel to occupied beds in Brazil are double those in the typical U.S. facility and two-thirds greater than in CQH facilities.

Intensive use of labor in Brazilian hospitals relative to international averages may be the result of low labor costs, low staff qualifications (e.g., intensive use of midlevel personnel in place of university-level staff), low productivity, or all three. An additional factor is the general absence or irregular application of standardized processes (e.g., scheduling) and clinical procedures such as practice protocols.

FIGURE 3.18
Total Personnel per Occupied Bed Ratio, 2002
(*N* = 588)

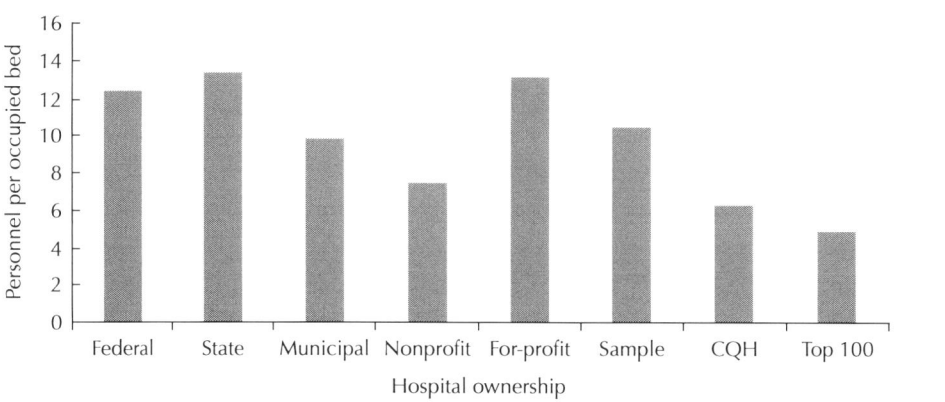

Source: Couttolenc et al. 2004.

Surgical Productivity

The rate of surgical inpatient admissions per operating room—a proxy for the ratio of surgeries per operating room—is another indicator that measures productivity of high-cost hospital services (figure 3.19). Low values suggest underutilization of operating rooms and of concomitant staff and equipment. The mean ratio per year is 173, or 0.66 surgeries per working day, suggesting very low productivity and utilization. The observed rates are associated with both size and technological complexity, increasing from 73 (0.31 per room per working day)

FIGURE 3.19
Surgical Patients per Operating Room per Year Ratio, 2002
(*N* = 588)

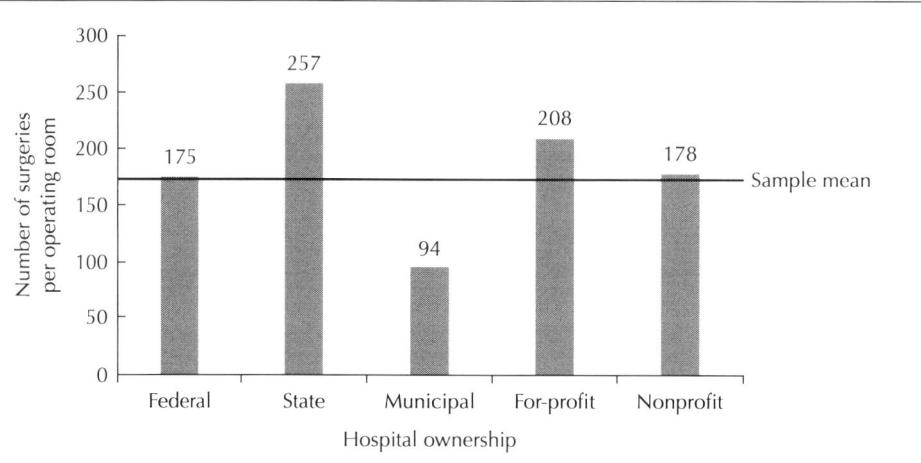

Source: Couttolenc et al. 2004.

in small hospitals to about 350 (1.5 per room per working day) for larger hospitals. The lowest ratios were found among municipal hospitals, which are often small, underused facilities. Unexpectedly, lower rates were found among federal hospitals than among private and state facilities, even through the former are usually large facilities.

Keeping an operating room open and in working condition implies sizeable equipment and personnel costs. Performing an average of 0.66 surgeries per day squanders resources, as it means long periods of staff downtime and underuse of expensive equipment. The overall low surgical and operating room rates may have several explanations. First, many hospitals are equipped with operating rooms but experience insufficient demand for them. Second, operating rooms may not be used when needed because of maintenance problems, lack of necessary inputs such as on-time diagnostic tests, or inefficient clinical management. Evidence from other research suggests that both factors contribute to the low utilization of operating rooms.[50] Low productivity also results from the generalized practice of performing scheduled surgeries in the morning—partly for clinical reasons, such as the need for patients to forgo food, and partly to adjust to physicians' personal time schedules. Operating rooms are nevertheless kept functioning with full ancillary staff around the clock to attend to a very small number of emergency patients.

Use of Technology

Use of technology in health care can help improve outcomes, but indiscriminate use can increase costs and decrease quality. To evaluate technology intensity in inpatient services and its effects, an index of technological complexity per bed was used as a proxy.[51] The results, shown in figure 3.20, indicate greater use of technology per bed in federal hospitals (index value of 1.29) and private for-profit hospitals (1.16) than in other types of facility. For federal hospitals, this result was expected, in view of the many university facilities in that group. In the second case, the high technological content of care seems to indicate that for-profit

FIGURE 3.20
Technological Complexity per Bed Ratio, by Ownership, 2002
($N = 588$)

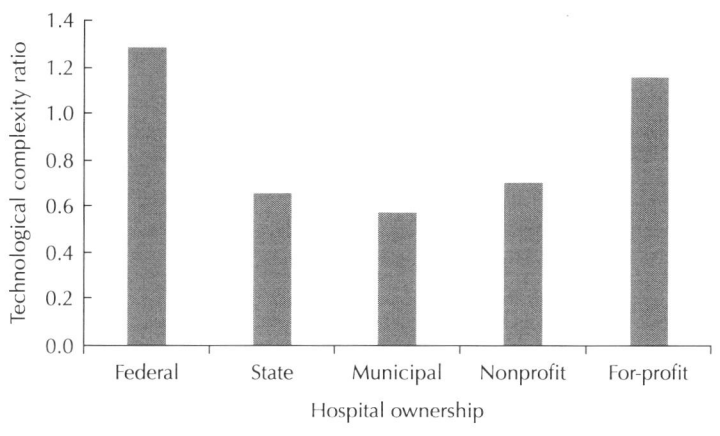

Source: Couttolenc et al. 2004.

hospitals, less dependent on SUS financing, have greater flexibility to focus on more lucrative types of care, often involving more intense use of technology. This behavior may reflect incentives embedded in hospital payment mechanisms. More interestingly, small hospitals are among the largest users of technology per bed, after the hospitals with 250 or more beds. This suggests that small hospitals make excessive use of technology for their size, perhaps without sufficient demand. In fact, the results indicate that a significant proportion of hospital technology available in Brazil is concentrated in small, specialized, for-profit facilities in a pattern reflecting economic incentives rather than efficiency or need.

These findings confirm the results of the DEA analysis. Hospitals that were deemed efficient on the basis of the DEA employ less technology. These facilities register lower technology per bed ratios, as well as more discharges in relation to technology. In contrast, inefficient hospitals show the opposite pattern; higher equipment per bed ratios and fewer discharges in relation to the technological index. The implication is that the average Brazilian hospital uses too much complex technology, resulting in inefficiency and probably higher costs.

Brazil's use of sophisticated diagnostic equipment is indeed high relative to international averages. Table 3.6 compares the density of some high-complexity, high-cost diagnostic equipment such as computerized tomography (CT) and magnetic resonance imaging (MRI) scanners in Brazil, in its state capitals, and in OECD countries. Equipment density for these two items is comparable to that in the much wealthier OECD countries.

Calil (2004) provides additional evidence of oversupply and overuse of medical technology in Brazil. The study looked at five types of imaging equipment (see table 3.7) and found that

TABLE 3.6
Equipment Density, Brazil and OECD Countries, 2002

(per million inhabitants)

Location	CT scanners	MRI scanners
Brazil	9.3	2.5
State capitals	13.2	7.2
OECD, lowest quartile	8.8	2.9
OECD	17.5	7.7

Source: IBGE 2003; OECD 2005.

TABLE 3.7
Supply of Imaging Equipment in Relation to Need, by Region, 2002

(percent of MS need parameter)

Equipment	North	Northeast	Southeast	South	Central-West
Radiology	154	146	303	243	273
Mammography	148	174	426	292	317
CT scanner	47	54	131	79	92
MRI scanner	65	44	121	84	100
Color ultrasound	116	112	226	166	198

Source: Calil 2004; need parameters from MS (Portaria 1101 GM/2002).

76 percent of the total was in private facilities. More than half of the equipment was in the richer southeast region, home to 43 percent of the population. Applying MS parameters for required density of this equipment, the study showed an oversupply in several regions (table 3.7). The equipment was heavily concentrated in large cities, and excessive supply in those cities coexisted with lack of access in secondary cities in much of the country. According to the study estimates, the excess equipment required US$112 million yearly in labor costs just for maintenance. The research also found that much of the equipment was dysfunctional as a result of grossly inadequate maintenance budgets.[52] This situation also compromised service quality.

Efficiency and Quality

Efficiency and quality are closely related. Efficiency can provide greater control and management of resources, which can affect quality. For example, efficient resource management such as the application of standardized practice protocols can narrow variations in treatment patterns and generate cost savings, but these measures can also help reduce hospital infections and other cost-inducing adverse events. Quality improvements can, however, result in inefficiencies through overuse of resources, resulting in higher costs; this phenomenon is known as "quality waste" (IoM 2001: 52).

Is there a trade-off between efficiency and quality? To answer this question, a quality indicator was computed from the available AMS variables.[53] This indicator was negatively correlated with the DEA total efficiency scores in the AMS sample (figure 3.21). But the dispersion observed in figure 3.21 suggests little association between efficiency and quality, as evidenced by an insignificant correlation coefficient ($r = -0.10$). No significant difference in quality was found between totally efficient hospitals (those receiving a TTE score of 1.0) and their inefficient peers.[54] These findings suggest that, at the very least, high efficiency does not impair quality. Thus, variability in both efficiency and quality may be more important than the relation between them.[55]

FIGURE 3.21
Quality and Efficiency in Brazilian Hospitals, 2002
($N = 428$)

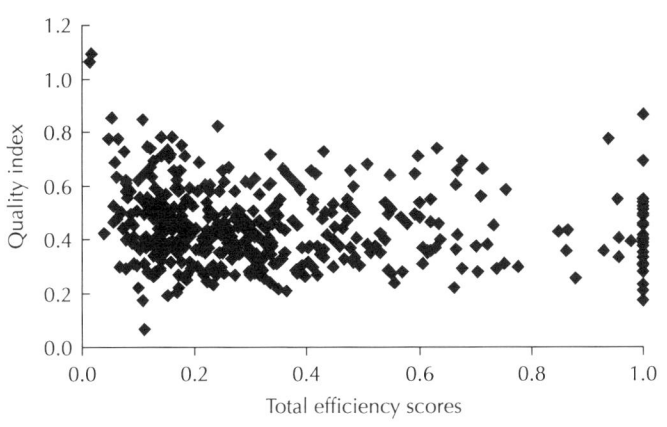

Source: Couttolenc et al. 2004.

Other Policy-Relevant Efficiency Analyses

This final section in the efficiency discussion attempts to fill some of the analytical gaps related to the studies reviewed in this chapter while presenting findings that complement and explain the results that emerged from the DEA and benchmarking analyses.

Linking DEA and Benchmarking

DEA and benchmarking have been employed in previous studies (described in the literature review above) to assess efficiency and performance in hospitals, but they have been used as alternative approaches. In this study, both were used simultaneously to complement and verify the consistency and robustness of the findings. Multivariate analysis was also applied to assess the simultaneous effect of factors affecting hospital efficiency.

To combine the results of the DEA and benchmarking analyses, the sample hospitals were grouped by their TTE scores given by the DEA, and the benchmarked indicators were computed for each group. The results illustrate the consistency of the findings (table 3.8).

TABLE 3.8
Summary of Benchmark Indicators, by Total Efficiency Level

Indicator	TTE, 1 (most efficient)	TTE, 0.999–0.666	TTE, 0.665–0.333	TTE < 0.333	Mean TTE
Hospitals (number)	25	24	109	270	428
Bed turnover (discharges/bed)	91.8	71.7	68.8	37.7	50.7
Occupancy rate (%)	34.4	38.1	44.6	25.6	31.7
Average length of stay (days)	2.2	2.6	2.9	3.1	2.9
Emergencies/discharge	4.6	3.4	0.8	0.8	1.2
Physicians/bed	0.5	0.6	0.6	0.4	0.4
Nursing personnel/bed	0.8	1.1	1.1	0.8	0.9
Other personnel/bed	0.8	1.1	1.2	1.1	1.1
Total personnel/bed	1.9	2.8	2.8	2.2	2.3
Technology points/bed	0.6	0.9	0.9	0.6	0.7
Discharges/personnel	286.0	246.4	107.2	51.8	116.0
Emergency procedures/ personnel	330.0	421.9	137.6	34.0	99.4
Discharges/technology points	1,229.0	664.3	812.3	431.0	587.8
Surgical admissions/ operating room	315.0	233.1	357.8	118.3	198.8
Mortality rate (unadjusted)	2.2	2.0	2.1	2.3	2.2
Mortality rate (adjusted for CMI)	1.4	1.2	1.3	1.5	1.4
Registered nurses/ nursing staff (%)	15.0	13.0	11.0	9.0	10.0
Quality index	0.4	0.4	0.4	0.5	0.5

Source: Compiled from Couttolenc et al. (2004); IBGE (2003).

Most of the productivity indicators and input use ratios are clearly superior in the efficient hospitals group and deteriorate as the efficiency score decreases. Importantly, and as noted above, the indicators relating to the quality of care—the hospital mortality rate, the proportion of registered nurses, and the general quality indicator constructed from the data—show little variation between high- and low-efficiency hospitals. If anything, efficient hospitals appear to have more favorable quality indicators, as measured by, for example, mortality rates and registered nurses, than their inefficient counterparts.

Both the DEA and the benchmarking analyses take into account a limited number of variables at a time. To assess the effect of several factors on efficiency simultaneously, the authors of this study ran a regression analysis, applying different combinations of variables to confirm the findings presented earlier in this chapter.[56] Drawing on the DEA and benchmarking datasets, the regression analysis used total technical efficiency scores as the dependent variable and the following independent variables: facility size, personnel per bed, bed turnover, ratio of emergencies to inpatient discharges, quality of care, technological complexity, teaching status, and ownership.[57]

Table 3.9 presents the results. Facility size (measured by the number of beds), bed turnover, and ratio of emergencies to inpatient discharges had a positive and highly significant effect on efficiency ($p < .001$). These findings confirm the results of the DEA and benchmarking analyses. Teaching status had no significant effect on total efficiency. This is also in line with previous findings because the impact of teaching status on efficiency was attributable to the large scale of teaching hospitals rather than to teaching status per se. Turning to ownership, only private status (for-profit and nonprofit) had a significant and positive effect on

TABLE 3.9
Tobit Regression Results, by Total Efficiency Scores

Variable	Coefficient	Standard error	t	P > |t|
Beds, number*	−0.016	0.003	−4.670	0.000
Bed turnover*	−0.074	0.008	−9.700	0.000
Physicians/bed	0.032	0.525	0.060	0.951
Nursing personnel/bed**	−1.508	0.521	−2.900	0.004
Other personnel/bed	0.239	0.344	0.700	0.486
Emergencies/discharge ratio*	−0.243	0.068	−3.580	0.000
Teaching status	−0.446	1.058	−0.420	0.674
Quality index*	17.299	1.693	10.220	0.000
State/federal dummy	−0.225	1.179	−0.190	0.849
Municipal/federal	−1.454	1.182	−1.230	0.220
For-profit/federal**	−2.679	1.243	−2.150	0.032
Nonprofit/federal**	−2.525	1.177	−2.140	0.033
Constant*	4.189	1.446	2.900	0.004

Source: Couttolenc et al. 2004.

Note: LR chi^2(12) = 235.23. The dependent variable was inefficiency (measured as 1 minus the efficiency score), so a negative coefficient implies a positive effect on efficiency.

*Significant at 1 percent.

**Significant at 5 percent.

total efficiency. Again, this confirms the DEA and benchmarking findings that private hospitals are generally more efficient than their public counterparts. Controlling for the other variables, whether a public hospital was federal, state, or municipal had no significant effect on efficiency.

In contrast to the benchmark findings, the quality indicator had a significant and negative effect on efficiency. This negative association seems to imply that there are limits to how much technical efficiency can be improved without hurting the quality of care as measured here. However, the limitations of the quality indicator constructed from the data have to be kept in mind.[58]

Hospital Admissions Sensitive to Ambulatory Care

An important hospital efficiency issue in Brazil is the high proportion of SUS hospital admissions that are for ambulatory care–sensitive conditions (ACSCs). These include several infectious diseases (e.g., tuberculosis, gastroenteritis, some forms of meningitis), nutritional deficiencies such as anemia, and respiratory infections, hypertension, and diabetes. These admissions could be avoided if the primary care network were more effective. The international literature suggests similar inefficiencies outside Brazil. ACSCs account for between 8 and 18 percent of all admissions in Spain (Caminal et al. 2002, 2004), 13 percent in New Jersey, United States (Vali 2001), and 18 percent under one large U.S. insurance plan (Axene and McQuillian 1999).

In Minas Gerais state, Brazil, research on hospital admissions found alarming results: 28 percent of admissions, representing 21 percent of AIH payments, could be avoided through effective primary care (SES-MG 2005). Application of similar methodology to nationwide data yielded similar results (figure 3.22).[59] About 30 percent of admissions and 28 percent of patient-days were attributed to cases that could have been more affordably treated at an ambulatory facility. Spending on these conditions was about R$4.5 billion (US$1.6 billion), or 21 percent of total estimated spending on inpatient care.

These avoidable admissions constitute the major part of inpatient care provided by small, low-complexity facilities. Hospitals with fewer than 50 beds account for 28 percent of SUS

FIGURE 3.22
Proportion of Inpatient Conditions Sensitive to Ambulatory Care, 2002

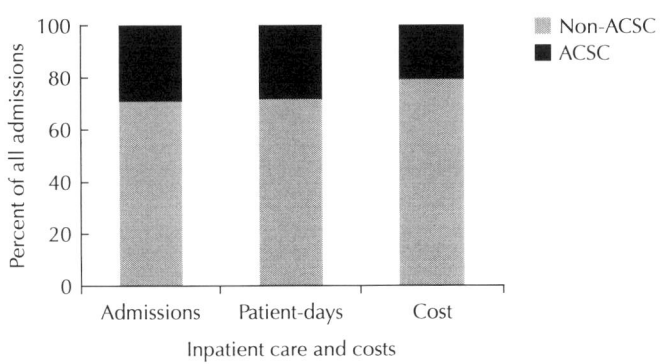

Source: Authors' estimates.

hospital admissions and consume R$4.4 billion (US$1.5 billion), or about 13 percent of SUS hospital spending. Most of these admissions are for conditions sensitive to ambulatory care.

These findings suggest that Brazil relies more than many other countries on hospital care for treating conditions responsive to ambulatory care. A considerable amount of resources spent on inpatient care for ACSCs could be saved by increasing the effectiveness of the primary care network. Closing these small, low-complexity hospitals, or converting them to ambulatory care centers, which provide treatments that do not require hospitalization would generate significant savings that could be used to extend primary care services.

Case Study: Whither the Small Hospital?

Between 1976 and 2005 the average size of public hospitals dropped significantly, from 124 to 55 beds. This reflected the growth in the number of small hospitals over the period; the public sector added over 1,600 mostly municipal hospitals, with an average size of 18 beds (IBGE 2000a, 2003).[60] With the founding of the SUS, which strongly emphasized municipal decentralization, expansion of municipal facilities responded to the political demands of newly empowered mayors and an explicit government policy favoring investment in public hospitals. Rational planning of a hospital network was of little concern. Over this same period the average size of private hospitals also declined, but less markedly, from 75 to 65 beds, reflecting the proliferation of small specialty and subspecialty facilities, particularly among for-profits. According to data from the 1990s, the average size of nonprofit hospitals stayed about the same (88 beds). Most nonprofits were already small, reflecting an earlier era of hospital expansion by charitable and philanthropic organizations, religious groups, and ethnic organizations.[61] Some observers suggest that nonprofits have been declining over the last three decades because of financial problems related in part to low SUS reimbursement (see chapter 4). Nevertheless, their numbers increased by one-third between 1992 and 2005, from 1,455 to 1,947, according to the IGBE/AMS surveys.

Not only do small hospitals provide inappropriate care, in that they admit many patients for conditions that can best be resolved at the ambulatory level, but they are also severely underutilized. They are often bypassed by users wanting larger facilities that offer a broad range of services. Hospitals with fewer than 100 beds report occupation rates of less than 30 percent, and rates drop to about 20 percent for smaller facilities in the sample.

Surgical production is also correlated with size: large hospitals (with more than 250 beds) carry out, on average, 349 surgeries per operating room per year.[62] Smaller hospitals produce many fewer: 73 and 108 surgeries a year for facilities with 0–24 and 25–49 beds, respectively.

Small hospitals are associated with poor quality of care, partly because of their low intervention volume. Considerable international evidence demonstrates that low-volume facilities and, correspondingly, low-frequency physicians have higher mortality rates, especially for complex treatments and surgical procedures. For example, in a review of 272 population-based studies conducted between 1980 and 2000, Halm, Lee, and Chassin (2002) found that for a wide range of surgical procedures and clinical treatments, better outcomes, usually measured in terms of lower mortality, were associated with higher-volume facilities and physicians.[63] Based on a large sample of 474,108 U.S. Medicare patients who underwent eight surgical procedures (cardiovascular procedures or cancer resections), Birkmeyer et al. (2003) reported a significant inverse relationship between operative mortality and volume. An editorial in the *New England Journal of Medicine* (Kizer 2003), summarizing the findings of outcome-volume studies for a large number of conditions, observed the public health importance of some of the studies. The findings demonstrated a similar volume-outcome association for higher-frequency conditions such as premature births, low-birthweight babies, some orthopedic procedures, cancer, and AIDS.[64]

As measured by a technological complexity index (annex box 3D.1), many small hospitals in Brazil offer high-complexity care, although volume is very low.[65] In a Brazilian study, higher mortality rates in coronary bypasses were found to be inversely related to patient volume, with much higher risk of death in hospitals with the smallest number of coronary surgery cases (Noronha et al. 2003; WHO 2003a). These findings, reported in table 3.10, are consistent with the above-mentioned international literature on hospital mortality rates for surgical procedures.

Health authorities in Brazil now acknowledge the irrationality of hospital infrastructure and supply distribution, and especially the scale diseconomies associated with the glut of small hospitals. They also recognize the poor quality and unsafe conditions in these facilities. The MS and at least one state are addressing this issue through hospital restructuring and conversion. An example is the Policy for Small Hospitals issued by the MS in 2004 (MS 2004f).[66] Instead of taking the politically difficult step of closing facilities, the policy attempts to change their role by adjusting the number of beds to local needs (which means removing nearly two-thirds of the beds); by reducing the services offered for low-risk deliveries, care in the four basic medical specialties, emergency dental care, and ambulatory surgeries; or by converting the facilities into emergency centers for the primary care network in areas where primary care coverage is high. Funding mechanisms for these converted facilities would be modified (e.g., a global budget) and linked to performance targets related to primary care (undefined as yet) and to performance indicators such as proportion of referred patients and utilization rates.

Although this policy is an important first step in acknowledging and addressing the issue of small, inefficient hospitals, it has several limitations. First, it is not mandatory, and municipalities can opt out. Second, it implies further investment to upgrade inefficient and underused facilities so they can fulfill their new role, with no guarantee that conversion will have the desired impact. Third, the main policy focus is on conversion of hospitals with fewer than 30 beds, but the broader issue involves irrational supply on an inefficient scale.

TABLE 3.10
Coronary Bypass Surgery, Brazil, 1995

Surgeries per hospital	Number of hospitals	Total operations	Total deaths	Mortality rate (%)
1–9	22	93	12	12.9
10–49	31	681	86	12.6
50–149	43	2,947	264	10.0
150–299	23	8,077	509	6.3
300+	5	4,269	228	5.2

Source: Noronha et al. 2003; WHO 2003a.

The policy does not address the issue of not-so-small, but scale-inefficient, hospitals with fewer than 100 beds, nor does it encourage horizontal integration of facilities into a network arrangement or rationalization of facilities across municipalities through establishment of municipal consortiums.[67] Moreover, the policy does not specify the role of hospitals that are not converted; will their funding be reduced?[68]

Closing hospitals is an unpopular policy in any country. In Brazil the remoteness and low density of many small municipalities and the poor state of the road network and public transportation make hospital closings more difficult and, when no alternative is available within a reasonable distance, infeasible.

Several countries have espoused more aggressive rationalization policies to reduce the supply of hospital beds. These include expanding day care programs, ambulatory surgery, and community aftercare programs to substitute for inpatient care; improving the appropriateness of hospital admissions, partly by reducing admissions below a severity threshold and concomitantly expanding primary care, home care, and special programs for the chronically ill; changing the configuration of the hospital system by closing redundant wards and underutilized or smaller facilities and adopting horizontal integration of services; and converting hospitals to convalescent or long-term care facilities.[69] Some of the results have been impressive. For example, France has implemented an investment consolidation policy affecting 380 hospitals (10 percent of the total), resulting in a 14 percent bed reduction over the last 10 years.[70] Australia, Canada, Italy, Sweden, and the United States have reduced ratios of beds per 1,000 population by 30 to 54 percent in the last 20 years, and the OECD as a whole has reduced them by 28 percent (Docteur and Oxley 2003).

Failure (or Lack) of Hospital Investment Policies

The surplus of small hospitals and the inequitable distribution of hospital resources described above are the results of inconsistent investment policies and practices in the hospital sector. Contributing factors include the absence of coordination between the public and private sectors, health authorities' inability to develop and enforce rational investment policies,[71] fragmented investment funding sources and mechanisms, and the influence of politics.

In Brazil the MS and subnational health secretariats theoretically have the authority to decide when and where to invest in hospital infrastructure and diagnostic equipment in the public sector, but they have little authority over investment by the private sector.[72] Even within the public sector, planning mechanisms such as the Investment Master Plans (Plano Diretor de Investimento) and the Multiannual Health Plans (Plano Plurianual) are often poorly prepared and hard to enforce. The MS has set parameters for the supply of hospital beds and equipment,[73] but investment policies and priorities remain unclear, and decisions are often made haphazardly and without any coordination among federal, state, and municipal governments.

Investment financing further complicates this situation. Rarely is investment financing included in annual health budgets at subnational levels.[74] Nor do hospital payment mechanisms (described in chapter 4) include financing for capital investment or depreciation. Instead, hospital investment relies on irregular extrabudgetary or parallel finance mechanisms that do nothing to encourage rational decision making and planning. For example, international loans by multilateral development agencies constitute a significant source of investment funding, but this lending is sporadic and is usually designated for specific areas and specific types of investment. Another and more common mechanism is the congressional amendment *(emendas parlamentares)*—bill riders or amendments supported by individual legislators for special projects in their electoral districts. The MS has attempted to offer guidance for these investments to make them compatible with health policies and priorities—but has not always been successful. Many small municipal facilities have been financed through this mechanism, usually to fulfill a political campaign promise. Few such facilities have benefited from supply-demand analysis of hospital services, and still less attention has been paid to how the proposed facilities may fit within an organized network.[75]

Another important weakness in investment policies is the lack of any link between investment decisions and funding to cover additional recurrent costs. As a consequence, health facilities may be built and equipped but remain unused for extended periods for lack of money to pay personnel and operating costs. For instance, several hospitals funded under the World Bank–funded São Paulo Metropolitan Health Program (Programa Metropolitano de Saúde) were only inaugurated 15 years after construction commenced because funds to finish construction, buy equipment, and cover recurrent costs were lacking.

In the absence of an effective mechanism for investment decision and allocation, political influence pervades the allocation process. First, local politicians are keen to build and equip health facilities—especially hospitals—because these facilities are vote-winners, whether or not they make technical or economic sense. Second, given the importance of intergovernmental negotiation and civil society participation in SUS decision making, political pressure influences the pattern of resource allocation in large investment projects.[76]

The MS and a few state governments are exploring strategies to give direction to allocation and investment decisions. For instance, the MS has started an initiative for rationalizing the allocation and use of high technology to reduce oversupply of some of these services. Such measures can contribute significantly to improved cost control and efficiency in health care, as several countries have discovered (box 3.5).

Conclusions and Recommendations

A consistent pattern emerges from the analyses of hospital costs and efficiency presented in this chapter: Many hospitals operate at lower efficiency and with higher costs than necessary. The costs of specific treatments and surgical procedures vary widely across hospitals and among patients within the same hospital. Use and occupancy rates for infrastructure and equipment also vary widely but are generally low.

These inefficiencies and the resulting costs are the results of shortcomings related to the scale of operations, distribution of infrastructure, variations in medical practices, overemphasis on hospital-based care, and lack of information on costs. At the same time, the results show that a subset of Brazilian hospitals is much more efficient than the average.

Summary Assessment

Scale

More than half of Brazil's hospitals are too small (with fewer than 50 beds) to operate efficiently, and most of them are overstaffed. Although small hospitals may be the only chance for medical care in remote municipalities, their sheer number, coupled with low utilization

Box 3.5
Making Rational Hospital Investment Decisions

While Brazil is considering the first steps toward allocating resources rationally in the SUS hospital network, many European countries have set up national planning systems for distributing investment in hospital infrastructure and technology. Funds for capital investment in publicly financed facilities—usually, public and private nonprofit—are available in most countries from the central or regional governments (in all 13 countries reviewed), from bank loans (in 9 countries), from private donations, and from hospitals' accumulated savings. Private finance is mobilized through direct loans to hospitals, loans to a regional health authority, or public-private partnerships (PPPs). The proportion of public and private financing varies widely across countries, with private funding representing up to 80–90 percent in the Netherlands.

In Germany and several other countries the regional health authority must approve private funding. In two-thirds of the countries, facility investment is subject to a national or regional investment plan, approval from the central government, or both, especially if government subsidies are sought. Because in most European countries public funds pay for almost the entire health system, hospital capital investment is usually subject to control and supervision by the health authorities. In England, Italy, and Spain recently established PPPs are responsible for a growing proportion of hospital investment and hospital operations, but even these investments are subject to prior approval and certification of need.

Source: Thompson and McKee 2004.

rates, suggests a flagrant waste of resources. Many were built in response to political campaign promises with little regard for factors such as health needs, institutional capacity, and financial sustainability.

Infrastructure

Hospital infrastructure and equipment are often oversupplied, underutilized, and irrationally distributed. The density of beds and diagnostic equipment is often at or above levels in some high-income countries. High-complexity imaging equipment, in particular, is oversupplied in metropolitan areas, and utilization rates are often low. In addition, bed occupancy rates, averaging less than 40 percent nationally, are among the lowest in the world.

Variations in Medical Practices

The absence of standards in medical procedures or treatment protocols is a major factor in cost variation and contributes to loose cost control, inefficiency, and low-quality care.[77] Limited application of case management or similar practices exacerbates these problems.

Hospital Focus

Brazil relies more heavily than most countries on hospital and inpatient care, partly because the primary care network is weak. Nearly 30 percent of hospital admissions are for conditions that could be treated in ambulatory care centers. Similarly, much ambulatory care is delivered in hospital emergency rooms, usually treating nonemergency cases. Although ambulatory surgery and other cost-reducing approaches are increasingly evident, inefficiency and costs resulting from overreliance on hospital care remain high.

Information on Costs

The general lack of information on costs hampers effective management and planning, control of resources, and monitoring and assessment of hospital performance. Inadequate patient documentation and information systems create significant obstacles to cost accounting and management, as well as to billing practices, payment, cost control, and quality control. They also inhibit meaningful analysis of costs and payment levels.

Efficiency

As seen in the DEA findings, some Brazilian hospitals, both private and public, are much more efficient than the average. Improving hospital efficiency and controlling costs could result in significant savings for the SUS. Although the available data do not permit a precise estimate of the cost of these inefficiencies, a simplistic estimate, based on the low occupancy rate alone, suggests that up to 40 percent of hospital spending could be saved or significantly reduced.[78] International literature also suggests room for considerable savings. Gaynor and Anderson (1991), for instance, estimated the cost of an empty bed in the United States at US$38,000 in 1987, or 18 percent of a hospital's inpatient costs. Since occupancy rates in Brazil are much lower (35–40 percent, against 65–70 percent in the United States), potential savings are likely to be greater. These savings could be used to expand primary care, improve the quality of hospital services, or both.

The analyses presented in this chapter suggest strategies for improving performance by promoting the characteristics of the highest performers. Efficient hospitals are generally larger; have higher bed turnover, higher occupancy rates, and shorter patient stays; use fewer nursing and, especially, nontechnical personnel; consume less technology per bed; and are more productive in terms of output per worker. There is no evidence that these efficient facilities scrimp on quality, but there is indirect evidence that their quality of care is superior to that of their inefficient peers. Improving resource allocation among inputs, reducing excess use of inputs (especially personnel and technology), and reducing the number of small hospitals are key elements in a new hospital policy. Identifying the best performers and analyzing managerial practices can help in drawing up strategies for feasible improvements in hospital performance.

Recommendations for Improving Hospital Efficiency and Cost Control

Improvement of hospital efficiency and better cost control depends on a broader policy framework, focused on the underlying structural factors that allow or provide incentives for current practices in hospital finance and operations. Most public hospitals have no autonomy to manage their resources according to their needs or to define goals, and the way hospitals are paid creates distortions and prevents achievement of an appropriate balance between efficiency, quality, and equity.

To improve hospital efficiency and contain costs, the following actions are recommended:

- *Develop a more aggressive national strategy for rationalizing the hospital network.* Set clear criteria for consolidating, converting, or closing hospitals that operate below capacity or that no longer satisfy local needs. This strategy should be developed as a national policy by the MS, but the state health secretariats should be responsible for adapting and implementing it.

- *Develop a national system for technology assessment,* with criteria and methodology for allocating technological resources. As a national system, the initiative should be undertaken under the leadership of the MS but should not necessarily be executed by the MS itself. International experience suggests that independent nongovernmental institutions (or a network of institutions) can exercise this responsibility better than a central government.

- *Develop and implement a national plan for the adoption of treatment protocols or guidelines.* Because this recommendation affects quality of care, as well as efficiency and cost control, it should be framed and developed within a broader perspective. The MS should lead this initiative with support from the states, but it would be most effectively executed by an independent institution such as one overseeing a national accreditation program.

- *Review or develop standards for the use and allocation of human resources* in hospital care in order to identify opportunities for cutting hospital personnel costs. The existing standards, written by nursing associations, pertain mainly to nursing personnel.

- *Improve hospital record keeping on patients.* Patient medical records should be standardized and eventually computerized to improve the reliability of patient and treatment information. Each hospital should have a functioning medical records committee; a records review process should be strongly encouraged.

- *Strengthen monitoring and evaluation systems,* particularly a nationwide hospital benchmarking system. Again, such a system would be better managed by an independent body, under the leadership and supervision of the MS, and should draw on experience in Brazil. This benchmarking system should be integrated with the proposed national accreditation program and the cost information system. Most important, the benchmarking results should be fully disseminated to allow identification of good practices and serve as references for pricing in the public and private sectors.

- *Develop and implement a standardized cost accounting system* in a sample of SUS hospitals, including public and private facilities. MS leadership is important in promoting and ensuring the use of a standard methodology in as many hospitals as possible. The methodology should not be limited to cost-center absorption costing but should be designed in a way that allows estimation and monitoring of hospital treatment and case costs. A key element of this initiative is to train managers and decision makers to use and interpret cost information in a cost-management framework.

- *Undertake further analytical studies on hospital efficiency and costs* to better inform efficiency improvement policies in hospitals. The MS and state health secretariats should promote and finance these studies.

Most of these actions require MS leadership in designing national policies and strategies. Nevertheless, the state health secretariats should play a key role in detailing these initiatives, as well as in coordinating and supervising their implementation at the regional and local levels. Independent regulatory bodies have also been shown internationally to be effective in coordinating such efforts.

Annex 3A

Cost Analysis Methodology:
The De Matos Cost Study Methodology

The De Matos (2002) study consisted of a sample of 25 hospitals and 107 procedures for inpatient care. The hospital sample was not representative of the Unified Health System (Sistema Único de Saúde, SUS) network, which includes a large proportion of university facilities, and it was too small to draw statistical inferences for subgroups of hospitals. These limitations may have biased cost estimates toward larger teaching hospitals and thus higher costs. The procedure sample included both medium-to-high-complexity and low-cost, high-frequency procedures. It covered 4.36 percent of the total number of SUS procedures, but these procedures account for 62.5 percent of the volume of Authorization for Hospitalization (Autorização de Internação Hospitalar, AIH) payments and 60.8 percent of all SUS payments for inpatient care. The sample included 16,482 cases or patients, randomly selected within each procedure, and their medical records were systematically reviewed, making up an average of 659 cases per hospital and 154 per procedure. Sample size was adequate overall, but for some less frequent procedures it was too small to allow for any reliable generalization of the results.

In the absence of a procedure-based cost information system, the general approach used to estimate procedure costs is usually based on two types of information: (1) cost information obtained from cost accounting systems—when they exist—or from indirect methods for estimating unit costs, and (2) a systematic review of medical records of the patients selected for sampling. The direct cost of treatment for each case is then estimated by multiplying the unit cost of the inputs or service components that enter into the treatment (derived through the cost systems or from market prices) by the quantity of each input or service used in that treatment, obtained by reviewing medical charts. General or overhead expenditures are estimated from the costing systems or, in their absence, by a proxy method. The mean cost of a particular treatment or procedure is then computed by averaging the costs of individual patients undergoing that treatment or procedure. When cost information is out of date, incomplete, or inconsistent, it can be updated using a health sector price index to adjust for changes in input prices or can be complemented by indirect estimation of input costs, based on market prices and available hospital financial information.

Ideally, in order for cost comparisons to be meaningful and to allow an efficiency interpretation, several assumptions must be met:

- The number of sampled procedures has to be sufficient to allow generalization.
- The quality of services provided in each facility has to be similar (or adjusted for).
- The clinical composition of the patients (the case mix) at all facilities has to be similar (or adjusted for).
- Input prices have to be similar across hospitals (or adjusted for).

Case-Mix Adjustment

Different hospitals treat different mixes of patients, which may vary by diagnosis, age or gender, risk factors, or severity. These differences have an important bearing on hospital costs. A tertiary hospital treating complex cases is expected to have a higher average cost for a given treatment or procedure than another, less complex hospital. Cost comparisons therefore need to be corrected for differences in case mix.

When applied to cost analysis, case mix is usually defined to control for differences in the patient mix that are reflected in differential resource utilization and thus treatment costs. Case mix can be measured in three main ways: simple unidimensional indicators usually related to facility characteristics and the type or complexity of services offered; patient classification systems that take into consideration patient severity or diagnostic groups and attempt to reflect differential risks; and measures of the intensity of resource use in treating different groups of patients.

Facility Characteristics

Simple proxy indicators of case mix include average length of stay (ALOS) and bed turnover. Both measures, however, can also be indicators of efficiency in bed use or differences in treatment practice rather than of inpatient characteristics or severity. The presence of high-technology diagnostic or treatment resources, including intensive care unit (ICU) beds, indicates that the facility can treat more severe or complex cases but not necessarily that these beds are actually being used to treat such cases. Despite these limitations, and in the absence of detailed information on patient characteristics, these simple indicators are often used as proxies for case mix.

Other facility-level, single-proxy variables can be used to indicate case severity or complexity. These include the proportion of medium-to-high-complexity procedures or cases in certain medical specialties to the total number of AIH procedures performed by the hospital. Such variables are more appropriate than the measures previously mentioned because they focus on the type of care actually provided, but they are limited in that they focus on one dimension or aspect and are not suitable for capturing patient-level differences.

A synthetic index of resource use can be constructed from a few easily observed variables such as ALOS, percentage of ICU days in ALOS, intensity (frequency) of diagnostic test use, points attributed to different surgical procedures by the Ministry of Health (Ministério da Saúde, MS) in defining AIH payment levels, and intensity of use of ortheses, prostheses, and special materials (expensive components of many high-complexity procedures). The simplest way of combining these indicators into one index is to measure each on a scale and take their simple average. A more elegant approach would be to perform a regression or a factor analysis of these variables to determine the weights to be assigned in constructing the resource use index.

Case-Mix Classification Systems

Patient classification systems are generally better indicators of case mix because they focus on the severity or relative risk (or both) of a group of patients. Such approaches, based on clinical characteristics of patients, relate to the clinical severity domain, which captures significant indicators of clinical needs and includes patient history, clinical conditions, and risk factors.

Regardless of the group under consideration, patient classification explains differences in outcomes through clinical assessment tools such as risk-adjusted mortality and risk-adjusted complications. Other methods, such as diagnosis-related groups (DRGs), correlate severity of illness with resource utilization.

Adjustment for severity or risk (or both), either for particular patients or for groups of patients, usually involves one of two approaches. The model-based approach relies heavily on regression models to predict health outcomes, service indicators, or costs, as measured by, say, probability of death, length of stay (LOS), or average cost. Two examples of this mode of analysis are the risk-adjusted mortality index and the risk-adjusted complications index. The other approach to severity adjustment is to group patients with similar levels of severity, using DRGs or similar patient classification systems.

The initial motivation for developing the DRGs was to create an effective framework for monitoring utilization of services in a hospital setting. Its widening use as a basic payment mechanism in several countries reflects the advantages of the approach, although implementation of the system usually requires adaptation to local characteristics.

The use of U.S.-based DRGs and weights for constructing a case-mix variable, as is done in several countries, such as Italy, is appealing, but in Brazil it would require extensive work to establish correspondence between the AIH system, based on the procedure performed, and the DRGs, based on diagnosis. A complicating factor is that information on diagnoses in the AIH system is often incomplete or unreliable, despite improvements in recent years. In addition, the validity of this approach relies on the assumption that hospital procedures and the input mix used are technically similar in the United States and Brazil, even though input prices can be very different.

A more feasible alternative would be to construct an indicator based on the medical specialties offered by each hospital or, better still, the mix of procedures or admissions, by specialty, produced by a hospital. Though appealing, this approach encounters the difficulty of attributing appropriate weights to each specialty or procedure group in constructing the case-mix variable. Using the SUS-defined reimbursement values is not a good choice because these are unrelated to actual costs—that is, they do not just underestimate cost.

Resource Use Classifications

The service utilization domain is the other case-mix dimension. It characterizes approaches that focus on the intensity with which different groups of patients use hospital resources and includes service indicators and provider characteristics as data elements. Two types of case-mix measures can be devised: direct measures of resource utilization, and relative costs of treating different patients.

Direct measures of resource utilization (e.g., personnel time, drugs, supplies), although technically best, are often not feasible because of the difficulty of obtaining such measures and combining them in a single index. A more feasible approach is to use the relative costs of treating different patients. In this case, the ratio to be computed is that between the cost of a particular procedure or facility and the average cost of all procedures or facilities included in the sample. The use of relative average cost as an indicator of case mix assumes that measured costs truly reflect the differential use of resources, that costs were correctly estimated, and that the costs estimated for the sample reflect the activity level and resource use for the other procedures (or facilities).

For the cost and efficiency studies undertaken as background papers for this volume, the three approaches outlined above were considered. However, the absence in the original REFORSUS study of information on patient attributes (e.g., severity of illness, risk of dying, prognosis, treatment difficulty, need for intervention) precluded any clinical notion of case mix and reduced the possible choice of measures. The database did, nevertheless, provide a fair basis for the concept of case mix as understood by administrators, economists, and regulators—that is, a measure based on resource utilization. A case-mix indicator based on relative costs rather than clinical complexity or risk was therefore chosen. The expected correspondence between the clinical approach and the resource-use approach implies that a hospital treating patients who require more hospital resources, and thus higher expenditure, would usually have a more complex case mix from a clinical/diagnostic perspective.

All costs were adjusted for differences in case mix, using an index based on the relative intensity of resource use (described in box 3.3). The case-mix index (CMI) used was empirically constructed as the ratio of the average cost for a given procedure and hospital—an indicator of resource intensity—to the average cost for all procedures and hospitals. It thus measures the relative resource intensity of patients cared for in a particular hospital, compared with that for the average patient in the sample. This approach is consistent with the one adopted for the DRGs in the U.S. Medicare patient classification system, and a preliminary comparison of DRGs and the cost-based variable applied to the sample showed very similar behavior.

Annex 3B
Supplementary Data

TABLE 3B.1
Comparison of the De Matos (2002) Sample and the AIH Database

	AIH				De Matos study				
Complexity	Value range (R$)	No. of procedures	Volume (%)	Spending (%)	CMI level	No. of procedures	Mean cost (R$)	Volume (%)	Cost (%)
Low	<250	570	41.51	16.13	<0.5	32	934.70	36.94	13.35
Medium-lower	<500	652	38.80	29.92	0.5–1	32	1,853.41	34.26	23.62
Medium-upper	<1,000	449	12.66	17.15	1–2	19	3,460.45	17.27	23.07
High-lower	<2,500	346	5.65	19.38	2–3	14	6,309.53	7.69	17.63
High-upper	>2,500	253	1.38	17.42	3+	9	22,310.78	3.84	22.33

Source: De Matos (2002); MS/Datasus.
Note: AIH, Autorização de Internação Hospitalar (Authorization for Hospitalization).

TABLE 3B.2
TOBIT Regression of Total Hospital Inefficiency, Using Governance Model 2

Variable	Coefficient	Standard error	t	P > |t|	[95% C.I.]	
Number of beds*	−0.013	0.003	−3.840	0.000	−0.020	−0.006
Bed turnover*	−0.073	0.008	−9.660	0.000	−0.088	−0.058
Physicians/bed	−0.102	0.530	−0.190	0.848	−1.144	0.941
Nursing personnel/bed*	−1.469	0.515	−2.850	0.005	−2.480	−0.457
Other personnel/bed	0.269	0.334	0.800	0.422	−0.388	0.926
Emergencies/discharge ratio*	−0.243	0.067	−3.650	0.000	−0.374	−0.112
Teaching status	0.298	1.060	0.280	0.779	−1.785	2.381
Quality index*	17.873	1.658	10.780	0.000	14.614	21.132
Direct public governance (DPG) (other)/direct public governance (health) (H)	2.213	1.387	1.600	0.111	−0.513	4.939
Foundation/DPG(H)*	−1.627	0.732	−2.220	0.027	−3.066	−0.188
Agencies/DPG(H)	−2.098	1.406	−1.490	0.136	−4.861	0.665
OSSs/DPG(H)*	−1.831	0.626	−2.930	0.004	−3.061	−0.602
Public corporation/DPG(H)*	−2.741	1.347	−2.030	0.043	−5.390	−0.093
Corporate/DPG(H)	−0.002	2.584	0.000	0.999	−5.082	5.078
Associations/DPG(H)	−1.185	3.248	−0.360	0.715	−7.570	5.200
Cooperatives/DPG(H)	−1.038	4.389	−0.240	0.813	−9.666	7.589
Unions/DPG(H)**	−1.486	0.778	−1.910	0.057	−3.016	0.045
Other/DPG(H)*	−1.590	0.801	−1.990	0.048	−3.164	−0.015
Constant*	2.908	1.003	2.900	0.004	0.936	4.879

Source: Couttolenc et al. 2004.
* *p* < .05. ** *p* < .10.

Annex 3C

Average Cost and Coefficient of Variation for Sample Hospital Procedures

Code	Procedure	Mean cost, unadjusted (R$)	Mean cost, adjusted (R$)	CV (%)	Range (R$)
31003052	Prostatectomy	1,818.47	2,017.58	26	787–3,724
31005055	Endoscopic resection of prostate	1,459.28	1,695.44	45	676–3,616
31802010	Kidney transplant (live donor)	6,161.90	5,687.50	221	2,266–14,888
32011016	Myocardial revascularization with extracorporeal circulation	9,994.28	10,810.79	30	6,200–19,829
32013019	Substitution of cardiac pacemaker	3,869.62	3,616.08	22	3,212–5,339
32015011	Cardiac pacemaker (intracavity)	5,282.21	5,789.77	60	3,732–10,818
32019017	Valvuloplasty	11,366.92	9,615.84	27	4,866–14,205
32020015	Implant of cardiac valvular graft	12,267.67	10,979.36	28	6,411–16,395
32021011	Surgical correction of congenital cardiac disorders	7,562.19	7,087.10	37	4,366–11,475
32023014	Coronary angioplasty	6,314.39	6,014.42	63	3,963–8,536
32040040	Resection of aortic arc with graft	5,400.37	14,658.98	*	*
33004080	Cholecystectomy	1,983.75	2,062.31	47	568–7,744
33005060	Appendectomy	1,024.68	1,097.36	48	257–1,928
33006067	Partial colectomy	3,718.27	3,859.09	38	940–8,825
33011117	Inguinal hernia surgery (unilateral)	838.40	957.16	40	271–1,999
33016119	Exploratory laparotomy	2,797.99	2,774.25	50	425–6,056
33021066	Enterostomy	4,624.13	4,946.30	63	823–7,309
33023069	Colostomy	3,644.83	3,660.28	40	877–9,248
34001042	Uni- or bilateral salpingectomy	1,372.26	1,264.40	29	363–2,304
34001050	Uni- or bilateral oophorectomy	1,370.80	1,414.25	40	612–2,844
34008020	Anterior or posterior colpoperineoplasty	1,143.39	1,210.41	40	412–2,779
34010033	Total hysterectomy	1,886.36	1,909.72	31	608–3,190
35001011	Normal delivery	619.27	884.31	33	329–1,130
35009012	Cesarean section	860.96	1,488.38	35	587–1,918
35014016	Postabortion curettage	661.49	722.47	56	186–1,437
36020052	Fasciectomy for intraocular lens implant	901.64	840.89	48	336–1,458
37040014	Cochlear implant	31,888.41	3,909.28	*	*

(continued)

Code	Procedure	Mean cost, unadjusted (R$)	Mean cost, adjusted (R$)	CV (%)	Range (R$)
38025019	Loss of skin substance— extensive superficial lesions	995.47	1,348.10	47	410–2,860
39003124	Arthroplasty of hip joint	5,777.33	4,115.26	56	1,638–11,168
39003140	Partial arthroplasty of knee	6,936.84	6,454.60	28	4,454–9,404
39004139	Amputation of the thigh	2,547.60	2,805.98	66	832–8,385
39009130	Surgical reduction of femur diaphysis fracture	3,124.69	3,073.81	27	688–6,140
39011151	Surgical reduction of tibia diaphysis, with immobilization	2,298.21	2,556.62	27	1,035–5,757
39011160	Surgical reduction of ankle fracture, with immobilization	1,475.90	1,529.60	33	445–2,607
39012131	Surgical reduction of hip joint fracture	2,550.67	2,720.41	29	729–3,852
39013081	Surgical reduction of forearm bones fracture, with immobilization	1,249.85	1,426.90	44	426–4,666
39013138	Surgical reduction of transtrochanterian fracture	2,956.48	2,564.93	32	858–5,351
39016129	Arthroplasty of hip joint with prosthesis	4,225.31	4,728.73	31	3,312–6,647
39022145	Total arthroplasty of knee, with implant	5,298.19	4,148.67	49	3,339–9,118
40001008	Conservative management of cranioencephalic trauma	513.24	619.75	70	168–906
40001040	Surgical treatment of epilepsy	7,762.45	3,481.43	30	5,722–10,823
40028011	Vascular intracranial microsurgery	6,705.90	8,729.59	20	6,528–7,445
40038017	Surgical treatment of subdural hematoma	3,334.23	3,041.09	87	1,524–15,249
40039013	Surgical treatment of extradural hematoma	5,548.97	4,825.35	23	1,163–6,846
40061019	Ventriculoperitoneotomy	8,825.35	7,081.01	38	3,119–18,802
42002079	Removal of breast tumor	691.86	623.10	45	254–1,456
42705070	Complete mastectomy with lymphadenectomy	1,877.57	1,607.60	55	653–2,697
46800018	Heart transplant	23,950.34	18,137.75	59	13,291–43,503
46800085	Liver transplant	25,123.16	15,535.85	54	12,870–45,067
46801014	Lung transplant	48,436.12	40,788.31	*	*
46814019	Allogenic kin bone marrow transplant	31,738.02	19,242.93	42	6,417–59,988
63001101	Treatment of psychiatric patient in general hospital	2,440.43	1,948.65	49	398–3,303
63001209	Treatment of psychiatric patient in day hospital	3,303.89	3,095.60	31	2,142–4,466

(continued)

Code	Procedure	Mean cost, unadjusted (R$)	Mean cost, adjusted (R$)	CV (%)	Range (R$)
63001403	Treatment of psychiatric patient in psychiatric hospital B	1,005.75	3,192.93	*	*
70000000	Treatment of AIDS	3,958.51	3,228.49	33	857–7,060
71300015	Prematurity	4,396.65	5,048.92	180	712–12,486
71300066	Acute pneumopathy	2,275.09	2,733.85	87	1,507–5,349
71300082	Neonatal jaundice	1,126.20	1,137.87	85	293–2,614
72300019	Acute dehydration (pediatric)	817.05	750.55	86	268–2,294
72500018	Acute dehydration (general medicine)	1,017.91	987.17	40	461–2,037
73500011	Malnourishment (general medicine)	2,045.15	2,645.85	44	634–3,900
74300113	Bacterial meningitis (pediatric)	2,386.45	2,151.88	44	308–4,175
74300237	Staphylococcus diseases (pediatric)	1,162.56	1,324.46	83	203–7,674
74300261	Septicemia (pediatric)	5,279.95	4,737.29	100	833–28,802
74300270	Entero infections (pediatric)	932.21	1,050.48	77	293–2,479
74500031	Pulmonary tuberculosis	3,108.12	2,225.14	59	478–4,584
74500201	Streptococcus diseases (general medicine)	929.80	1,148.95	47	216–2,509
74500244	Septicemia (general medicine)	3,166.52	3,308.18	85	636–6,125
75500027	Peptic ulcer	885.04	981.20	66	325–1,921
75500035	Gastritis and duodenitis	906.37	958.41	57	280–2,418
75500124	Digestive hemorrhage	1,124.63	1,184.00	76	422–6,336
75500213	Hepatic cirrhosis	2,837.15	3,069.17	48	572–5,108
75500272	Acute cholecystectomy	875.67	1,014.40	45	335–1,705
76300056	Acute bronchiolitis	997.97	976.79	82	146–2,647
76300064	Staphylococcus pneumonia	2,257.28	2,641.82	53	900–4,632
76300072	Other pneumonia	1,382.83	1,577.24	43	479–3,314
76300080	Bronchopneumonia	1,220.51	1,165.02	52	203–3,148
76300102	Asthmatic crisis	733.29	804.25	45	247–1,530
76300188	Acute respiratory insufficiency	3,144.94	3,056.29	83	399–9,259
76400077	Infant pneumonia	1,866.72	2,320.37	62	566–3,933
76400085	Infant bronchopneumonia	1,454.10	1,803.01	106	208–2,603
76400271	Infant entero infections	1,304.76	1,421.49	80	223–2,959
76500063	Unspecified pneumonia	1,404.85	1,513.02	44	372–2,950
76500071	Bronchopneumonia	1,672.52	1,691.31	43	318–3,530
76500080	Pulmonary emphysema	1,807.67	1,736.55	70	544–8,977
76500110	Unbalanced cor pulmonale	6,959.76	5,742.48	74	267–17,322
76500128	Asthmatic crisis	1,136.71	1,121.31	71	347–3,419

(continued)

Code	Procedure	Mean cost, unadjusted (R$)	Mean cost, adjusted (R$)	CV (%)	Range (R$)
76500225	Chronic obstructive pulmonary disease	1,836.07	2,241.12	43	513–3,485
76500233	Acute respiratory insufficiency	2,305.10	2,691.80	59	703–5,722
77500024	Acute myocardial infarction	2,951.50	3,113.84	48	902–6,055
77500032	Acute coronary insufficiency	1,669.56	1,739.29	85	543–3,342
77500113	Cardiac insufficiency	1,688.12	1,815.79	50	573–3,080
77500121	Hypertensive crisis	816.26	672.59	79	271–2,401
77500164	Acute pulmonary edema	2,607.67	2,646.56	82	642–10,270
77500180	Arrhythmias	1,244.65	1,260.97	31	310–2,289
77500202	Peripheral vascular disease	1,804.30	2,169.86	61	510–6,573
79700896	Hospitalization for chronic leukemia in acute phase for chemotherapy	3,978.11	3,686.61	50	1,601–10,997
80500072	Pyelonephritis	892.55	1,031.82	39	316–1,780
80500110	Renal colic	556.59	585.40	95	115–2,258
80500170	Chronic renal failure—metabolic acidosis	1,378.27	1,587.22	57	327–2,766
80500218	Other diseases of genitourinary system	784.43	778.66	52	268–2,130
81001010	Diagnostic exploration of epilepsy	7,342.94	3,252.09	38	3,823–9,620
81500106	Acute stroke	1,684.73	1,933.24	39	687–5,266
82500053	Diabetes mellitus	1,283.93	1,321.38	56	383–5,373
83500022	Acute back pain	915.66	958.96	73	278–3,684
85500755	Long-term care of patients with neurological disorders	2,475.98	2,313.02	107	2,134–2,510
85500879	Clinical intercurrent conditions in oncological patients	1,528.45	1,595.92	50	594–2,580
	Full sample mean	2,606.83	2,515.32	55.5	115–59,988

Source: De Matos 2002; Dias, Couttolenc, and De Matos 2004; for codes, Datasus SIH (Sistema de Informação Hospitalar, Hospital Inpatient Information System) database.
Note: * = insufficient number of cases.

Annex 3D
DEA Methodology

In its production process, a hospital combines various inputs such as manpower, drugs, supplies, and equipment to produce multiple outputs, including inpatient discharges or patient-days, outpatient consultations, and diagnostic tests. The relation between the quantity of inputs used to the quantity of outputs produced indicates the efficiency of the production process. Efficiency and effectiveness are different but related concepts. *Efficiency* gives the capacity to reach the best result with the minimum amount of resources; *effectiveness* indicates the capacity to produce a desired result (Grassetti, Gori, and Bellio 2003).

Concepts of Efficiency

Efficiency is thus a relation between the result or output obtained and the amount of resources used to achieve it. An efficient firm produces more output relative to the inputs used than an inefficient firm. But a number of factors may be involved: better managing and optimizing the production process itself, combining inputs in the most appropriate proportion so that none are wasted, or producing on a sufficiently large scale to minimize fixed costs. These factors correspond to different types of efficiency, as shown in figure 3D.1 and described in the next paragraphs.

FIGURE 3D.1
Relation Between Different Types of Efficiency

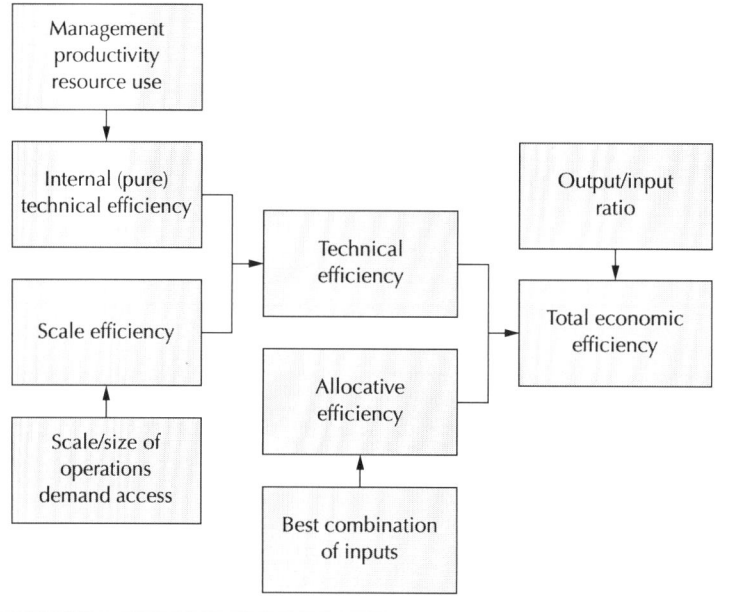

Source: Authors' elaboration.

Technical efficiency is a firm's ability to obtain the maximum output for a given set of inputs, and *allocative efficiency* is the firm's ability to use the inputs in optimal proportion for a given price and technology (Farrell 1957). In other words, when two firms produce the same amount of output but firm A uses less inputs than firm B, firm A is said to be more efficient, from the technical efficiency point of view. Alternatively, if A and B use the same amount of inputs but A manages to produce more output, then, too, it is more technically efficient. However, for efficiency, a given production process may require the combination of two inputs P and Q—say, labor and equipment—in a particular proportion. If firm A uses these inputs in less than optimal proportions, resulting in higher costs, it will be inefficient in the allocative sense. The combination of the two measures—technical and allocative—gives *total economic efficiency.*

Figure 3D.2 provides a graphic explanation of these concepts. In this example, the firm uses two inputs (x_1 and x_2) to produce one output (y). The SS' line (the isoquant) represents the fully efficient firms in the sense that these produce a given quantity of product using the minimum possible quantity of inputs x_1 and x_2.[79] Technical efficiency would be represented in the graph as follows. A firm represented by point D uses a given amount of x_1 and x_2 to produce y output; in this case it lies away from the fully efficient firms on line SS', and the inefficiency of the firm is represented by the distance to that line, *DC. DC* is the proportional amount by which input use could be reduced holding output unchanged.

The technical efficiency of the firm is then measured by the ratio

$$\text{TE}_i = OC/OD$$

where TE_i is a value between zero and one and indicates the degree of technical inefficiency of firm i. A value of 1 means that the firm is totally technically efficient, while a low value (close to 0) indicates a high degree of inefficiency.

A fully efficient firm in the allocative sense will be located at the point where allocative efficiency (AE) = 1, that is, at point C', where the isoquant SS' and the isocost (the line joining

FIGURE 3D.2
Technical and Allocative Efficiencies

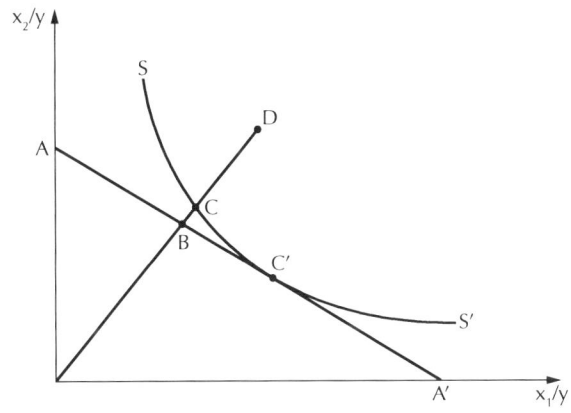

all points with similar costs) AA' are tangent. The distance between B and C represents the cost reduction implied if the firm is to operate with both allocative and technical efficiency (i.e., at point C' instead of the technically efficient but allocatively inefficient point C).

The product of TE_i and AE_i gives total economic efficiency (EE_i):

$$EE_i = TE_i \times AE_i = OB/OD.$$

An important topic in analyzing efficiency is its relation to the scale of operations. In many production processes, efficiency increases as the volume of production increases because fixed costs are being spread over larger quantities of output. For instance, small hospitals may be inefficient because they are too small to compensate for the fixed costs of equipment and installations. Returns to scale (RTS) reflect the degree to which a proportional increase in all inputs used increases output. Constant returns to scale occur when an increase in all inputs produces the same increase in output—when, for instance, doubling labor and equipment doubles the volume of output produced. When an increase in inputs results in a more than proportional increase in output, the firm is said to operate with increasing returns to scale, and when the increase in output is less than proportional, RTS is said to decrease. When the size of the firm is such that it experiences gains in efficiency (i.e., minimizes the costs of production), it is said to experience scale efficiencies.

In the economic literature, various methods have been used to estimate efficiency. Some require knowledge of the particular form of the production process (parametric methods); others do not (nonparametric methods). A peculiar hospital characteristic is the joint production of multiple outputs (e.g., inpatient discharges, ambulatory consultations, emergency procedures, diagnostic tests) that cannot be easily summarized in a single measure. This makes methods that do not require specification of the production process a convenient approach for handling efficiency measurement. One of these methods, data envelopment analysis (DEA), used in this study, is described below.

Data Envelopment Analysis

DEA is a method for estimating efficiency that involves the use of linear programming to rank firms according to a score of relative efficiency. It is based on the idea that production units—or decision-making units—seek to maximize their output for a given quantity of inputs or, alternatively, minimize the quantity of inputs for a given output. The method was originally proposed in a paper by Farrell (1957). The term data envelopment analysis, however, first appeared in an article by Charnes, Cooper, and Rhodes (1978) that expanded on Farrell's idea by creating a model which became known as the CCR DEA model, from the names of its authors. The great advantage of the CCR model is that it allows for multiple inputs and outputs—a plus in hospital analysis. It relies on the construction of an efficiency frontier that joins all the possible points for a fully efficient firm to produce a given output. Firms (or decision-making units, the recognized term in the DEA literature) that minimize the ratio of inputs to outputs are said to be efficient, are located on the frontier, and receive a score of 1. The inefficient ones are below the frontier and receive a score between 0 and 1.

Various models of DEA have been developed to accommodate different situations and assumptions. The CCR model estimates efficiency under the assumption of constant returns to scale (CRS) and shows how firms seek to maximize the combined quantity of outputs subject to the feasible combination of inputs used. However, the use of the CCR model when not all firms operate with constant return to scale may result in measures of technical efficiency that are confounded by scale efficiencies. Observing this fact, Banker, Charnes, and Cooper (1984) suggested an extension to the CCR model. Their BCC model estimates efficiency, assuming variable returns to scale (VRS), by including an additional constraint.

Total technical efficiency (estimated under CRS) can be decomposed into two components: scale efficiency and pure, or internal, technical efficiency (given by the VRS model). To calculate the scale effect, both the model with constant returns to scale (CRS) and the model with variable returns to scale (VRS) should be run. Then scale efficiency is just the ratio between the scores estimated under these two models:

$$\text{Scale efficiency} = \text{CRS}_e/\text{VRS}_e = \text{TTE}/\text{ITE}$$

where e is the efficiency score produced by each model.

Alternatively,

$$\text{TTE (under CRS)} = \text{ITE (under VRS)} \times \text{SE}$$

In this volume the more intuitive term "internal technical efficiency" is used instead of "pure TE" because this form of efficiency is associated with factors internal to the decision-making unit, such as management practices, organizational structure, and the production process. Scale efficiency, by contrast, is related to external or environmental factors such as demand and sector policies, which often determine the size of operations. Total technical efficiency scores are generally smaller than those for internal technical efficiency because they combine both efficiency in operations (internal technical efficiency) and external conditions (associated with scale efficiency), both being less than 1. A decision-making unit that has a high internal technical efficiency score but a low total technical efficiency score is said to be locally efficient (i.e., for its size or considering only its internal organization and operations) but globally inefficient because it operates below its most productive scale size.

The DEA can produce an input-oriented measure or an output-oriented measure. The former indicates how much an input can be proportionally reduced without a change in total output produced. Output-oriented measures indicate by how much outputs can be increased holding input quantities constant. These two measures are equal when the firms have constant returns to scale.[80]

Several variations of and alternatives to the basic CCR and BCC models have been devised, although the basic models continue to be the most used. The models' characteristics and uses are presented in the literature review summarized in annex 3E. Different model specifications can lead to different results for the same sample. The model to be used is thus an important issue (Webster, Kennedy, and Johnson 1998). Similarly, DEA should in principle be applied to decision-making units that use the same production process. In this sense, and because results are specific to the sample used, it is usually applied to homogeneous samples. Little is said in the literature about the implications of applying DEA to nonhomogeneous samples.

A relevant aspect in DEA models is the relation between sample size (the number of firms) and the number of variables (inputs and outputs). The larger the number of variables relative to the sample size, the larger the proportion of efficient firms will be. A too small sample size will affect both the ability of the model to rank from the more efficient to the less efficient firms and its robustness.[81]

The DEA analysis was performed in four main steps: classification of hospitals, DEA separated by group using the DEA Excel Solver, DEA on the full sample using the DEAP software, and regression analysis.

Classification of Hospitals

To obtain more homogeneous subsamples, the hospital units were first grouped and classified according to several institutional variables: ownership, size (number of beds), governance style, and level of technological complexity.

DEA Separated by Group Using the DEA Excel Solver

A DEA was initially run for each subsample, and the results were analyzed. This was done to circumvent the limitation of the software to only 200 DMUs at a time. DEAs were run assuming variable returns to scale and also under constant returns to scale in order to be able to separate internal efficiency from scale efficiency.[82]

Then, for each classifying variable, the efficient hospitals in each subsample were combined in a single sample, and their projected points (targets) were used in a new DEA for the purpose of identifying possible differences in efficiency according to ownership, number of beds, and other variables.

DEA on the Full Sample Using the DEAP Software

In this step the analysis was run on the whole sample, after excluding hospitals with fewer than 25 beds, which have different characteristics and often can hardly be called hospitals. The final model used the other variables mentioned: inpatient admissions, emergency procedures, full-time equivalent personnel by category, equipment complexity, number of beds, and number of consultation rooms.

To test the validity of this model, several alternative models were run with different input and output variables, including or dropping the potentially troublesome ones, and with or without adjustment of the output variables for service complexity. All of these models gave similar results, indicating stability of the results. The analysis was also run separately for hospital groups by size and other criteria. Excluding hospitals with fewer than 25 beds or those with fewer than 50 beds did not change the results, which proved, overall, consistent and robust across models and specifications. The results presented below refer to the final model only. ANOVA and Mann-Whitney tests were run to assess the significance of the differences observed across hospital groups.

Regression Analysis

Finally, as recommended by Coelli, Rao, and Battese (1999), a regression analysis was run of the efficiency scores on explanatory variables, including ownership and governance, to estimate the effect of these variables and confirm the DEA results.

Box 3D.1
Measuring Hospital Complexity, Case Mix, and Quality from a Facility Survey

Hospital output, efficiency, and costs are strongly affected by three factors that are difficult to measure: the mix of patients (or case mix), the level of technology used in delivering services, and the quality of care. In this volume an attempt was made to measure these variables with the limited information available in the AMS dataset.

A technological complexity indicator was used as an input variable. It was constructed as a weighted sum of diagnostic and other equipment available at the hospital, with the weight representing relative complexity and cost and being assigned empirically as an index varying between 1 and 4. The index was computed as the logarithm of the points achieved and was then adjusted to lie in the 1 to 10 range.

A case-mix proxy was constructed on the basis of the availability of resource-intensive services, such as the number of intensive care units and operating theaters and the proportion of patients treated in nonbasic medical specialties (i.e., other than general medicine, surgery, obstetrics and gynecology, pediatrics, and psychiatry) and in especially high-complexity procedures. The complexity index was then logged and adjusted to vary between 1 and 10 and was used as a case-mix proxy to adjust the product variables.

The quality indicator was constructed based on the three variables available in the dataset and often shown to be associated with quality: the mortality rate adjusted by the case-mix proxy, the rate of nursing personnel per bed, and the proportion of graduate nurses to total nursing personnel. Each variable was transformed into a 0 to 1 indicator, and their unweighted mean constituted the quality indicator.

Source: Authors' elaboration.

To adjust for differences in hospital complexity, case severity, and quality of care, three indicators were constructed from the AMS data and were then applied as described in box 3D.1.

DEA and Provider Payment Mechanisms (PPM)

The DEA results on the impact of PPMs on hospital efficiency could be influenced by confounding variables and by differences among the hospital groups other than the payment mechanism. For example, PPM groups are highly correlated with ownership and organizational arrangements. Variation in hospital size could also distort the efficiency results (see the discussion on scale in the text of this chapter). However, applying multivariate analysis and also controlling for size did not materially alter the results. Additional factors could have confounded the efficiency results, including case mix, clientele (SUS vs. private) and technological complexity. Separating the effects is difficult because a PPM is often an integral component of an organizational arrangement, particularly for public hospitals.[83]

Annex 3E

Brazilian Studies on Hospital Efficiency

Author	Sample	Objective	Model, sample size, and regression variables	Input variables	Output variables	Main results
Marinho 2001a	Public and private hospitals	Compare DEA methodology with performance indicators	*Model* • AP model *Sample size* • 6 hospitals	• Number of beds • Number of staff • Number of doctors	• Number of inpatients • Number of outpatients • Number of patients treated	• DEA has a more consistent result. • Efficiency ranges from 15.89% to 310.5%.
Marinho 2001b	18 municipalities, state of Rio de Janeiro, 1998	Assess regional differences	*Model* • CCR + Tobit *Sample size* • 390 hospitals *Regression variables* • GDP • Population • ALOS	• Number of beds • Ambulatory capacity • Average value of reimbursement per patient-day • Average value of ambulatory procedure	• Number of inpatients • Number of ambulatory procedures • Mortality ratio (quality)	• No regional pattern. • 83.7% average efficiency. • Overall excess supply. • Adjusted beds. • Bigger hospitals have lower efficiency score. • GDP is positively correlated with efficiency. • ALOS is negatively correlated with efficiency.
Marinho 2001c	Brazil Federal Teaching Hospital, five semesters from 1998	• Evaluate in each semester • Evaluate for all semesters and units	*Model* • CCR + fixed effect panel data *Sample size* • 45 hospitals *Regression variables* • Occupancy rate • Turnover rate • ALOS	• Built area • Number of rooms (ambulatory, surgery, and emergency) • SUS financial resources • Number of nurses • Number of doctors • Number of adult beds and ICUs • Number of teachers	• Number of surgeries • Number of outpatients • Number of inpatient visits • Number of general tests • Infection rate • Inverse of number of general deaths • Number of general discharges • Number of interns	• Efficiency: 93.9% Model 1; 84.2% Model 2. • No tendency over time. • North more efficient. • Not affected by size. • ALOS negatively related to efficiency.

Study	Setting	Evaluation	Model / Sample size	Inputs	Outputs	Results
Marinho and Façanha 2001	Brazil Federal teaching hospital, 1996	Evaluation	*Model* • BCC *Sample size* • 43 hospitals	• Built area • Number of teachers (paid by MEC) • Financial resources • Number of staff • Number of beds • Number of intern physicians • Number of physicians (paid by MEC) • Number of resident physicians • Number of ambulatory rooms • Number of ambulatory and surgery rooms • Number of surgery rooms	• Number of surgeries • Number of outpatients • Number of inpatients • FIDEPS	• Increase inpatients, surgeries, and FIDEPS. • Bigger hospitals are less efficient.
Calvo 2002	Mato Grosso state, 1998	Compare public and private facilities	*Model* • BCC *Sample size* • 40 private • 40 public	• Number of physicians • Number of beds • SUS financial resources	• Number of discharges	• No difference between public and private hospitals.
Pereira, Tusi, and Lanzer 1995	Federal teaching hospital, Santa Catarina	Temporal evaluation of hospital surgery clinic	*Model* • FDH and window analysis *Sample size* • 1 hospital, 8 periods	• Total cost • Patient-days • Number of surgery-hours	• Number of surgeries	• First and last periods were efficient, working as reference point for managers.

(continued)

113

Author	Sample	Objective	Model, sample size, and regression variables	Input variables	Output variables	Main results
Prefeitura da Cidade de Rio de Janeiro 2002	General hospital of Rio de Janeiro city, 2000	Evaluate general medicine and surgery clinic	*Model* • CCR *Sample size* • 19 general hospitals, general medicine • 18 general hospitals, surgery	*Clinic* • Mortality ratio • LOS *Surgery* • Mortality ratio • LOS	*General medicine* • Infectious and parasitic diseases • Respiratory diseases • Digestive diseases • Circulatory diseases • Endocrine, nutritional, and metabolic diseases • AIH value *Surgery* • % of high-risk surgeries • Value of AIH	• Mortality ratio and LOS diminished, holding constant disease pattern and resources.
Holanda, Pettrini, and Nogueira 2004	Municipalities of Ceára, 2002	Regional differences	*Model* • BCC (nonincreasing) + Tobit *Sample size* • 163 municipalities *Regression variables* • Municipal population as % of microregion population • Municipal GDP as % of microregion GDP	• Health professionals/1,000 inhabitants • Number of pieces of equipment in use/1,000 inhabitants • Number of hospital beds/1,000 inhabitants	• Number of outpatient visits/1,000 inhabitants • Number of inpatients/1,000 inhabitants	• Best-quality municipalities attract patients from other regions? • Excess of input in some regions? • Concentration of high-cost and high-complexity resources in high-efficiency municipalities. • High scores positively associated with high population and GDP.

Note: AIH, Autorização de Internação Hospitalar, Authorization for Hospitalization; ALOS, average length of stay; AP, Anderson and Petersen DEA model; BCC, Banker, Charnes, and Cooper DEA model; CCR, Charnes, Cooper, and Rhodes DEA model; DEA, data envelopment analysis; FDH, Fundo de Desenvolvimento Hospitalar (Hospital Development Fund); FIDEPS, Fator Incentivo ao Desenvolvimento de Ensino e Pesquisa em Saúde (payment to university hospitals for teaching and research); GDP, gross domestic product; ICU, intensive care unit; LOS, length of stay; MEC, Ministério da Educação e Cultura (Ministry of Education and Culture); SUS, Sistema Único de Saúde (Unified Health System).

Notes

1. On the United States, see Schneiter, Riley, and Rosenthal (2002); NCSL (2003). On Europe, see WHO (2000b, 2000c, 2000d, 2000e).
2. Sources for this section include World Bank (2007) and Couttolenc et al. (2004).
3. As discussed below, analysts have attempted to estimate these costs on the basis of existing cost accounting systems.
4. Appropriation is the process of distributing the cost of general administrative and support cost centers to the cost of final products (e.g., a medical consultation or an inpatient stay). Different criteria can be used for this purpose; for example, administrative costs can be allocated according to the number of personnel working in each cost center.
5. Many small and medium-size hospitals are managed centrally (by the health or other secretariat) and thus spend only a small proportion of their expenditure directly.
6. The AIH system is described in chapter 4.
7. "Procedure" (*procedimento*) is the general term used in Brazil to mean a patient's treatment, as opposed to "service" (*ato medico*); it includes all medical services used to treat a patient or case.
8. Although biased toward more expensive procedures, the sample distribution of procedures by cost range was not unlike the distribution of all inpatient procedures and spending in the national AIH system. (See annex 3B, table 3B.1, for a comparison of the AIH database and the De Matos sample.)
9. Many high-frequency but low-cost procedures, together with a few low-frequency but high-cost procedures, accounted for a large proportion of total expenditure. The procedures contributing the largest expenditure in the sample (above R$1 million) were mostly low-volume, high-complexity procedures: bone marrow transplants and myocardial revascularizations with extracorporeal circulation (both over R$2 million); valvular prosthesis implants; liver transplants; coronary angioplasties; treatment of pediatric septicemia; premature births; and cardiac pacemaker implants. These eight procedures accounted for 8.3 percent of volume but for 28.4 percent of spending.
10. For a discussion of case-mix adjustment and the construction of a case-mix index, see annex 3D.
11. The coefficient of variation is a measure of relative differences, defined as the ratio of the standard deviation to the mean. (Standard deviation is a measure of variation around the mean.) For instance, the appendectomy procedure had a mean cost of R$1,056 and a standard deviation of R$628, resulting in a CV of 59 percent across all cases. Annex 3C provides CVs for all sampled procedures.
12. For instance, a mix of more severe cases treated in a given facility when compared with another will push up the mean cost of any procedure or case in that facility and can thus distort any comparison of mean costs. Mean costs therefore have to be corrected for differences in case mix.
13. SUS authorities claim that many severe cases covered by private insurance plans are dumped into public facilities to avoid expensive treatments. Available data suggest, however, that this practice may not be as widespread as claimed. The number of patients identified as covered by private insurance and treated in an SUS facility (823,000 between 1999 and 2005) is a very small proportion of care provided to privately insured patients (155 million consultations and 7 million hospital admissions per year). Also, although systematic data are lacking, not all these cases are for high-complexity care. For example, the National Agency for Health Insurance (Agência Nacional de Saúde Suplementar, ANS) reported that 44 percent of claims in the first six months of 2006 were for obstetric care, including normal births and cesarean sections (ANS 2006b).
14. The issue of underpayment by the SUS for most hospital procedures relative to costs and the distorted incentives embedded in this payment mechanism are discussed in chapter 4. Public hospitals are funded through a budget that includes but is not limited to the amount paid through the federal AIH system and the Ambulatory Care Information System (Sistema de Informação Ambulatorial, SIA) while private facilities rely essentially on these latter payments. Private facilities therefore have fewer financial resources for funding treatment of SUS patients.

15. As seen in figure 3.4, the intrahospital group of cases does not include adjusted CVs because, by definition, case-mix adjustments are performed across hospitals.

16. Individual case severity was not controlled for in the sample because collection of diagnostic information was beyond the scope of the De Matos (2002) study.

17. Three of these low-variation procedures are surgical procedures. Considerable clinical standardization exists for normal delivery.

18. The AIH billing and payment system consists of six main components: hospital services (including nursing and all general support and administration services): professional services (payments to physicians): diagnostic tests: drugs and medical supplies: special drugs and supplies (mostly high-cost items): and special procedures (usually high-cost ones).

19. The ANS is the national regulatory agency that oversees private health insurance plans. UNIDAS is the trade association for corporations that offer their employees direct coverage (self-managed plans).

20. The comparatively low costs of the OSS hospitals for inpatient care is an important finding and suggests that the private-public partnership on which the OSS model is based is robust, at least in terms of efficiency. See chapters 5 and 6 for a discussion of OSS hospitals.

21. These figures take into account the whole population. Counting the population that uses SUS services regularly, the number was 8.3 per 100 in 2005.

22. Procedures classified as high complexity are in the areas of orthopedics, transplants, cardiology, renal diseases, oncology, and neurosurgery, among others.

23. Quality of care was not controlled for in most of this research.

24. See, for instance, IHBF (2005); Brosi et al. (1997); Englert, Davis, and Koch (2001); Auton (1994); McKee (1997).

25. Methods recommended to correct for low degrees of freedom include window analysis and bootstrap analysis.

26. AIH payments for inpatient care are in most cases well below actual costs, but complex procedures tend to be well paid.

27. One of these methodologies is proposed by the ANS Programa de Qualificação da Medicina Suplementar for measuring the quality of private health insurers.

28. The analysis was conducted by the Brazilian Census Bureau (Instituto Brasileiro de Geografia e Estatística, IBGE). Several data sources have been used for analysis of hospital efficiency in Brazil, and all of them proved to have important limitations in coverage, data quality, or both. Alternative data sources considered included the Ministry of Health (Ministério da Saúde, MS) Health Facility Registry (Cadastro Nacional de Estabelecimentos de Saúde, CNES), the Datasus hospital database, and the 1998 AMS survey (IBGE 2000a). The first two are limited to hospitals providing services to the SUS, and a number of public and private hospitals are not in the registry. The 1998 AMS survey allowed identification of individual hospitals but had fewer variables than the 2002 edition.

29. The DEA model used two output variables: inpatient discharges and emergency procedures. Outpatient consultations, another hospital output, were not available in the dataset. Input variables included six input variables: three capital inputs (number of beds, number of consultation rooms, and the log of the equipment-based complexity index), and three labor input variables (physicians and interns combined, nursing personnel, and other personnel). Both output variables were adjusted by a service complexity index, a proxy for case mix. The methodology, including the definition of proxy indicators used to measure complexity, case mix, and quality, is described in annex 3D. Because facilities with fewer than 25 beds cannot be considered comparable, the final models were applied to a subsample of 428 hospitals with 25 or more beds.

30. The IBGE defined a hospital as a facility providing inpatient care for more than 24 hours.

31. Distribution by ownership and governance arrangements was not so representative. Reflecting SUS priorities, the number of for-profit hospitals was intentionally undersampled, and public federal hospitals were oversampled.

32. Hospitals with fewer than 25 beds were dropped from most analyses or were analyzed separately. These facilities reported few inpatient stays and could thus have distorted the results.

33. An index of technological complexity was generated and was used as a proxy for complexity. It is based on the availability of medium-to-high-complexity equipment and is measured on a scale 1 to 10, then divided into six categories (0 to 5).

34. The high proportion of non-SUS patients in federal hospitals in the sample—much higher than for federal hospitals as a whole—is attributable to the number of federal facilities treating "closed clientele," that is, civil servants and military personnel, included in the sample.

35. This is because TTE is the product of internal efficiency and scale efficiency.

36. The analysis was also performed with the sample reduced to hospitals with 50 beds or more to check whether small hospitals (25–49 beds) were affecting the results. The conclusions were not significantly altered.

37. When only hospitals with 50 or more beds were considered, the pattern of results was similar. The smallest category included showed the highest internal efficiency score but the lowest scale efficiency and the lowest total efficiency.

38. Organizational arrangements in public hospitals are discussed in chapter 5.

39. The references are (1) the mean value for all SUS hospitals (obtained from the MS/Datasus data bank), (2) the median for hospitals enrolled in the CQH quality accreditation program in São Paulo, (3) the mean for OECD countries, and (4) the median value from a U.S. "top 100 hospitals" benchmarking study (see box 3.4).

40. Variables follow different definitions depending on the country. The year and scope of the data are not the same, and information sources use different categories (for instance, the term "nurse" means different levels of personnel in different countries, and so does the scope of what is defined as the health sector and health expenditure). In its Health Data project—a comparative database of all member countries—the OECD is attempting to make data more comparable, but there are considerable difficulties.

41. The lower value for the OECD may be attributable to the longer ALOS associated with an elderly population and the high incidence of chronic diseases.

42. As shown below, some of these inpatient stays could be treated in an ambulatory setting.

43. An occupancy rate of 100 percent does not allow for spikes in demand and emergency care and can result in overcrowding and the use of makeshift arrangements such as placing beds in corridors.

44. The figure from the sample, 29 percent, was not used because patient counting in the sample was carried out on December 31, biasing the OR estimate downward. However, the general pattern observed in the sample was similar to the one based on SUS data.

45. The proportion of hospitals with low OR was inflated in the sample because the patient counting was done on December 31, but even the MS/Datasus data indicate a large number of hospitals with low occupancy rates.

46. This does not always hold, however, because many complex procedures can be performed during a short stay, using new surgical technology.

47. Staffing ratios are also used as a proxy for quality, especially in the case of nurses.

48. Staffing ratios were adjusted to full-time equivalents (FTEs).

49. Efficient hospitals, with DEA scores of 1.0 for total efficiency, use 20 percent less personnel per bed than the average hospital in the sample.

50. Based on a survey of facilities, 17 percent of surgeries were reported canceled mostly because of nonclinical factors (unrelated to the patient's status) such as physician absenteeism, malfunctioning equipment, or the unavailability of a particular supply (World Bank 2007).

51. The index was derived by calculating the ratio of the technological complexity index for a given hospital—computed as explained in annex box 3D.1—to the number of beds.

52. World Bank (2007) presents additional evidence of the irrationality of equipment allocation and management.

53. The main limitation of the method (described in box 3D1) is its bias toward input use rather than outcomes.

54. Other DEA studies have found an important positive relation between quality and efficiency, but this depends on how quality variables are defined. For example, applying DEA analysis and introducing

nosocomial infections as a quality output, Prior (2006) found a positive relation between quality and productivity in Spanish hospitals. The AMS database did not allow specification of a quality output indicator. For a review of evidence on the relation between (poor) quality and (higher) costs, see Institute of Medicine (1999).

55. High efficiency scores do not imply personnel ratios that could reduce quality. Efficient hospitals (in the TTE sense) had a total personnel per bed ratio of 1.9 and a nursing personnel per bed ratio of 0.77. These values approximate international averages.

56. The regressions were performed using the Tobit model (see annex table 3B.2) because of the censored distribution of the efficiency scores.

57. In the main model (model 1), ownership and size were used as explanatory variables. The other models (model 2 is shown in table 3B.2) included governance instead of ownership, and technological complexity in place of size. It was not possible to include both complexity and size, or both ownership and governance, because of the high correlation between these pairs of variables, which could generate a multicollinearity problem. Excluding hospitals with fewer than 50 beds from the regression did not change the results significantly, indicating that the presence of small hospitals (25–49 beds) in the sample did not

58. As mentioned previously and discussed in box 3D.1, the quality indicator was constructed on the basis of two inputs—the number of nursing personnel per bed, and the proportion of graduate nurses to total nursing personnel—rather than output variables. This may have biased the results because the resulting quality indicator was by construction negatively correlated, although lightly, with efficiency scores. Direct quality output indicators were unavailable in the AMS database, and the hospital mortality indicator may have been insufficiently adjusted for case mix.

59. In this study the MS/Datasus AIH inpatient database was used to identify ACSCs (as defined in Caminal et al. 2004), and data were collected on hospital admissions and patient-days for these conditions. Estimates of the cost incurred by the SUS for inpatient treatment of these conditions were based on the unit costs of hospital procedures estimated in De Matos (2002).

60. AMS data show that the number of municipal hospitals more than doubled, from 875 in 1990 to 1,831 in 2005.

61. Time series data on the number of nonprofit hospitals are unavailable. Chapter 5 discusses the historical roots of the private, nonprofit hospital sector.

62. As mentioned earlier, the number of surgeries was proxied by the number of surgical admissions.

63. The study also found that the magnitude of the outcome-volume association varies greatly.

64. In chapter 7 the association between quality of care and neonatal and perinatal mortality in Brazilian hospitals is addressed.

65. As a group, private, for-profit, specialized hospitals are generally small facilities offering more high-complexity care.

66. Small hospitals (defined by the MS as having between 5 and 30 beds) represent 40 percent of all SUS-funded hospitals. Sixty-five percent are located in small municipalities (fewer than 30,000 inhabitants), where they may be the only alternative for inpatient care. However, more in-depth spatial analysis is required to determine the extent to which this is so.

67. Regulation of municipal consortiums was revised by Law 11.107/2005, which proposed a clearer framework for public consortiums.

68. Minas Gerais state adopted a strategy of upgrading and improving the quality of 120 (out of 720) publicly financed hospitals after an exhaustive analysis of hospital service access, supply, and demand. The other 600 hospitals, all small facilities, were deemed unnecessary. These are mainly municipally owned facilities or nonprofits supported in part by the state. Gradually the state will withdraw this support, leaving the facilities to fend for themselves. The Minas Gerais experience is discussed in chapter 8.

69. On the European experience regarding hospital restructuring, see McKee and Healy (2002); Saltman and Figueras (1997).

70. The policy promoted the expansion of day hospitals, ambulatory surgery, and other alternatives to inpatient care (DREES 2005).

71. This in fact relates to the rigidity and formalism of the planning and budgeting process, coupled with weak local managerial capacity, discussed in chapter 2.
72. The SUS can refuse to contract with a private provider if its services in a specific area are not needed, but this leverage is rarely used.
73. These parameters are given in Portaria MS/GM 1101 of 2002.
74. See World Bank (2007) for an analysis of subnational budgeting and budget execution processes in health.
75. Chapter 8 discusses organized provider networks.
76. Political criteria applied to investment allocation can scatter both efforts and resources, as described in World Bank (2004a).
77. Treatment protocols do exist for a number of procedures, and more are under development, but they are irregularly applied.
78. The estimate is based on the mean occupancy rate of 40 percent in this study, relative to an optimal target of 80 percent, and assumes for simplification that the cost of inpatient care is similar in all hospitals. This calculation is likely to overestimate the waste of resources resulting from unused beds, but as shown in this volume, other important sources of inefficiencies have important cost implications.
79. An isoquant is a line joining all possible combinations of inputs that can be used to produce the same given level of output.
80. Coelli, Rao, and Battese (1999) argue that the choice between models is of only minor importance and point out that both output- and input-oriented models estimate the same frontier and identify the same set of firms as being efficient. It is only the efficiency measures associated with the inefficient firms that may differ.
81. As a rule of thumb, Cooper, Seiford, and Tone (2002) provide a formula for empirical studies: $n \geq \max\{m \times s; 3(m + s)\}$ where n is the number of hospitals, m is the number of inputs, and s is the number of outputs in the model.
82. Following Coelli, Rao, and Battese (1999), internal technical efficiency is defined as the ratio of VRS efficiency and scale efficiency.
83. These results are reported in chapter 4.

4

Hospital Payment Mechanisms and Contracting Arrangements

Provider payment mechanisms (PPMs) are means by which purchasers compensate health care providers for their services. They are used to pay provider organizations, such as hospitals, and individual providers, such as physicians. Examples of PPMs for hospitals include line-item budgets, fee-for-service payments, per diem payments, and case-based payments. Through incentives, PPMs shape hospital behaviors and therefore their performance. Each type offers both advantages and disadvantages, but all PPMs are powerful levers that institutional purchasers such as government and private insurers can use to induce providers to respond to policies and priorities such as improving quality, raising efficiency, expanding access, and containing costs. In addition to the incentives embedded in PPMs, practical considerations are important. For example, overcomplex PPMs may tax the administrative capacity of both purchaser and provider or result in high transaction costs.

This chapter examines PPMs used to pay for hospital services in Brazil, their embedded incentives and administrative characteristics, and the effects of both on hospital behaviors. It reviews the experience of Brazil's Unified Health System (Sistema Único de Saúde, SUS) with contracting hospital, clinical, and nonclinical services, including a promising contracting innovation that links payment to performance.

A well-designed PPM is based on robust data and is implemented within an enabling institutional and regulatory environment. It is an instrument that policy makers can use to address several system and performance shortcomings related to hospital service delivery in Brazil, including bed and facility overcapacity, overemphasis on inpatient care, cost shifting and patient dumping, equity gaps (as manifested in, e.g., a two-tier system), overstaffing, productivity inefficiencies, low quality, and lack of decision-making accountability for hospital managers (Murray 2006).

An essential element of a PPM is rate setting—pricing a service or package of services. PPMs constitute the process and methods for determining rates and allocating financial resources to hospitals on that basis. They are an essential driver of performance because health care providers respond to the incentives embedded in specific payment mechanisms. Although there is no perfect PPM, a carefully designed payment system can go a long way toward promoting efficiency, cost consciousness, and quality. The main effects of different PPMs on efficiency, quality, and costs are summarized in annex 4A.

Payment mechanisms to hospitals are also directly or indirectly related to payments to physicians. Medical practice affects how care is delivered and is a major determinant of resource use. Physicians in Brazil are paid either on a fixed salary (when they are employed in a public facility) or on a fee-for-service basis, which is the case in most private hospitals. Salary payment—especially when lower than expected—leads to low physician productivity, work shirking and absenteeism.[1] Fee-for-service payments without other kinds of controls, however, often encourage physicians to overprovide or to specialize in the best-paid procedures and cases, contributing to Brazil's oversupply of high-technology services and equipment (see chapter 3)

PPMs that effectively drive performance improvement are data intensive and contain rate structures based on sound information on hospital cost, volume, and case mix. Budget-based payment mechanisms, for example, are generally not information intensive or based on any inherent rate structure and are therefore usually the weakest method of influencing hospital behaviors. Many countries are reorienting their budgetary systems toward PPMs that standardize payments and outputs while at the same time providing incentives to promote efficiency and effectiveness in hospital service delivery. The proliferation of diagnosis-related group (DRG) models in Europe is an example of this reorientation. Securing the data needed to develop PPM models is a major challenge for all countries seeking to change the way hospitals are paid.

Brazil has experimented with alternative ways of paying for hospital services, and debate on the effectiveness of PPMs used by the SUS continues. For example, the Authorization for Hospitalization (Autorização de Internação Hospitalar, AIH) system is a PPM that sets case rates for inpatient procedures and treatments. Most private insurance plans in Brazil use a fee schedule developed by the Brazilian Medical Association (Associação Médica Brasileira, AMB). Despite modest initiatives to use PPMs to support policy priorities, payment mechanisms remain essentially an unused policy instrument in the public sector. The use of payment mechanisms to influence hospital performance is even less developed in the private sector. Tackling the inefficiencies discussed in the previous chapter entails designing a more rational and proactive incentive structure—and, invariably, rethinking current payment mechanisms.

Payment Mechanisms for Hospital Care in Brazil

Health service purchasers in Brazil (the SUS and private plans) use an array of mechanisms for paying hospitals. For this discussion, PPMs are classified along two dimensions: by their use in the public and private sectors, and by their pricing method and whether the amounts are defined before (prospective) or after (retrospective) care is provided (Wouters, Bennett, and Leighton 1998; Barnum, Kutzin, and Saxenian 1995; Bitrán and Yip 1998). The main features of the PPMs applied in Brazil are summarized in table 4.1.

Public Sector

Five types of PPM are used in Brazil's public sector: prospective line-item budget, with its variants decentralized budget and prospective global budget; prospective case-based payment; and prospective fee-for-service payment.

Prospective Line-Item Budget
In this traditional form of PPM, the budget is fixed annually and is allocated in advance by functional and line-item categories. Budget formulation is not information intensive and is generally based on historical values. Budgets are managed directly by government, and hos-

TABLE 4.1
Main Features of Hospital Payment Mechanisms Used in Brazil

Mechanism	Source of funding	Providers paid	Services paid	Basis for payment
AIH, Authorization for Hospitalization	Federal	Private only (increasingly included in federal transfers to states and municipalities)	Inpatient care	Fee schedule per case, unrelated to costs
SIA, Ambulatory Care Information System	Federal	Private only (increasingly included in federal transfers)	Ambulatory care	Fee schedule per service, unrelated to costs
Additional incentives, support, emergency funds (paid to hospitals)	Federal	Public and nonprofit	Teaching and research facilities, emergency care, high-cost care	Service based
Budget	Federal, state, municipal	Public	Payroll plus part of other expenses	Historical trend
Fee-for-service	Employers, individuals	Mostly private	All	Negotiated fee schedule (not based on cost)
Out-of-pocket	Individuals	Private (especially for-profit), some public	All	Fee schedule

Source: Authors' elaboration.

pitals have little flexibility or managerial autonomy to reallocate resources. In addition, the government is the residual claimant, which means that any savings hospitals achieve revert to the government—but the government also absorbs budget overruns. This is the chief public hospital model.

In Brazil there are two variants of line-item budget: the decentralized budget and the prospective global budget.

- *Decentralized budget.* Less than 10 percent of public hospitals are considered budgetary units and therefore have their "own" budgets. They include all federal hospitals and hospitals under "indirect administration."[2] Managers may have a modicum of financial and managerial autonomy, but usually only for buying consumables such as drugs and supplies. Because purchases by decentralized hospitals follow the same procurement rules as central units, from a management perspective there is little difference between decentralized and line-item budgets.

- *Prospective global budget.* This PPM consists of a negotiated global payment allocated monthly or quarterly. As implemented in Brazil, global budgets are attached to a management contract with predefined performance targets (e.g., service volume, coverage, and quality). A proportion of the budget is at risk if the facilities fail to achieve the targets. The facility is also responsible for cost overruns but may keep any savings. This model, which is applied in a handful of public hospitals, allows facility managers much more flexibility; accountability requirements are more stringent.

Prospective Case-Based Payment
Under this PPM, payment is based on predefined episodes of care, treatment, or disease, which include all or most of the individual services or procedures performed for that episode. Values are usually based on average or expected costs. Brazil's AIH system is a prospective procedure-based PPM used mainly by all levels of government to pay for inpatient care in private hospitals.[3] As a prospective, case-based PPM, the AIH system is similar to the DRG PPM used in the United States and, increasingly, in other countries, but unlike the DRG, in which rates are related to diagnoses, the AIH is based on service-related case rates (i.e., treatments performed). The SUS reimburses hospitals for predefined and standardized services authorized for each treatment or major procedure within predefined values for each service.[4] Specific lengths of stay are authorized for each standard procedure; if any extra stay is needed, a complementary AIH must be submitted with an appropriate justification.

Prospective Fee-for-Service Payment
Under this system, hospitals are paid for each service provided under a predefined fee schedule. The Ambulatory Care Information System (Sistema de Informação Ambulatorial, SIA) pays for outpatient care on a mostly fee-for-service, prospective basis. As in the case of the AIH system for inpatient care, the SIA is funded by the federal government and is used mainly to finance ambulatory care in private facilities, including hospitals.

Private Sector

Two types of PPMs are used in the private sector: prospective fee-for-service payment or prepayment, and out-of-pocket fee-for-service payment.

Prospective Fee-for-Service Payment (Prepayment)
This is a service-based mechanism by which the cost of individual services provided is reimbursed. It can be based either on the cost incurred or on a previously agreed fee schedule. Service units can be packaged in aggregated measures such as per diem, treatment episodes, admissions, or discharges. This is the main PPM used by institutional purchasers in the private sector. Most private insurance plans pay providers according to a fee-for-service schedule developed by the AMB. Most of the agreements *(convênios)* negotiated between insurers and providers, especially for medical and diagnostic procedures, consist of a predefined but discounted fee schedule based on the AMB-recommended fee. Large public referral facilities also maintain contractual relationships with private health insurers and derive revenue through this PPM.

Out-of-Pocket Fee-for-Service Payment
For private, uninsured patients, the main form of payment is out-of-pocket. Payments are based on fee schedules, which are defined, usually prospectively, by each facility and are generally much higher than the fees negotiated between health plans and providers.

Critical Review of PPMs in Brazil

This section examines the potential and major shortcomings of the main PPMs used to pay Brazilian hospitals. It focuses on AIH and SIA systems applied by the SUS and, to a lesser extent, on the prospective fee-for-service system used by private payers.[5] The section concludes with a comparison of AIH reimbursement rates and actual costs.

The AIH System

The AIH system classifies cases by the main procedure or treatment performed within medical specialties. Its classification scheme includes about 2,300 medical procedures, grouped in 524 procedure groups and medical specialties. Some represent small variations of other procedures.

The AIH uses service or procedure case rates and therefore can be considered a rough form of DRG. Whereas patient diagnosis is the basis for the DRG classification system, AIH rates are based on procedure or treatment classifications (box 4.1). The AIH does, however, record the patient's primary and secondary diagnoses, but these are not used for classification

Box 4.1
The AIH and the DRG: Similarities and Differences

The development and implementation of the hospital payment system in Brazil took place at the same time as the diagnosis-related group (DRG) system was being implemented in the United States. Both systems are similar in their prospective nature and in the standardization and grouping of individual services and inputs into broader cases or procedures. The primary difference is that the AIH focuses on the main procedure performed, while the DRG focuses mostly on the patient's diagnosis. According to Chiyoshi and Moura (1989), two mostly practical factors explain why DRGs were not adopted in Brazil. First, DRGs are based on the International Classification of Diseases, which was not used at that time by the Social Security Medical Institute (Instituto Nacional de Assistência Médica da Previdência Social, INAMPS), the institute then in charge of curative medical care. Second, the DRG system, which is computerized and centrally managed, requires terminals in each hospital, which Brazil's INAMPS could not afford. In addition, DRGs require cost information on treatments and procedures, which neither the public system nor the private sector possessed.

Another key difference is the relation to costs. DRGs are based on the relative use of resources (and thus cost), but the AIH structure and value are not linked to actual costs or resource use. As designed, however, the system was supposed to reimburse the cost of procedures (see annex 4B.)

Since the inception of DRGs, most European countries and a growing number of other countries have adopted or are adopting some version of the system. They use it either as a direct basis for payment or as a basis for adjusting global budgets according to the activity level. The DRG's focus on diagnosis allows more direct linkage of resource allocation to disease patterns and better payment adjustment for differential risk.

Source: Authors' elaboration.

purposes. Another important difference is in design: the DRGs were designed for measuring resource use, and the AIH was designed to be a billing system.

Reimbursement for each AIH is calculated separately for four major categories of service: hospital services (e.g., room and board, equipment and operating room fees); physician fees; drugs and supplies; and diagnostic tests and therapeutic procedures.[6] Physician fees are usually paid directly to physicians; payments for the other categories are made to the hospital. Hospitals receive a flat rate per admission according to the procedure group in which the patient is classified. Expensive supplies and high-technology procedures require specific authorization and are paid separately. Authorization and control, once the responsibility of auditing units in the Ministry of Health (Ministério da Saúde, MS), have been decentralized to the state and municipal health authorities. The payment process has also been decentralized to state and municipal health secretariats that have demonstrated capacity to assume this responsibility.

The AIH system represents a major advance over the previous fee-for-service system. As a prospective, case-based payment system, it avoids the incentive to overproduce services and simplifies the billing process. Because hospitals receive a fixed fee for each procedure, providers have an incentive to contain costs and produce efficiently. But the low reimbursement rate for most procedures undermines this incentive. Moreover, under the AIH, hospital managers have an incentive to reduce length of stay and increase admissions. However, attempts to reduce resource use may jeopardize the quality of care.

The AIH suffers from other limitations that compromise its theoretical incentive structure. According to Martins and Travassos (1998), the main problem is that the system classification has not been systematically updated or revised since its creation in 1981. The current system, replete with distortions, duplications, and inconsistencies, is the result of accumulated ad hoc and partial revisions and additions of new medical procedures and technologies.

Another limitation of the AIH system is the poor recording of diagnoses. The system's design as a billing system based on existing classification of medical procedures makes it an unreliable and imprecise source of diagnostic information. Several studies have shown that AIH information on the primary diagnosis is often inaccurate and distorted, especially for certain diagnostic classes such as external causes, which are greatly underreported. In addition, Veras and Martins (1994) have shown that secondary diagnoses often go unrecorded in the AIH; they were recorded in only 19 percent of cases in an AIH sample, against 42 percent in patients' medical charts.[7] Since accurate diagnostic information is essential for assessing case severity, the system does not lend itself to risk adjustment.

The quality of AIH data is also compromised. First, patient and treatment information recorded in medical charts is often unreadable, and missing information is common. Second, the fact that the AIH is primarily a billing system affects its reliability because most hospitals record information in a way that facilitates billing or increases payment amounts. The system is also subject to fraud, mostly through "ghost patients" or "upcoding" of the treatment or procedures performed.[8] The auditing system is meant to reduce this behavior but succeeds only partially because of its legalistic focus.[9]

Widespread inconsistencies between AIH bills and procedures performed are most often interpreted as signs of fraud by hospitals. In some cases they may be, but hospitals' day-to-day reality is often more complex. The AIH schedule structure contains rigid guidelines (e.g., regarding length of stay for each procedure or treatment) that are frequently out of date with current medical practice.[10] They may also be inconsistent with general accounting practices.[11] Often, the AIH bill cannot reflect the procedures actually performed or the associated complications and is unaligned with accounting categories. Because of these rigidities, hospitals have to "fit" the actual treatment to the AIH guidelines, whether medically appropriate or not. It is thus common for a hospital to "upcode" (and sometimes "downcode") or otherwise change the procedure in the AIH bill, to generate more revenue, or to avoid suspension of payments and the resulting requirement for further justification during auditing—and further payment delays.

In contrast to DRGs, which explicitly include adjustments for risk, comorbidity, and case mix, the AIH contains no such adjustment mechanism. Any additional care in response to case severity that results in a longer stay or in greater use of resources needs to be justified and presented in a second bill.[12] As a result, some hospitals are penalized for factors beyond their control or for treating severe or chronic patients. This encourages them to practice risk selection.

Perhaps the most serious flaw in the AIH is the low and distorted reimbursement rates (see below). As originally designed, the fee schedules or rates were based on average costs of procedures (Chiyoshi 1989). The initial parameters, however, were determined from a small and unsystematic sample of hospitals with poor-quality cost information. Furthermore, Brazil's economic difficulties in the 1980s and 1990s led health authorities to adopt a cost containment strategy based on adjusting the schedule below the inflation rate. Rate adjustments were introduced haphazardly at irregular intervals, often in response to pressure from interest groups representing hospitals, physician specialty groups, or equipment manufacturers. Lobbying and political pressure have been influential in determining rate and adjustment setting because no systematic cost information is available to inform rate setting. No systematic revision of the schedule has been undertaken since its inception in the 1980s.

Consequently, large gaps have accumulated between service costs and the SUS reimbursement rates for most hospital procedures. Additional payments for specific items such as special materials and extended stays have partly compensated for these gaps but still do not cover the full delivery costs for most procedures. Short-changed, hospitals are driven to refuse SUS patients, use fraudulent billing practices, shift costs from higher-rate payers such as private health plans, or seek special government bailouts (discussed below). Adjustments through the years have introduced new distortions and inconsistencies because they were either linear for all procedures (the most common policy until the late 1990s) or selective but inconsistent.[13]

The SIA System

The Ambulatory Care Information System (SIA) is the main system for recording and paying SUS ambulatory care services, both nonemergency and emergency. Payments are based on a predefined fee-for-service schedule. In other words, the SIA compensates hospitals for specific individual services or medical procedures. The list of services is detailed, ranging from simple primary care procedures performed by an auxiliary nurse to high-complexity ambulatory and emergency procedures. Documentation consists of claim and payment forms, and diagnoses are not recorded. Nor does the system permit aggregation of units of care or services by patient. These shortcomings limit the SIA's usefulness as an information system for monitoring volume and utilization patterns.

Starting in the mid-1990s, the MS launched a capitated block grant system that transfers funds to municipalities to pay for primary care provided at public facilities (e.g., Basic Care Grant, Piso de Atenção Básica, PAB) and program-specific transfers (e.g., Family Health Program, Programa de Saúde da Família, PSF), based on meeting specific targets. This system has gradually replaced the SIA in public facilities. Nevertheless, the SIA continues as a general SUS information system on ambulatory care and as a payment mechanism for private facilities under contract with the SUS.

Because of its fee-for-service nature, the SIA system encourages providers to increase production of specific services, which can be helpful in expanding supply. But the multiplication of individual services often takes place at the expense of the comprehensiveness of care, and providers have little incentive to control costs.

Block Grants and the Expansion of Line-Item Budgets

Line-item budgets are now the main PPM for public hospitals, but this was not always true. Until the mid-1990s, most public hospitals were paid through both line-item budgets drawn from federal, state, and municipal treasuries; and through AIH/SIA reimbursements paid by the MS. By 2005, however, all federal funds were being channeled to states and municipalities through block transfers.

The block grant monies are combined with state and municipal treasury funds to finance public facilities' line-item budgets and are channeled to private facilities, mainly through the AIH. The MS no longer pays facilities directly except for its own facilities funded through the federal budget. Additional payments to compensate for the cost of teaching, research activities, and emergency care (originally through an additional percentage over AIH rates) have been recalibrated as fixed amounts and included in the block transfers to states and municipalities. Again, these funds are incorporated in facility line-item budgets by states and municipalities.

Because nearly all states and municipalities are now responsible for the organization and management of health services, the line-item budget has become the sole PPM for most public facilities. The AIH and SIA persist, nonetheless, as payment mechanisms for private hospitals and as information systems.

Line-item budgets offer the great advantage of simplicity and require little information. (Historical data are often used as the basis for establishing a new budget.) These budgets make it easy to control total expenditures, but because they are not linked to performance, they do little to promote efficient delivery.

The inclusion of public hospitals for production-based payments through the AIH/SIA in the late 1980s had a dubious effect. Although it introduced a productivity focus in public hospitals and encouraged public providers to expand production and coverage to increase revenues, it allowed state and municipal governments to freeze or cut hospital budgets and save their own revenues for other purposes. The ultimate impact of introducing AIH/SIA payments at the time is unclear. The progressive inclusion of AIH/SIA payments in block transfers to states and municipalities beginning in the early 2000s withdrew the productivity incentive, and again, the impact of this step on hospital finance is still uncertain. Whether states and municipalities are increasing hospitals' budgets to compensate for the rechanneling of AIH/SIA payments is unknown.

Expenditure Limits

In an attempt to control volume and contain overall hospital spending, since the mid-1990s the MS has defined annual expenditure ceilings (*tetos*) for inpatient and outpatient care for each state. In turn, many states set ceilings for municipality- and state-financed hospitals. These ceilings, based mostly on historical trends, generally rely on per capita estimates of demand for inpatient and outpatient care. The ceiling may vary with available funding and fiscal constraints at any or every level of government. Consequently, the quantity of services billed (and of revenues received) by a hospital does not necessarily reflect its actual production. In fact, production often exceeds billing because hospitals do not bother to bill for services that will not be reimbursed.

Prospective Fee-for-Service Payment in the Private Sector

Payment mechanisms in the private sector suffer from several of the problems and distortions found in the SUS. The incentives embedded in the fee-for-service payment mechanism used in the private sector are similar to those attached to the SIA system. They encourage providers to increase the production of services, sometimes leading to oversupply of the most lucrative services. The high supply and use of complex and expensive technology by for-profit hospitals, documented in chapter 3, illustrate this point.

Rates paid by private health plans are set mostly through negotiations between the health plans and providers; the above-mentioned AMB rates are reference points only.[14] Price negotiations between private health plans and providers are based on interest group pressure and bargaining power rather than on objective information regarding resource use and costs.[15] As in the SUS, the lack of reliable cost information results in wide discrepancies between rates and costs. Most of the fee schedules used in the private sector lack a solid cost basis and are largely arbitrary.[16] This situation has invited bitter disputes between physicians and hospitals, on the one hand, and insurance companies, on the other, over appropriate fees. The financial problems faced by some health plans and private hospitals stem partly from the lack of alignment between provider payment mechanisms and costs. These problems also have important implications for the SUS and health authorities, not only because the National Agency for Private Health Insurance (Agência Nacional de Saúde Suplementar, ANS) is responsible for regulating and supervising the private health insurance sector but also because any failure in that sector would shift large numbers of users to the SUS, creating additional demand that would further stretch public resources.

In recent years payers and providers have been negotiating payment by "packages"—broadly defined medical procedures or treatments (e.g., deliveries).[17] This process has accelerated since 2000 in an attempt to keep costs within the limits imposed on premium increases by the ANS. But fee-for-service payment remains the main PPM in the private sector.

Out-of-Pocket Fee-for-Service Payment

Out-of-pocket fee payments from individual patients are an important source of income for for-profit and some nonprofit hospitals. For example, while the average provider was paid R$26.20 by health plans for a medical consultation in 2004 (against the AMB reference fee of R$42.00), the market price for private out-of-pocket patients ranged from R$50 to R$500.[18]

Distribution of PPMs across Facility Types

The potential impact of incentives embedded in any PPM also depends on its importance relative to a hospital's total revenue. For example, the incentives related to a PPM representing 90 percent of revenues would have a greater impact than a PPM accounting for only 10 percent. Because no systematic information was available on hospital revenues by PPM, the sample used in this study was derived from the AMS national survey of health facilities (IBGE 2003).[19] Facility revenues were estimated on the basis of distribution of inpatient admissions by patient category (e.g., the SUS, health plans, private out-of-pocket patients). Drawing on this classification, the proportion of financing from different sources or payment mechanisms was then estimated.[20] The findings for PPMs that contribute a significant share of revenue are reported in figure 4.1.

The figure shows that the PPM composition of the sampled facilities varies with ownership. With the exception of federal hospitals, most public hospitals rely heavily on traditional line-item budgets as their main source of funding. Because many federal facilities in the sample are university hospitals or facilities catering to the armed forces or civil servants (and thus functioning under indirect administration or established as autonomous units), 20 percent of their revenue comes from the decentralized budget and nearly 50 percent from private health plans through prospective fee-for-service payments.[21] Nonprofit facilities are heavily dependent on AIH/SIA prospective payments from the SUS, which account for 63 percent of their revenues. Although for-profit hospitals rely on private prepayment plans for nearly half of their funding, the SUS AIH/SIA payments constitute 25 percent of their revenues.

SUS Prospective Payment Rates and Costs

The extent to which payment rates correspond to actual costs of care influences provider behavior and can enhance or weaken the incentives inherent in payment mechanisms. Rates far removed from costs may result in distortions such as under- or oversupply of services, "cream skimming" whereby providers avoid treating sicker patients, inappropriate referral patterns, inadequate quality, and informal payments by patients (Waters and Hussey 2004).

FIGURE 4.1
Hospital Funding, by Payment Mechanism, 2002

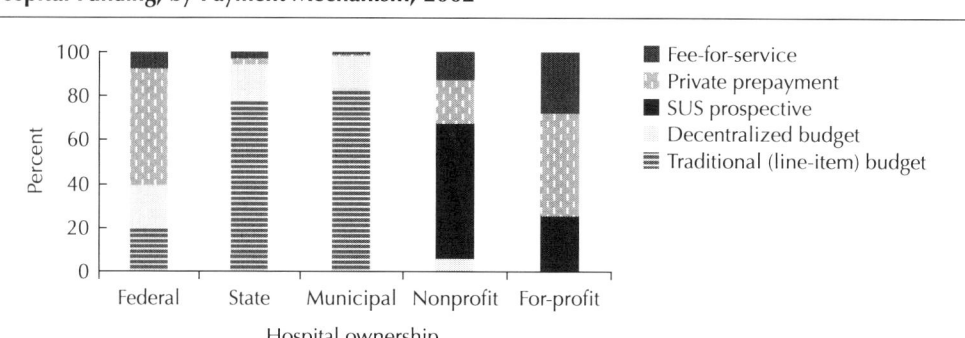

Source: Couttolenc et al. 2005.
Note: Because no precise information is available on sources of revenue, service costs, and payment mechanisms by hospital category, the data presented in this figure are approximations.

SUS payments for hospital care are not based on the cost of services and do not reflect actual costs. Attempting to estimate the relation between costs and AIH rates, De Matos (2002) analyzed the costs of 107 procedures in 25 hospitals. Comparing these costs with the AIH payment schedule in effect at the time of the study, De Matos found that AIH payments covered only 43 percent of the average cost of these procedures.[22] The SUS complements the fee schedule with additional outlays for "special procedures" such as extended stays and high-cost drugs, tests, and medical supplies. Together, these adjustments raise total payments by about 50 percent over the base schedule. Accounting for these adjustments, SUS prospective payments covered 53 percent of procedure costs in 2002, compared with 34 percent (weighted mean) if only the AIH schedule rates were considered.

To differentiate the gap between rates and costs by type of procedure, in this study the 107 procedures from the De Matos (2002) dataset were grouped by level of complexity, and the mean ratio of AIH rates to actual costs was calculated for each group.[23] Two distortions are evident, as seen in figure 4.2. First, most procedures are reimbursed well below cost: low-complexity procedures at 24 percent of their actual cost (range, 11–46 percent); medium-complexity procedures at 32 percent (range, 12–132 percent); and long-term care at about 40 percent (range, 22–77 percent). Second, high-complexity procedures in the sample are on average paid markedly above costs, at 127 percent (within a wide range of 23–332 percent).[24] Again, payment adjustments correct partially for these distortions, increasing the mean AIH/cost ratio for low-complexity and medium-complexity procedures to 41.9 and 55.6 percent, respectively, while reducing the ratio for high-complexity ones (to 112.9 percent). The adjustments, however, do not dramatically change the picture.

The first distortion—reimbursement of hospitals far above costs for high-complexity care—provides a strong incentive to specialize in expensive, technologically intensive services. (This was confirmed in the benchmarking and DEA analyses.) Although overuse of complex technology is not confined to the SUS network, the distortion in the payment

FIGURE 4.2
Mean Ratio, SUS Schedule/Cost, by Procedure Complexity, 2002
($N = 107$)

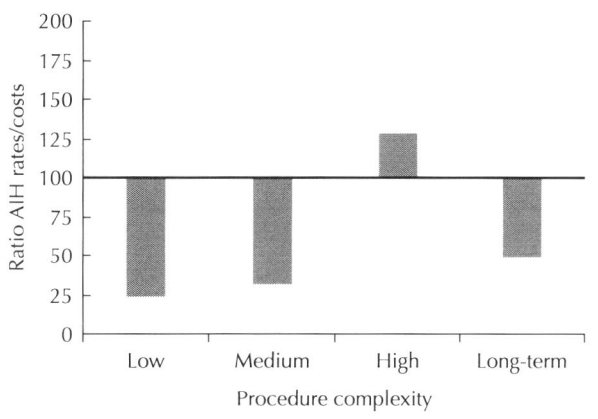

Source: Dias, Couttolenc, and De Matos 2004.

mechanism provides a strong incentive for the proliferation of advanced diagnostic equipment and contributes to the high density of such equipment in large Brazilian cities. Such overabundance may contribute to the excellence achieved by some private and university hospitals in transplants and other high-cost procedures, but it puts a heavy load on health costs.[25] This result contrasts with the prevailing view that SUS rates are too low across the board. The findings suggest that hospitals specializing in high-complexity procedures are likely to make tidy profits from the SUS. This in turn seriously distorts SUS resource allocation and equity by encouraging facilities to cut back on low- and medium-complexity procedures and to specialize in well-paid, high-technology services.

In contrast, hospitals such as nonprofits that specialize in low- and medium-complexity care services for which there is greater demand, and that are heavily dependent on SUS/AIH payments, have a hard time making ends meet. They are forced to diversify revenues by catering to health plans that pay higher rates (thereby allowing them to shift costs), or to seek bailout payments through political contacts in government—or to shut down.

Finally, the wide variation in rates (figure 4.2) is evidence of the absence of a consistent basis and methodology for setting and adjusting payment values. This is partly a consequence of the nonexistence of procedure- or diagnosis-centered cost information. In lieu of this information, irregular, across-the-board adjustments to compensate for inflation are the rule, perpetuating the built-in distortions.

SUS payment systems do not cover the cost of capital—nor are they meant to. For public hospitals, capital is funded through irregular and unsystematic specific budget allocations managed centrally. An undetermined number of private facilities under an SUS contract may also receive periodic lump-sum budgetary supplements, usually linked to a bailout payment or allocation (see next section). But most must fend for themselves and mobilize additional funds from other sources, such as donations and revenues from private patients.

In several countries payment mechanisms cover the cost of capital. This may not be feasible or appropriate in Brazil in the short and medium term because many facilities (and local governments) lack the capacity for investment planning and purchasing. Furthermore, addressing imbalances in infrastructure allocation requires specific priority-setting criteria, which are lacking in many jurisdictions.

The Plight of Private Hospitals under the SUS

The future of nonprofit hospitals operated by philanthropic and charitable organizations is uncertain in Brazil. Although these usually small nonprofits are still the backbone of the SUS-financed hospital system, many of them are severely underutilized, highly indebted, and verging on bankruptcy. Most nonprofit private hospitals under contract with the SUS rely almost exclusively on AIH/SIA payments from the SUS for their funding (see figure 4.1). Some private for-profit facilities are also heavily dependent on these payments. The gap between SUS payment rates and actual costs has resulted in severe indebtedness and closures of nonprofit facilities.

It is important to keep in mind that nonprofit hospitals do not obtain complementary regular public budget revenue from subnational governments, unlike their public counterparts and although the SUS considers them quasi-public institutions. Nonprofits are therefore funded at significantly lower levels than their public counterparts for the same set of services. For example, the value of federal AIH/SIA payments channeled to public hospitals by subnational governments represents less than 35 percent of the hospitals' budgets.[26] In contrast, these payments are the sole source of public financing for SUS patients treated in private facilities (World Bank 2007). Except for large facilities in urban centers, most nonprofits do not tap additional revenues from health plans or private patients. They thus often depend on ad hoc bailouts from federal, state, or municipal governments to avoid bankruptcy.

Although systematic information is lacking, press reports and pronouncements from trade associations suggest that a serious financial crisis is overtaking many nonprofit hospitals.[27] The Confederation of Philanthropic and Benevolent Hospitals (Confederação das Santas Casas de Misericórdia, Hospitais e Entidades Filantrópicas, CMB), a trade association representing nonprofit hospitals, estimates that the accumulated debt of SUS-funded nonprofit facilities owed to suppliers and social security was R$1.8 billion (US$0.8 billion) in recent years.[28] In one high-profile case a large nonprofit hospital in a low-income suburb of São Paulo city that treated more than 3,000 patients a day reported a monthly deficit of R$3 million (CREMESP 2005, CREMESP data). More than 30 nonprofit hospitals have been taken over (*intervenção*) by federal, state, or municipal authorities. Five nonprofits closed their doors in 2005.

Because private hospitals are the main providers of SUS-financed hospital care, their financial instability undermines the stability of the entire SUS. An undetermined number also receive irregular lump-sum bailouts from subnational governments to forestall bankruptcy and closure, such as the R$70 million received by a large hospital from the São Paulo government in 2005.[29] In 2005 the São Paulo state government also paid R$15.8 million to bail out highly indebted nonprofit hospitals throughout the state,[30] and it planned to spend R$48 million to do the same in 2007.[31] The financial plight of nonprofits is also evident in other states.[32] In Paraná state special allocations from state lottery revenues are under consideration for financially distressed nonprofit facilities.[33]

The total amount of public funds used for bailouts is difficult to estimate, but press reports suggest that it may be substantial. In chapter 2, figure 2.9, "unidentified" funding sources, which probably consist mostly of bailouts, were estimated at 11 percent of public hospital funding. Bailouts—usually in response to political pressure and influence—are short-term remedies that provide few incentives for the facility to improve quality or efficiency.[34] They just allow the distressed hospitals to continue limping along.

Financial instability may be impairing the quality of care because nonprofits cannot afford to maintain or replace plant and equipment and retain a large enough professional staff to handle their case loads. This was confirmed in a recent survey of structural conditions in hospitals in São Paulo state by the regional medical council (CREMESP 2004a). The findings revealed that nonprofit hospitals had the worst ratings in terms of availability of equipment, personnel, and infrastructure.[35]

A first step toward addressing the financial plight of nonprofits was the MS policy initiative of 2005 for restructuring the SUS-financed nonprofit sector.[36] That initiative proposes a new contract mechanism based on achieving predefined targets. The MS will pay a nonprofit R$200 million on signing a contract, and it will extend to nonprofit providers some special payments previously reserved for public providers, such as the incentive for providing health care to indigenous populations. How large the expected revenue increase will be beyond the initial payment is not clear, however, and, as discussed later in this chapter, the new contracting mechanism is a significant step toward strategic purchasing, as long as contracting and payment do not become automatic and contracts are monitored and evaluated.

Payment Mechanisms and Performance

The impact of hospital payment mechanisms can be assessed in terms of efficiency, costs, and quality of care. In general, policies for reforming payment mechanisms attempt to improve performance along one or all of these dimensions. This section examines the association between PPMs and efficiency, costs, and quality in Brazilian hospitals, drawing on the AMS survey, DEA research, the cost study by De Matos (2002), and other research described in chapter 3.

Effects on Efficiency

To study the relation between PPMs and efficiency, two analyses were performed. The first involved grouping the hospitals sampled from the AMS survey[37] by PPM and then determining and comparing their DEA scores for total technical efficiency (TTE). The second compared the same PPM groups according to the benchmark indicators presented in chapter 3.[38]

The DEA results by PPM group are presented in figure 4.3. Hospitals financed mainly by private prospective prepayment and fee-for-service displayed markedly higher total efficiency scores: 0.456 and 0.437, respectively. All hospitals in these groups are private. Hospitals that are dependent on line-item budgets—all of them public facilities—are the least efficient, with a score of 0.270. Public hospitals constituting the decentralized and SUS prospective (AIH/SIA) PPM groups occupy an intermediate level of efficiency, with TTE scores approaching the sample average of 0.341. Hospitals paid through global budgets, consisting of public hospitals under autonomous management arrangements, achieve scores (0.398) that approximate those of privately funded facilities.

Table 4.2 presents the findings of the benchmarking analysis by PPM group. Bed turnover was highest among private prepayment hospitals (60), followed by traditional (line-item) budget facilities (53) and global budget facilities (52). The other groups registered

FIGURE 4.3
Total Efficiency Scores, by PPM[a], 2002
(N = 428)

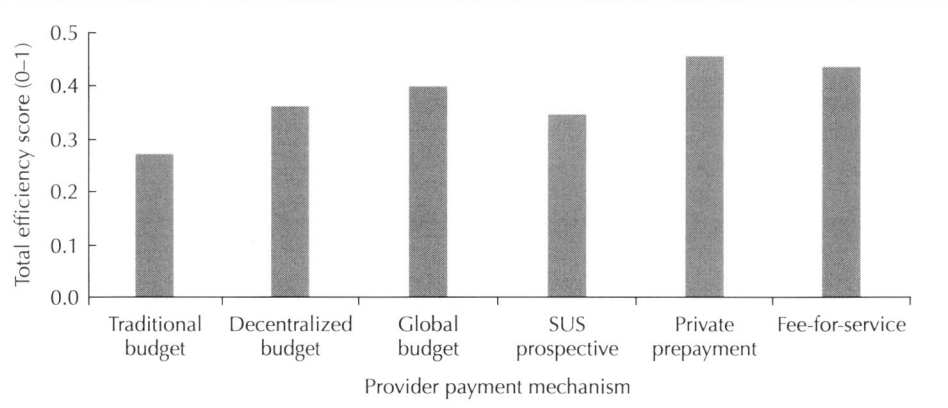

Source: Dias, Couttolenc, and De Matos 2004.
a. Account for at least 50 percent of facility revenue.

similar values, about 45. Average length of stay (ALOS) was highest among the line-item and decentralized budget hospitals and lowest among the fee-for-service group. Hospitals in the SUS prospective and global budget groups also had low ALOS. These findings are consistent with the benchmarking results by ownership reported in chapter 3. The SUS prospective, fee-

TABLE 4.2
Efficiency and Productivity Indicators, by Payment Mechanism[a]

(N = 428 facilities with 25 or more beds)

Indicator	Public			Private[b]		
	Traditional budget	Decentralized budget	Global budget	SUS prospective	Prepayment	Fee-for-service
Characteristics						
SUS inpatients (%)	98.1	93.7	86.8	87.0	12.4	12.8
Complexity level (index)	3.7	5.4	5.1	4.4	5.4	4.0
Emergency procedure/ discharge (ratio)	7.7	1.1	0.4	1.0	0.8	0.3
Efficiency and productivity						
Bed turnover (ratio)	53.4	45.0	51.7	44.1	59.9	45.8
Occupancy rate (%)[c]	33.5	40.4	38.0	21.2	30.4	6.3
ALOS (days)[c]	3.5	3.9	2.4	2.0	2.3	0.6
Discharges/personnel (ratio)	21.8	20.5	29.5	38.8	23.8	41.0
Emergency procedures/ personnel (ratio)	18.8	12.6	7.9	37.1	10.2	8.1
Personnel use						
Medical personnel/ bed (ratio)	0.6	0.6	0.6	0.3	1.5	0.7
Nursing personnel/ bed (ratio)	1.1	1.2	0.8	0.5	1.1	0.5
Other personnel/ bed (ratio)	2.0	1.5	1.0	0.6	1.6	0.6
Total personnel/ bed (ratio)	3.8	3.5	2.5	1.4	4.3	1.8
Graduate nurses (% of all nursing personnel)	10.0	11.9	9.9	8.7	13.3	8.7
Equipment use						
Equipment/bed (ratio)	0.6	0.9	0.7	0.5	1.6	1.4
Quality						
Unadjusted mortality rate (%)[d]	2.1	2.8	1.9	1.9	1.8	0.7

Source: Couttolenc et al. 2004.
a. Account for at least 50 percent of facility revenue.
b. The SUS prospective group consists mostly of nonprofit hospitals heavily dependent on SUS financing, but it also contains some for-profit facilities and decentralized public facilities.
c. Occupancy rate and ALOS are underestimated in the AMS data and may be distorted, as explained in chapter 3.
d. Deaths per 100 admissions.

for-service and, to a lesser extent, global budget groups are the most productive, as measured by discharges per bed and in relation to personnel use. Line-item and decentralized budget groups and hospitals under prospective prepayment are the least productive.

Turning to human resources, hospitals with prospective prepayment as their main source of income show the highest use of overall personnel (total personnel/bed ratio, 4.3), followed by traditional budget and decentralized budget (3.8 and 3.5, respectively). Hospitals dependent on SUS prospective payments have the lowest personnel ratio. As suggested below, the below-cost AIH payments may lead these hospitals to reduce personnel use. Interestingly, global budget–funded facilities exhibit much lower personnel per bed ratios than the average public hospital. The fee-for-service hospital group also appears to optimize personnel use.

The use of technology, measured by the equipment points per bed ratio, is much higher among hospitals funded through prepayment and fee-for-service PPMs. This suggests that these hospitals use more technology in the services they provide, either to signal differential quality to consumers or because high-technology services are more lucrative.

Effects on Costs

Using data from De Matos (2002) to assess the effect of PPM on costs, the average procedure cost was computed by PPM group. Because of dataset limitations, only four PPMs were included in the analysis: line-item or traditional budget, decentralized budget, SUS prospective payment (AIH/SIA), and prospective prepayment by private health plans.[39] The unadjusted and case mix–adjusted findings are displayed in table 4.3.

Before adjustment for case mix, the mean procedure cost was highest for public hospitals (several of them university hospitals) under traditional budget and decentralized budget PPMs and lowest for private hospitals funded either through the SUS prospective system or private prepayment PPMs. The high values observed for public hospitals, especially those under decentralized budgets, were expected because most university and teaching hospitals are classified in that group and overall treat a more severe case load than private hospitals, as shown by the CMI (table 4.3, column 2). After adjusting for case-mix differences, the relative costs changed significantly.[40] The decentralized budget group displayed the lowest

TABLE 4.3
Average Cost of Typical Procedures, by PPM Group, 2001

Payment mechanism	Mean cost unadjusted (R$)	Mean CMI	Mean cost-adjusted CMI (R$)	Mean cost ratio[a]
Traditional line-item budget	2,924.24	1.105	2,718.40	114.35
Decentralized budget	2,883.72	1.525	2,129.10	77.99
SUS prospective payment	2,037.52	0.851	2,691.25	102.92
Private prepayment	2,011.29	0.851	2,830.29	100.05

Source: De Matos 2002; Dias, Couttolenc, and De Matos 2004.
Note: No hospital in the sample belonged to the fee-for-service group. US$ = R$ 2.35 (2001). CMI, case-mix index.
a. The mean cost ratio is unweighted and thus does not equal the ratio of columns 3 and 1.

procedure costs, while hospitals under private prepayment displayed the highest, followed by public hospitals under traditional line-item budgets. The large change introduced by case-mix adjustment in the decentralized budget group was mostly attributable to the presence of several teaching and referral hospitals.

To illustrate the relative costs between hospital groups, a ratio of the PPM-adjusted mean cost to the overall mean cost was constructed. This ratio appears in the last column of table 4.3. The traditional line-item budget group displayed the highest relative cost and the decentralized budget group, the lowest. Private hospitals, whether funded through SUS prospective payment or private prospective prepayment, showed similar relative costs around the sample mean.[41] Taken together, results on costs and relative costs suggest that when adjusted for case mix, facilities under the traditional budget PPM are relatively costly.[42]

The findings in this section are consistent with the DEA and benchmarking results. Public hospitals under traditional line-item budgets are not only the least efficient group but also have higher costs after adjusting for case mix. Public hospitals funded through some form of decentralized budget, including the social organizations paid under global budgets, are both more efficient and less costly (after adjustment) than traditional public hospitals. Private hospitals owe some of their efficiency and cost advantage to their less severe and costly case load. These results are in line with the economic incentives imbedded in each PPM, as described above. The rigidities of the traditional line-item budget do not encourage efficiency and cost containment, but flexible budgets, associated with managerial autonomy, do. Prospective payment systems based on production (case based and fee-for-service), as implemented in Brazil, appear to provide only limited incentive for cost control. This smaller-than-expected impact likely stems from the fact that in both the SUS and private sectors, payments are unrelated to costs, and distortions encourage providers to specialize in the more lucrative procedures.

Effects on Quality

Payment mechanisms must be judged not only by how much they encourage efficiency and are amenable to cost control but also by how they influence quality. Although controlling for quality of care in efficiency analysis is a necessary step, it is usually not an easy one because of the empirical difficulty in measuring quality and the lack of data for doing so. This section reports on a preliminary analysis of the effect of PPM on quality.[43] The findings, presented in table 4.4, should be interpreted with caution because of the limitations of the quality index as computed from the dataset, as well as the small number of hospitals in some categories.[44]

On average, hospitals funded through traditional and decentralized budgets achieved higher-quality scores (around 0.5) than those in the other categories. The hospitals funded through the SUS prospective payment system and fee for service had the lowest values. These results suggest an inverse relation between efficiency and quality, although this tradeoff appears weak in the benchmarking analysis in chapter 3.

The results presented in this section suggest that hospitals funded mostly through private prepayment plans are more efficient, while maintaining an acceptable level of quality. Hospitals depending on SUS payments or funded mostly through fee-for-service payments are efficient but may provide low-quality care. In the case of hospitals dependent on SUS

TABLE 4.4
Quality, Payment Mechanism, and Ownership, 2002
(N = 428 hospitals with 25 or more beds)

Ownership	Traditional budget	Decentralized budget	Global budget	SUS prospective	Private prepayment	Fee for service
Sample mean	**0.507**	0.502	0.458	0.386	0.453	0.355
Federal	**0.600**	0.555	—	—	0.441	—
State	0.547	**0.575**	0.458	—	—	—
Municipal	0.473	0.461	—	—	**—**	—
Nonprofit	—	0.452	—	0.385	**0.457**	0.412
For-profit	—	—	—	0.388	**0.451**	0.324

Source: Authors' elaboration from IBGE 2003 (AMS 2002) and the DEA analysis in chapter 3.

prospective payments, low quality may be attributable to severe resource constraints, inasmuch as the SUS pays well below the cost of most procedures. Autonomous hospitals under global budgets achieve good scores on efficiency, apparently without compromising quality. Hospitals funded through traditional budgets are the least efficient overall, although their high personnel use allows them to attain high scores in the quality index.[45]

Hospital Contracting Arrangements in the SUS

The financial relationship between payers and hospitals often involves contracting—selectively purchasing health services rather than allocating a budget to pay for services in a specific facility. Contracts define the relationship between purchasers (e.g., government) and providers (e.g., hospitals). They accompany many payment mechanisms because they specify the terms and conditions of payment. Contracts are the instrument by which the purchaser specifies the range and volume of goods and services to be provided, as well as the desired performance (in terms of a population's health, efficiency, and quality) during a defined time period. This arrangement contrasts with public direct management systems, which allocate resources on the basis of inputs—such as facilities and staff—with little regard for the volume or quality of services produced. When properly executed, and when the necessary regulatory framework is in place, contracting can improve the performance of health service providers.

Most goods and services in the health sector can be produced efficiently with good quality by the private sector (Preker and Langenbrunner 2005). The United States and Canada have a long history of contracting hospital services from the private sector. Countries that finance health through social insurance systems (e.g., France, Germany, Singapore, South Africa, and Switzerland) also have a tradition of contracting. During the last 15 years United Kingdom, Italy, Spain, Sweden, and other European countries have introduced contracting among public agencies and between public agencies and private providers.

Contracting also suggests that governments must do business differently. Consequently, it carries some risks. To contract effectively, government must develop the infrastructure to prepare, manage, and monitor the contract. This includes capacity to prepare and conduct bidding, provide financial oversight and cost analysis, monitor outputs and results, and enforce contract provisions. Developing such capacity takes time, but without it, performance gains may be elusive.

This section reviews contracting experiences in the SUS, focusing on government contracting with private hospitals, public hospitals, and clinical and nonclinical service providers. It concludes with a brief assessment of an innovative contracting experience in the state of São Paulo.

SUS Contracting with Private Hospitals

Contracting with hospitals, in Brazil as in many other countries, is used nearly exclusively to buy services from the private sector. The SUS has a long history of outsourcing medical and nonmedical services in public facilities, contracting private for-profit hospitals, and entering into agreements with private nonprofit hospitals for inpatient and outpatient care for public patients. Yet the contracting arrangements themselves are rudimentary.

As practiced by the SUS, purchasing is a passive, poorly managed activity. The SUS maintains a global legal agreement (*convenio padrão*) with nonprofits holding a certificate of nonprofit status.[46] Although private providers receive 56 percent of SUS hospital spending, the convenio is a global, pro forma, legalistic instrument used to distribute AIH/SIA-based payments among private hospitals historically affiliated with the SUS.[47] The only requirements are to furnish information already required by the AIH system and to provide services. Thus, the convenios are not tools for modifying or even influencing provider behaviors regarding service mix, volume, or quality. Although a minority of states and municipalities has established special terms with a subset of nonprofit facilities, most convenios lack service specification and output definition. Performance, if specified, is unrelated to financing, pricing is unrelated to costs, and convenio management and monitoring by public purchasers are sporadic.

For most publicly financed nonprofit facilities, the relationship with the SUS consists of annual negotiations with municipal, state, or federal authorities over budgetary caps. The annual expenditure limits, which are applied to all SUS-funded hospitals, are often adjusted during the year, depending on the fiscal situation of the government partner. Throughout the fiscal year, nonprofit facilities present bills to the SUS for AIH/SIH reimbursement within the allowable budget cap. The only apparent requirement is to report output information already required by the AIH/SIH system for reimbursements. Although the caps are nominally based on across-the-board MS estimates of demand (e.g., admissions and specialty consultations per 1,000 population), these estimates are based on historical data rather than on demand or need, while actual payments are often determined by the availability of public funds in government health budgets. In a sense, the caps are a type of revenue guarantee for facilities traditionally linked to the SUS. It is worth repeating that financing is unrelated to demand, costs, or performance indicators such as production, productivity, or quality.

The MS has attempted to link financing for nonprofit hospitals to performance. In 2001 the federal government initiated the INTEGRASUS program, in which nonprofit facilities selected by state health secretariats could receive additional financing in return for compliance with a set of rules and performance indicators.[48] On the supply side, the facilities were to reserve at least 70 percent of beds and five intensive-care beds for SUS patients, ensure that at least 70 percent of outpatient consultations were for SUS patients, and serve as referral centers for nearby municipalities. As for performance, the program called for maintaining cesarean rates agreed with local authorities and assuming coresponsibility with local health officials for reducing infant and maternal mortality and hospital infection rates. Participating hospitals also had to score at least 60 percent compliance with (mainly structural) indicators included in the National Hospital Evaluation Program. In 2004 nearly all nonprofit hospitals were receiving additional funds through INTEGRASUS. There is no evidence, however, that the MS monitored INTEGRASUS or hospital compliance with program performance indicators. In effect, all hospitals received some payment through INTEGRASUS.

Following up on the enactment in 2004 of MS regulations introducing contracting arrangements in public hospitals (described below), representatives from CONASS, CONASEMS, the MS, and philanthropic societies formed a working group to develop guidelines for crafting performance-oriented contracts between the SUS and nonprofit hospitals. In August 2005 the working group drafted a regulation to establish a program for restructuring and contracting nonprofit hospitals (CONASS 2005).[49] Unless the MS and the states develop capacity to monitor and assess contract compliance, this measure is likely to increase financing for private hospitals without any impact on performance.

Outsourcing in Public Hospitals

Contracting-out gained popularity in the 1990s, driven by spending limits placed on public employee payrolls.[50] Many public hospitals outsource some hotel, security, and maintenance services. According to Ferreira (2004), difficulties in managing in-house, statutory personnel charged with executing these functions was another contributing factor prompting hospitals, states, and municipalities to outsource. Outsourcing is, for the most part, managed directly by local government rather than by the facility. Management of the contracts is lax, however. A health expenditure tracking survey (World Bank 2007) found that most contracts for hotel and support services in state and municipal hospitals lack production targets, quality indicators, or sanctions for nonperformance. The contracts themselves are rarely updated.

Although the volume of contracting in medical services is more limited, medical outsourcing is also evident in public hospitals. The most common form is contracting out specific services to professional cooperatives. Cooperatives consist of groups of specialists, usually with significant market power or monopoly positions (e.g., orthopedists, neurosurgeons, and anesthesiologists), that are legally organized to sell services to public facilities. The main objective is to achieve higher salaries or payments than the members would receive as civil servants or as individual contractors. Cooperatives help attract medical personnel to public facilities because they generally pay higher salaries (but no benefits). They relieve public managers of the task of managing specific services or medical staff. For example, a cooperative can be contracted to provide physicians and nurses for an entire facility or service, such as anesthesiology.

There is no evidence that performance-based contracts are applied in such arrangements. A few state governments (e.g., Rio de Janeiro and Amazonas) contract out a high volume and broad range of health care. In Amazonas cooperatives have led to higher spending with no evidence of health impact (box 4.2). Cooperatives are paid per staff-hour provided, which is unrelated to costs, productivity, or quality.[51] Similar to nonmedical services, these contracts are managed directly by local government and are irregularly monitored or enforced.

Box 4.2
Two Case Studies: Outsourcing Medical Care in the SUS

Outsourcing Hospital Care in Amazonas State

The Amazonas state government makes extensive use of cooperatives to staff publicly financed hospitals, diagnostic centers, and emergency facilities. The state has contracted 19 cooperatives to provide services in 36 ambulatory and hospital facilities, representing about 20 percent of state spending on health. Physician cooperatives (by specialty) represent the dominant form, followed by nursing cooperatives.

A recent assessment sheds light on some of the issues facing local governments interested in expanding outsourcing (Sanigest International 2005). Fifteen years ago, the first cooperative was formed as a means of ensuring high income for specialized physicians providing only specialized services. By 2004 the contracted cooperatives accounted for about 42 percent of state-financed hospital procedures but consumed 52 percent of spending. Facilities under direct administration, which are managed directly by the state, with services provided by public employees, accounted for the difference. On average, surgical, clinical, and pediatric procedures produced by medical cooperatives constituted 35, 43, and 24 percent, respectively, of such procedures produced by SUS in the state. Cooperative-produced care, however, was found to be more expensive than similar procedures delivered in direct administration facilities. Furthermore, although some cooperatives were more productive than others (for example, surgery and pediatrics registered nearly double the production of obstetrics and internal medicine), no significant differences in productivity were found when medical staff hired under cooperatives and public employee arrangements were compared.

The higher costs are related to the monopoly position held by the cooperatives, the payment mechanism, and weak monitoring and contract management by the state government. As is typical of public contracting throughout the SUS, the contract is of an administrative nature and does not specify services or promote quality. The contracts are managed directly by the state government rather than by the facility. In short, there is no labor or managerial relationship between cooperative doctors and the facilities. Production targets, based on historical patterns, are set in the contract; the cooperatives are given a fixed monthly payment for a fixed number of four-hour shifts (*plantão*) to meet specified global production targets. The relation between production and (per shift) payments appears arbitrary. Payments are not based on costs, which are unknown, but on the fees for plantões, negotiated between parties. This system is cost inducing because it provides an incentive to maximize the time (paid plantão) required to meet the production ceilings. Any unanticipated additional production means paying for more shifts. All financial risk associated with meeting service demand is transferred to the state government. State monitoring centers on financial statements and production ceilings. Quality of care, patient satisfaction, or continuous care coverage of at-risk groups (e.g., hypertension, diabetes) is not considered.

Outsourcing Primary Care in the Municipality of São Paulo

The Health Care Plan (Plano de Atendimento à Saúde, PAS) implemented by the municipality of São Paulo between 1993 and 1996 was an innovative but controversial model for organizing and managing health care provision. It was based on analyses that identified structural problems in the system at the time—overcentralization, lack of coordination across providers, low efficiency and quality, and low productivity and responsiveness on the part of public sector workers—and that pointed out the need for alternative models (FIPE 1994).

(continued)

Box 4.2 *(continued)*

Designed by a group of academics from the University of São Paulo, the model originally proposed was based on the following principles:

- Regionalization of health facilities and services in territorial "modules" (subdistricts), with registration of the population to be covered in each module.
- Flexible labor management through the organization of health workers' cooperatives, combined with extended managerial autonomy.
- Partnership between the municipality (which retained ownership of facilities and equipment) and private entities. The latter were worker cooperatives responsible for managing the modules under contract through convênios.
- Prospective capitated payment and some implicit risk equalization. (Low-income groups were prioritized through an income-based per capita adjustment.)
- Supervision and oversight by the municipality to provide management support and avoid the distortions associated with the new payment mechanism (e.g., minimizing the quantity of services produced or referring patients to providers outside the cooperative).
- Gradual implementation, starting with a pilot project in one district.

In early 1995 the municipality prepared three successive versions of the project that altered the original model somewhat and resulted in Municipal Law 11866/95. From the early official documents through passage of the law to its implementation, PAS was strongly resisted and was repeatedly challenged in court by health worker unions, public health professionals, opposition political parties, and others who regarded the plan as an unconstitutional privatization of the public health system. The federal government also considered the new model incompatible with basic SUS principles and cut off federal funding to the municipality for PAS, so that the city had to fully fund the program.

Two main issues were critical to the design and implementation of PAS. First, following a transition period municipal health workers were given the choice of taking an unpaid leave of absence and joining the cooperative, or remaining in the civil service and being relocated to another work site. (Additional workers were later hired through a new cooperative.) Second, because of their weak managerial expertise, the cooperatives contracted out private firms to manage the module or individual facilities.

Aside from the heated political debate and the overrapid implementation of the plan (all 14 modules were operational nine months after passage of the law), PAS exhibited four main weaknesses that impaired its performance and were critical in its demise and dismantling after the change in municipal government in 2000:

- The governance structure was complex, involving one leading cooperative formed by university-level professionals, a second cooperative of midlevel workers, and three representative councils and boards; the cooperatives in turn subcontracted private firms for management functions.
- A number of civil servants opted out of PAS and were shifted to jobs for which there was little work. Yet they continued to receive their public salaries for doing little or nothing, thus inflating the final cost of the model.
- The municipal information systems, which were weak to start with, were basically dismantled and replaced with a new but ineffective monitoring and control system.
- Weak managerial control resulted in inflated operating costs, well above those originally planned, amid denunciations of fraud.

Source: FIPE 1994; Cohn and Elias 1999; Harvard Medical International 1998; Sanigest International 2005.

Outsourcing of medical services has recently come under criticism and has lost some momentum. Discussions are highly politicized. Employee unions and politicians criticize outsourcing as a veiled form of privatization. Charges include inflationary distortions of payment systems, monopoly price gouging, corruption, conflict of interest, and weak government capacity to manage the contracts and monitor service delivery (see box 6.3). More recently, the federal attorney general's office (Ministério Público) has been cracking down on states and municipalities that evidently handpicked the cooperatives instead of applying competitive bidding practices, as specified by national procurement legislation (Law 8666). The labor ministry is also investigating allegations of unfair labor practices. Finally, a 2003 modification in the federal tax law eliminated the tax advantages of contracting professionals through cooperatives, significantly raising their costs to purchasers. A number of states and municipalities are canceling contracts with cooperatives.

Contracting Innovations in São Paulo State

A purchasing model that is being implemented in São Paulo state in public hospitals managed by private nonprofit health social organizations (*organizaçoes sociais de saúde*, OSSs) points the way toward more robust contracting arrangements as governments become interested in implementing similar arrangements to improve the performance of both public and SUS-financed private hospitals.[52] The management contract (*contrato de gestão*), fine-tuned over a period of nearly 10 years, is a distinguishing feature of the OSS model. The contract and its link to a global budget are two elements of an accountability arrangement that drives the superior performance results reported in chapter 5.

OSS contracts specify volume targets by type of service (e.g., inpatient, outpatient, emergency, diagnostic, and surgical procedures). These service categories are further broken down by specialty, specific procedure, type of diagnostic test, and so on. The contract mandates the establishment and functioning of medical record systems and facility-based commissions for reviewing mortality data, ethics issues, and infection control. It also specifies monthly and annual reporting requirements for activities, costs, payroll, spending, AIH (coding and billing), and patient surveys.[53] The OSSs are subject to yearly audits by the state comptroller general and the state health council. In 2001 the state set up an assessment commission to review OSS compliance with performance indicators in the contracts.

All payments are specified in the contract and are linked to per-service and activity production targets, as well as to a set of reporting requirements and quality indicators. Ninety percent of the budget is allocated in monthly disbursements and is linked to compliance with 85 percent of the production targets. Failure to meet the target leads to reduction of the subsequent allocation. For example, if only 75 percent of the target is reached, the OSS can lose 10 percent of the payment. If production falls below 75 percent of the target, a facility can lose up to 30 percent of the monthly allocation.

Ten percent of the budget is retained by the state but is allocated quarterly. This funding is tied to performance indicators agreed between the state and the facility. The indicators used may vary across facilities but they fall into four assessment categories: information quality, efficiency, quality of care, and patient satisfaction. Examples of indicators and weights used in 2002–4 are presented in table 4.5. For each indicator, quarterly targets are negotiated and assessed by an independent state evaluation commission.

TABLE 4.5
Performance Indicators Linked to the Variable Financing Component of the OSS Global Budget, São Paulo State, 2002–4

Category and weight	Indicator
Information quality/0.10	• Medical records contain secondary diagnoses.
	• Place of residence codes completed in patient records.
	• Reason for cesarean sections provided.
Efficiency/0.10	• ALOSs for specific services (without secondary diagnoses) remain within predefined ceilings.
Quality of care/0.70	• Mortality, ethics, and infection control commissions fully operational.
	• Percentage of deaths analyzed by mortality commission.
	• Percentage reduction in hospital infection rate.
Patient satisfaction/0.10	• Percentage of patient complaints addressed.
	• Completion of patient satisfaction survey.

Source: Health secretariat, São Paulo state.

SUS Contracting with Public Teaching Hospitals

Building on the OSS experience, the MS recently moved to implement more robust contracting arrangements in some public hospitals. In 2004 the MS launched a program to restructure and improve the quality of public teaching hospitals by introducing performance-based contracting.[54] By June 2006, the MS had signed contracts with 86 (of 220) teaching hospitals and had transferred R$270.3 million (US$123.9 million) to these facilities. The program has yet to be evaluated.

The program has several innovative features. It consolidates three separate federal grants into a single block grant to form a global budget. In the case of teaching hospitals run by states and municipalities, the global budget also consists of subnational budgetary sources.[55] The program also introduced a financing scheme consisting of fixed and variable parts. The fixed transfer augments the total value of the formerly separate transfers that these facilities already receive from the MS; it is not tied to performance.[56] The variable part, 15 percent of the value of the global budget, is linked to process, volume, and quality indicators. The variable payment is to increase annually by 5 percent until it reaches 50 percent of the value of the total (fixed and variable) global budget. The regulations call for four performance levels, each linked to a percentage-based payment of the value of the variable transfers.[57] The MS directly manages the global budgets and contracts for the 48 federal teaching hospitals, while states and municipalities do the same for the remaining 172 facilities.

Table 4.6 compares major contracting features of OSS contracts with the model convenios for teaching hospitals, many of which are similar to those implemented by the OSSs. As in the early years of OSS contracting, the lack of specificity of some of the proposed MS arrangements described in the table is a consequence of the lack of government experience with contracting.[58]

Although the initiative suggests that the MS is serious about contracting and views it as a means of improving performance, this contracting effort faces three problems. The first

TABLE 4.6
Comparison of Summary Features of the OSS Contract with the Draft Contract between the SUS and Teaching Hospitals

Key elements in contracting process	Proposed convenio for public teaching hospitals	Management contract, OSS/São Paulo
Objectives	Defined generally in terms of "integration" into the SUS system and guaranteed access for people from surrounding municipalities.	Combination of general and specific clauses.
Service specification	The facility is responsible for complying with the operational plan. Whether volume targets are specified depends on the contract.	Detailed in terms of volume of inpatient discharges, specialty outpatient consultations, emergency consultations, and laboratory exams.
Incentives	Fifteen percent of value of transfer (variable part) linked to process, volume, and quality targets in annual operational plan.	Defines compliance bands for each production target, linked to percentage of fixed payment.
		Defines performance indicators for 10 percent variable payment (issued quarterly).
Payments	Both fixed and variable amount specified. Payment made monthly.	Fixed payments specified by area of production (e.g., inpatient, outpatient, emergency). Payment of fixed part made monthly; variable part, quarterly.
Performance indicators	Specified in terms of production, quality, access, and utilization. Some are difficult to measure.	Specified in terms of production and quality (outputs and outcomes).
Reporting requirements	Four reports specified: monthly service volume reports; bills (AIH) for services rendered; annual report on contract execution; and timely provision of data to MS information systems.	Monthly production reports by nearly all service areas.
		Quarterly cost reports.
		Monthly reports on quality on compliance indicators.
		Annual financial balances and human resource ledgers.
Monitoring and evaluation	Contracting municipality or state is to establish monitoring commission to monitor compliance. If local government fails to form the commission, the national auditing system will monitor compliance. MS monitors federal teaching hospitals.	Specifies roles of • Independent assessment commission—verify compliance with production targets and quality indicators and produce an annual report; and • Health services contract coordination unit of state secretariat—perform contract management functions, including issuing payments, monitoring production, and analyzing costs.
Sanctions	Nonspecific: convenio can be rescinded by local government if conditions not fulfilled.	Specified at three levels: warning, fine, and suspension
Dispute resolution	Either party can challenge contents of convenio within 120 days of signature.	OSS has five days to challenge any sanction. Dispute resolution process not specified.

Source: Model convenio prepared by MS; OSS contract.

relates to autonomy. Experience with public systems in Europe and elsewhere suggests that hospital independence in modifying the scope of services, managing inputs, and negotiating prices and resource flows with the payer is a key determinant of successful contracting (Preker and Langenbrunner 2005; Preker and Harding 2003). Most public hospitals have very limited decision-making authority regarding these functions. This is particularly the case for hospitals operated by states and municipalities. Federal teaching hospitals have more freedom to manage their budgets and nonlabor inputs.

The second problem concerns the large number of performance indicators and subnational capacity to manage the convenios. Thirty indicators of various weights were defined in the 2004 regulations. Although the MS reduced this number to 17 in subsequent (2006) regulations, some facilities have proposed convenios with an unmanageable 60 indicators. Others have proposed a more reasonable number of indicators with weighted targets. The indicators themselves consist of a wide range of processes and outputs, most of them setting minimums for bed availability by care level, bed occupancy rate, ALOS, production, and supply of equipment. Other provisions mandate the establishment of an array of human resource formation, training, and continuing education programs. Many of the indicators are difficult to benchmark and measure, and others may not be implemented without significant increases in financing. Of equal concern, many municipalities and states do not have the capacity to monitor these convenios.[59] The risk is high that this instrument will become a mechanism for distributing budget directly to hospitals, similar to the global agreement applied to private facilities.

The third problem relates to incentives for performance. The MS has mandated that future increases in spending be linked to performance, as specified in annual service agreements (*convênios de assistência*). Whether this mandate will be fully enforced is uncertain. Significantly, the MS has withheld part of the variable financing to an undetermined number of hospitals for failure to comply with one or more of the performance indicators. As the variable payment increases vis-à-vis the fixed payment, the hospitals will face stronger incentives for performance compliance.[60] Municipal and state authorities, however, are resisting any link between finance and performance; how far this aspect will continue to be implemented is unclear.

Conclusions and Recommendations

Provider payment mechanisms for hospitals attempt to change behaviors to improve performance. This can involve a combination of raising efficiency, increasing equity, improving quality, and lowering costs. The mechanisms can also create incentives to stimulate organizational change that can further affect performance. A well-designed PPM depends on a series of inputs and enabling factors, including information on costs, volumes, outcomes, and patient characteristics such as diagnosis and case severity (Waters and Hussey 2004; Langenbrunner and Wiley 2002).

How this information is collected and measured is another important consideration. Because many PPMs involve some form of rate setting, they are dependent on providers' characteristics and their relations with purchasers (e.g., provider autonomy, use of contracts, negotiation, and regulation). As in many middle-income countries, many of these enabling factors are absent or not well developed in Brazil.

Major Findings

As applied in Brazil, PPMs appear to stimulate performance only weakly, and some may actually drive poor performance. The main factors contributing to the limitations of hospital PPMs in Brazil are summarized below.

Diluted Incentives and Adverse Behaviors

The diversity of the Brazilian hospital sector and the large number of payers contributes to a multiplicity of PPMs.[61] The typical private hospital, and an increasing number of public facilities, receive revenue from several public and private sources. Each funder applies one or more PPMs. This situation results in diluted and sometimes conflicting incentives that fail to affect efficiency and quality. For example, many private hospitals derive an important share of revenue through three or more PPMs (e.g., AIH, SIA, discounted prospective fee-for-service, fee for service). Any cost control or efficiency-enhancing incentives inherent in one may be offset by another. Instead of stimulating hospital managers to allocate revenues efficiently, the lack of uniformity in PPMs may encourage undesirable hospital behaviors such as marking up prices to shift costs from lower-rate payers such as the SUS to higher-rate payers such as private health plans. In turn, this may encourage inequity by creating a two-tier system even within the same facility, with care that is more responsive (e.g., shorter queues) and probably higher quality for patients affiliated with high-rate payers such as private health plans, and less responsive and probably lower quality for patients affiliated with lower-rate payers. In both cases, hospitals seek to maximize revenue from high-rate payers to compensate for revenue "loss" from low-rate—but high-volume—payers.

Absence of Cost Information

The situation described above is closely related to a major systemwide shortcoming: in every case, PPMs are unaligned with underlying costs and therefore do not reflect resource use. As a result, they do not provide hospitals with incentives to use resources efficiently. Distorted rate-to-cost ratios also offer incentives to overprovide or underprovide specific services. The AIH payment schedule is a case in point. The heavy distortions in rate-to-cost ratios, overpaying relatively low-volume, high-complexity procedures while severely underpaying high-volume, low- and medium-complexity care, encourage private hospitals to behave inefficiently (but probably rationally). These hospitals have developed financial survival strategies such as further diversification of payers and specialization in well-paid procedures and specialties. Other, less transparent strategies include risk selection and fraud.

PPMs are unrelated to underlying costs partly because there is almost no hard information on costs in Brazilian hospitals. Few hospitals have cost accounting systems, and information is seldom comparable or available in those that do have them. Lack of reliable and systematic cost information is the main constraint on improving current case-based PPMs (such as the AIH) and developing alternative PPMs with greater potential to influence performance. The absence of information on treatment costs also precludes adoption of or migration toward a DRG-based payment system.

Failure to Adjust for Case Severity

None of the payment methods used for financing hospitals in Brazil makes or allows payment adjustment for case severity or case mix.[62] Line-item budgets, the main payment mechanism for public hospitals, do not account for differences in case mix. Although the AIH requires that diagnoses be recorded, this information is not used for risk adjustment. The SIA does not record diagnosis or case severity, either; rather, ambulatory services are classified as basic, medium, or high complexity. None of the PPMs used by the private health plans adjusts for case mix. Considering the importance of risk adjustment in the design of PPMs, the lack of case-mix adjustment is an important limitation on hospital payment mechanisms in Brazil.

As in the case of costs, adjusting for case mix is constrained by the general absence of reliable patient information at the facility level. This is related to poor recording in medical charts, lack of standardized medical practices, and near nonexistence of systematic case review. The inconsistent registering of primary and especially secondary diagnoses is particularly problematic because diagnoses are an important basis for case-mix adjustment.

Expansion of Line-Item Budgets in Public Hospitals

The federal government's decision to replace AIH/SIA payments with grant transfers to subnational governments has resulted in the expansion of line-item budgets as the overriding PPM for public hospitals. The potential incentives in volume-based payment mechanisms (such as a reformed AIH/SIA mechanism) are thus lost to public hospitals. This is worrisome. Although line-item budgets provide predictable funding for hospitals and are easy to administer, the rates paid (e.g., budgets) are based on historical funding patterns. Budgets provide few incentives to increase productivity and quality, adapt managerial innovations, stimulate managerial flexibility, decrease excess capacity, or establish a robust information environment. Because of these limitations, most high-income countries that once used line-item budgets to pay hospitals have implemented more sophisticated PPMs such as DRGs, per diem payment, and performance-based global budgets.[63] Hospitals funded through line-item budgets are among the less efficient and more costly in Brazil. The line-item budget PPM contributes to the observed low performance in public hospitals.

Outdated Case-Based PPM

The AIH system is a big improvement over the fee-for-service based system of the early 1980s. Its case-based structure groups many individual services and inputs into major procedures or treatments. In theory, the system has the potential to contain cost escalation. It also can allow for better control of the volume of procedures performed because of its prospective nature and can help hospitals better plan and control expenditure. It suffers, however, from several limitations and distortions that have accumulated over the years. Outdated procedure lists and rules, time-consuming and ineffective auditing, poor recording of diagnose in the AIH system, mismatch between AIH bills and medical records, and dissociation from resource use and cost are the main factors limiting the reliability of the AIH both as an information system and as a payment system.

Unfair Competition

The SUS compensates public hospitals at much higher rates (remunerated through public budgets) than private providers, whose SUS revenues are limited to AIH/SIA payments from the federal government. As mentioned, AIH/SIA payments cover only a portion of actual costs, except for some high-complexity treatments and procedures. This distorts competition and does not encourage efficiency among public or private providers.

Passive Contracting

Although the SUS has a long history of contracting private hospitals to deliver hospital services, it applies a passive instrument (convenio) that does not specify functions, define outputs, or indicate performance targets in return for funding. The convenios are essentially legal instruments for distributing budget to private providers traditionally linked to the public system. As a contracting tool, the convenio is devoid of accountability and is not used as a means of creating incentives to improve the production, quality, and efficiency of hospital services.

Recommendations

To improve the hospital payment system in Brazil, both short-term and medium- to long-term policy changes are recommended. In the short term, given the difficulties and time lag involved in reforming information systems, emphasis should be placed on improving and upgrading systems and expanding successful models of payment mechanisms. In the medium to long term, payment mechanisms should evolve to support the new organizational arrangements proposed in chapter 5 and incorporate systematic diagnostic and cost information.

Reliable diagnostic and cost information is basic for designing provider payment mechanisms that give appropriate incentives for delivering efficient and high-quality health care. It is also needed if performance is to govern provider selection and payment and if efficiency in resource allocation is to be encouraged.

Short-term policies and activities include the following:

- *Developing and testing alternative payment systems* that stimulate efficiency and quality and support new organizational arrangements in public hospitals. The contract-based, performance-based global budget applied to new public hospitals in São Paulo state (see chapter 5) could serve as the reference. These global budgets should include a fixed part linked to targets (coverage, production) and a variable part linked to performance indicators (efficiency, quality, and targets exceeded) and to participation in initiatives such as accreditation and costing systems. The expansion of performance-based global budgets should be coupled with strategic purchasing policies that include the use of management contracts, more autonomous organizational arrangements, monitoring of compliance with performance targets, contract management, and impact evaluation.
- *Improving patient and service information systems* both in hospitals and at the national level. The AIH/SIA systems can serve as building blocks because they include an established data series and allow monitoring of service production and use. These systems should, however, be reviewed to eliminate inconsistencies and distortions in the procedures list and to adjust payments to remove distortions from overpayment and underpayment of different procedures. Although the AIH and the SIA are no longer used to pay public hospitals and

the MS is considering paying nonprofit hospitals through a PPM akin to global budgets, both the AIH and the SIA remain key information sources. Once improved, these systems can provide the information inputs for determining the global budgets.

- *Developing and testing a diagnosis-based system for measuring and adjusting for case mix.* In the short term such a system could use the diagnostic information recorded in the AIH, despite its limitations. As the system is upgraded, case-mix adjustment techniques should be applied to refine diagnostic information.

- *Developing a nationwide standardized hospital costing system* that allows for estimation of treatment or case costs.

- *Promoting fair competition and a level playing field for public and private hospitals alike* by harmonizing payment systems and incentives. This would contribute greatly to eliminating current distortions in resource allocation.

- *Evaluating the impact of ongoing programs and initiatives* such as performance-based contracts with public teaching hospitals.

Medium- and long-term policies and activities include:

- *Migrating the AIH/SIA toward a DRG-like system,* to function as a solid information system and as the basis for defining and monitoring global budgets and treatment costs. An in-depth study should be undertaken to assess which elements of these systems can and should be retained and adapted from the AIH/SIA and which should be abandoned and replaced. Key elements of the migration include revising the AIH schedule and linking AIH procedures to diagnoses (this work has been undertaken by isolated researchers and has proved feasible);[64] introducing adjustments for severity and case mix; and rolling out a robust cost accounting system to generate information on treatment costs.

- *Stimulating a level playing field among all payers of hospitals,* including the SUS and private insurers and plans, through regulation by the ANS and adoption or development of similar payment systems. This would facilitate comparisons and cooperation between the SUS and the private insurance sector. As a preliminary step, an in-depth study of private payment systems in Brazil should be undertaken, assessing their strengths and weaknesses and taking into account international experience.

Payment mechanisms and their inherent incentives influence provider behavior. A hospital can respond to these incentives only within the limits defined by its organizational arrangements, as will be seen in chapter 5.

Annex 4A
Characteristics and Effects of Main Provider Payment Mechanisms (PPMs)

Payment method	Payment unit	Prospective or retrospective	Description	Efficiency	Quality and equity	Management and information systems	Financial risk
Line-item budget	Functional budget categories	Either	Budget is allocated by specific categories of resources or functions, usually annually. Budget categories include salaries, medicine, equipment, food, overhead, administration.	Little flexibility in resource use. Tendency to spend entire budget, even if not required, to ensure maintenance of at least that level of budget support.	Rationing may occur if budget is too low. If rationing occurs, complex cases may be referred out.	Relatively simple.	Provider = LOW Payer = LOW
Global budget	Health facility: hospital, clinic, health center	Prospective	Total payment is fixed in advance to cover specified period of time. Some end-of-year adjustments may be allowed. Various formulas can be used: historical budgets, per capita rates with various adjustments (age, gender), utilization rates for previous year.	Flexibility in resource use. Spending set artificially rather than through market forces. Not always linked to performance indicators (e.g., volume, quality, case mix). Cost shifting possible if global budget covers limited services. Provider may refer patient to another provider outside purview of global budgets to minimize own global budget expenditures.	Rationing may occur if budget is too low. If rationing occurs, complex cases may be referred out. Case-mix adjustments in global formulas link budget amounts to complexity of cases. Other adjustors may be used to adjust payment for special population groups.	Requires ability to track efficiency and effectiveness of resource use in different departments, and mechanisms to switch resources to most effective uses.	Provider = HIGH Payer = LOW

(continued)

Payment method	Payment unit	Prospective or retrospective	Description	Efficiency	Quality and equity	Management and information systems	Financial risk
Capitation	Per person per year	Prospective	Payment is made directly to health care providers for each enrollee. Payment covers costs of defined package of services for specified time period. Provider may sometimes buy from other providers services it cannot (or declines to) provide itself.	Flexibility in resource use. The broader the service package, the narrower is the scope for cost shifting. Resources are closely linked to size of population served and its health needs.	Providers may sacrifice quality to contain costs. Rationing may occur if capitation is too low. Capitation may encourage providers to enroll healthier patients and exclude less healthy. Patient choice of provider is generally restricted. Adjusters in capitation formula can adjust payment to special population groups.	Management systems are required to ensure registration of each beneficiary with one provider. Utilization management and quality assurance programs are essential to prevent underservicing. If payment covers primary and secondary services, providers at different levels of system must establish contractual links with each other.	Provider = HIGH Payer = LOW

Payment method	Unit	Timing	Description	Advantages	Disadvantages	Requirements	Risk
Case-based payment	Per case or per episode	Prospective	Fixed payment covering all services for a specified case or illness. Patient classification systems (such as DRGs) group patients according to diagnoses and major procedures performed. Most frequently applied to inpatient services, although outpatient groups are being developed.	Flexibility in resource use. Tendency for hospitals to inflate cases (by increasing or double-counting admissions) to increase revenue. Patient classification systems can be used to monitor performance.	Case-based payment links payment directly to case complexity.	Providers need ability to record and bill by defined case, which generally entails collecting a large volume of reliable information on patient characteristics, diagnoses, and procedures.	Provider = MODERATE Payer = MODERATE
Per diem	Per day for different hospital departments	Prospective	Aggregate payment covering all expenses incurred during one inpatient day.	Flexibility in resource use. Tendency for hospitals to increase length of stay to increase revenue.	Per diem rates allow longer stays for more complex cases.	Need to track inpatient days by department and ensure costs are covered.	Provider = LOW Payer = HIGH
Fee for service	Per unit of service	Retrospective	Separate fees for different service items (e.g., medicines, consultation, tests).	Flexibility in resource use. Tendency for provider to increase number of services to increase revenue.	Payment is directly related to intensity of service. Tendency to overservice or provide unnecessary interventions.	Providers must record and bill for each medical service transaction.	Provider = LOW Payer = HIGH

Source: Wouters, Bennett, and Leighton 1998.
Note: DRG, diagnosis-related group.

Annex 4B
History of Government PPMs for Hospitals in Brazil

The first national system for paying for hospital services in Brazil was set up by the Social Security Institute (Instituto Nacional de Seguridade Social, INSS) when organizing purchases of private services for its beneficiaries. The system was based on a fee-for-service payment mechanism. Under a standard contract, payments authorized by the INSS were made according to a schedule of medical services, procedures, and products at prices specified in service units (*unidade de serviço*). In 1975–77 the Hospital Admission Form (Guia de Internação Hospitalar, GIH) was introduced, and DATAPREV, the Ministry of Social Security data processing unit, began computerizing the medical billing system (Castro, Travassos, and Carvalho 2002).

In the early 1980s the Ministry of Social Welfare and Social Assistance (Ministério de Assistência e Previdência Social, MPAS), implemented a new system, the Social Welfare Hospital Assistance System (Sistema de Assistência Médico Hospitalar da Previdência Social, SAMPHS). The system authorized higher payments as a financial incentive to providers of higher-complexity care, as specified by the Hospital Incentive Index (Indice de Valorização Hospitalar, IVH). The IVH was introduced experimentally in Paraná state in 1981 and was extended to the rest of the country starting in 1983, with the publication of the first Schedule of Hospital Procedures. The new computerized system introduced validation filters and checks, greater standardization of prices and procedures, and auditing of bills and hospital visits. It could generate automatic error reports, and it established the grounds for refusing to pay part or all of a hospital bill. A scoring system for reimbursements was used, and payments were broken down into medical supplies, professional services, per diem, and diagnostic and therapeutic services.

The SAMPHS and GIH systems were still based on fee-for-service payments, and this contributed to the financial and structural crisis of the mid-1970s (Lebrão 1999). By retaining the previous system of paying for individual procedures, it encouraged hospitals to overproduce inpatient services, leading to distortions, and it was open to fraud because of weaknesses in the process of checking and verifying hospital claims—suspected fraudulent bills were usually checked manually (Chiyoshi 1989; Levcovitz and Pereira 1993).

The move to the current system, based on prospective payment through the Authorization for Hospitalization (Autorização de Internação Hospitalar, AIH), was made in 1983–84 by the AIH Commission. The commission, which was convened to address problems in the GIH system, included representatives from the Brazilian Medical Association, the Confederation of Philanthropic and Benevolent Hospitals (Confederação das Santas Casas de Misericórdia, Hospitais e Entidades Filantrópicas, CMB) university hospitals, and the Brazilian Hospital Federation (Castro, Travassos, and Carvalho 2002). The new model was designed for reimbursement of hospital expenses after checking the provider invoice against predefined parameters based on expected use of inputs to treat a particular condition or to undertake a particular medical procedure (Levcovitz and Pereira 1993). Maximum values were set, for each medical procedure, for number of patient-days, medical materials and drugs used, and other parameters. To ease the transition into the new system and maintain compatibility, the focus of classification in the new system was on treatment and on the main medical procedure performed rather than on patient diagnosis.

Beginning in the mid-1980s two important changes were introduced: responsibility for managing the AIH system—up to that point, under the MPAS and its regional offices—was transferred to the state health secretariats, and, starting in 1990, public hospitals were brought into the system (Levcovitz and Pereira 1993).

Annex 4C
Provider Payment Mechanisms Used by the SUS

Type and program

A. *Payments for services rendered*
   1. Ambulatory care (SIA)
   2. Inpatient care (SIH/AIH)

B. *Transfers, intermediate and high complexity*
   3. AIDS—strategic interventions
   4. Posttransplant follow-up—strategic interventions
   5. Hearing deficiency—strategic interventions
   6. Human leukocyte antigen (HLA)
   7. Assistance to municipalities facing natural disasters
   8. Hospital and ambulatory care, intermediate and high complexity (MAC)
   9. Ophthalmology campaigns—strategic interventions
   10. Campaign for follow-up of hearing deficiencies
   11. Campaign for follow-up of posttransplants
   12. Campaign for cardiovascular surgeries
   13. Campaign for cataract surgery
   14. Campaign for prostate surgery
   15. Campaign for inguinal hernia surgery
   16. Campaign for epilepsy
   17. Campaign for prenatal care
   18. Campaign for chemotherapy
   19. Campaign for radiotherapy
   20. Campaign for diabetes retinopathy
   21. Campaign for vaccinations
   22. Campaign for antirabies vaccination
   23. Varicose vein surgery
   24. Craniofacial deformity surgery
   25. Breast surgery
   26. Cancer surgery
   27. Elective surgeries—strategic interventions
   28. Cofinancing of HIV viral load and TCD4/CD8
   29. Cofinancing for funding of MS facilities
   30. Additional finance ceiling, full management
   31. High-complexity compensation mechanism
   32. Uterine cancer—strategic interventions
   33. Craniofacial deformity—strategic interventions
   34. Resetting factor 25% (full management)
   35. Financing of registration and evaluation of health facilities
   36. High-risk pregnancy, over ceiling
   37. Full management of municipal system—high complexity

Type and program
38 Full management of municipal system—intermediate complexity
39 Histocompatibility—strategic interventions
40 Delivery humanization—strategic interventions
41 Impact of psychiatry
42 Incentive (MAC) for services to indigenous population
43 ICU beds, over ceiling
44 MAC sanitary surveillance
45 High-cost drugs to chronic patients
46 High-cost drugs for transplants
47 Neurosurgery, over ceiling
48 Orthodontics—strategic interventions
49 National plan for tuberculosis control
50 Program for fighting uterine cancer
51 Program for humanization of prenatal care and delivery
52 Program for radiotherapy/chemotherapy
53 Prostate—strategic interventions
54 Burns—strategic interventions
55 Rehabilitation—strategic interventions
56 Renal therapy
57 Extraordinary transfers
58 Transplants
59 Transplants—strategic interventions
60 Tuberculosis—strategic interventions
61 Emergency care, over ceiling
62 Varicose veins—strategic interventions
63 PNASH inspection—strategic interventions
C. *Transfers, basic care*
64 Support to indigenous population
65 National registry of SUS users
66 Epidemiology and disease control
67 Basic drugs
68 Additional incentive for program for attracting health professionals inland
69 Incentive for sanitary surveillance basic interventions
70 Incentive for fighting nutritional deficiencies
71 Incentive for decentralization of FUNASA facilities
72 Incentive for dental care
73 Drugs for mental health
74 Basic care flat fee (PAB fixed)
75 Health community agents program
76 Family health program (FHP)
77 Project similar to FHP
78 Polio vaccination

Source: Ministério da Saúde/Datasus.
Note: AIH, Autorização de Internação Hospitalar (Authorization for Hospitalization); FUNASA, Fundação Nacional de Saúde (National Health Foundation); ICU, intensive care unit; MS, Ministério da Saúde (Ministry of Health); PAB, Piso de Atenção Básica (Basic Care Grant); PNASH, Programa Nacional de Avaliação dos Serviços Hospitalres (National Hospital Services Assessment Program); SIA, Sistema de Informação Ambulatorial (Ambulatory Care Information System); SIH, Sistema de Informação Hospitalar (Hospital Inpatient Information System); SUS, Sistema Único de Saúde (Unified Health System).

Differential Increases in Reimbursement Rates, 1995–2001

Treatment or procedure	Adjustment (%)
Identification and contact of possible organ donor	300
Extraction of organ for transplant (several procedures)	300
Amigdalectomy	133
Clinical treatment of brain contusion	113
Eclampsia (severe pregnancy disease)	107
Anaphylactic shock	105
Schistosomiasis	86
Myocardial infarction	77
Resection for urothelial tumor, multicentric and synchronic	75
Total cystectomy	75
Prostatectomy	75
Ureterocystoneostomy	75
Total cystectomy and simultaneous derivation	75
Prostatovesiculectomy	75
Transplant (all organs)	75
Pancreatitis	75
Peritonitis	75
Abortion threat	73
Acute dehydration	71
Renal abscess	70
Total nose reconstruction	70
Endoscopic resection of prostate	69
Drug intoxication	66
Rheumatic diseases	64
Intestinal obstruction	63
Acute liver insufficiency	60
Liver cirrhosis	60
Conservative treatment of osteomyelitis	59
Appendectomy	58
Videolaparoscopic cholecystectomy	55
Spine fracture	54
Diverticulitis	53
Acute renal insufficiency	51
Cholecystectomy	50
Infectious hepatitis	49
Measles	49
Infant pneumonia	48
Acute bronchitis	48
Gastritis and duodenitis	48
Hypertension crisis	47
Inguinal hernia surgery	46

Source: MS 2004b.

Annex 4E
From the AIH to DRGs

Over the last two decades a number of countries have adopted some variant of the diagnostic-related group (DRG) method as their main hospital provider payment mechanism (PPM). Originally designed and implemented in the United States in the early 1980s, variations of DRG schemes have gradually been implemented in Australia (starting in 1985) and in several European countries, in most of them, during the 1990s. More recently, middle-income economies such as Hungary, the Republic of Korea, Taiwan (China), and Thailand have begun to adopt DRG. Most of these countries have implemented DRGs within a general shift from fee-for-service and per diem mechanisms for financing hospitals toward global budgeting and case-based payment systems (Schneider 2007). DRG implementation is often part of a broader package of health sector or hospital reforms (Fidler et al. 2007).

Why Use DRG?

Briefly, DRG is a case classification scheme that groups cases requiring similar resources and treatment processes. It is a hierarchical classification system: for example, under a particular form, APR-DRG, it lists 25 major diagnostic categories (MDCs) based on body system/medical specialty; over 400 DRGs based mainly on diagnosis; and approximately 1,500 subclasses based on risk factors and secondary diagnoses (see figure 4E.1).[65]

The DRG method's increasing popularity is related to a number of factors. It has been shown to contain hospital costs, mainly through the reduction of length of stay (Cashin, Samyshkin, and O'Dougherty 2005). It is a flexible tool: the core DRG system has been adapted in different country settings according to particular needs and available information

FIGURE 4E.1
DRG Hierarchical Structure and Classification Criteria

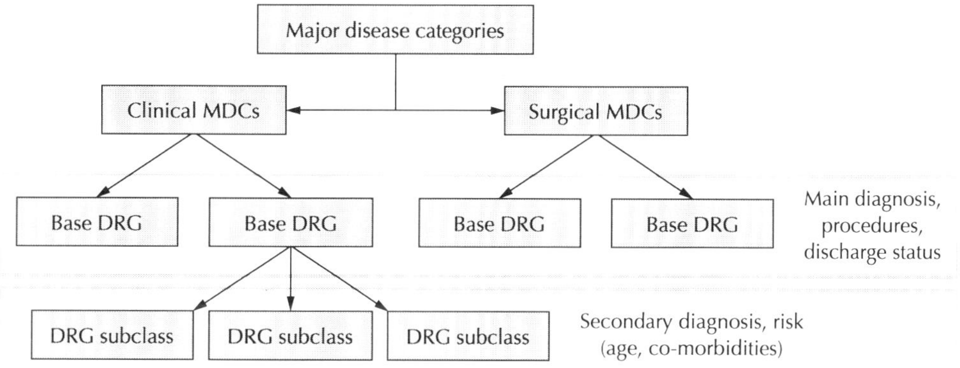

Source: Adapted from Schneider (2007).

systems.[66] Another reason for its popularity is that the system is useful not only as a payment mechanism but also for determining resource allocation, managing care, promoting quality assurance, and monitoring performance. Furthermore, it allows for adjustment for case mix and for risk factors such as age and severity, which can raise costs.

Any PPM should reflect the cost of care. Since DRG is a classification system based on the relative intensity of resource use, it requires extensive and reliable cost information. The system also relies on diagnostic information, including primary and secondary diagnoses and comorbidities, as well as information on hospital activities.[67] In most countries, DRG classifications are revised and updated regularly, often on an annual basis, and therefore require timely and updated information, which can further strain information systems.

In addition to intense information requirements, DRGs require considerable oversight and quality control. Fraudulent practices such as early discharges and readmissions and upcoding are constant problems faced by DRG systems.[68] Since payment is case based, DRGs may stimulate hospitals to increase the number of inpatient cases, resulting in escalating expenditures. Countries have responded to this potential distortion by combining DRGs with global budgeting and case-mix adjustments (Docteur and Oxley 2003).

Although Brazil's inpatient payment mechanism (AIH) system shares several similarities with DRGs, the latter offers several advantages. Table 4E.1 compares the major features of these systems, highlighting the major advantages of DRGs. Brazil implemented the AIH case-based PPM for hospital care in the mid-1980s at about the same time earlier adopters were implementing DRGs, but the AIH system followed a different approach, as described in annex 4B.

As stated in the chapter text, the AIH system needs an in-depth revision of classification and structure in order to correct existing distortions.[69] Such a revision represents a critical opportunity to develop and initiate a process of migration toward a DRG-based system. Compared with other countries that recently adopted DRGs, Brazil (and its Unified Health System, the SUS) have an advantage because of the related features of the AIH system. These include a case-based information and payment system for inpatient care that records a subset of the information needed for a DRG system, and a central unit, Datasus, that already collects and processes this information. What is missing in the AIH system is information on costs and diagnoses.

Finally, Brazil would benefit most from an approach combining global budgeting and DRGs, as demonstrated by experience in several European countries (Docteur and Oxley 2003). Global budgeting is a fixed payment, usually paid in advance, to cover aggregate expenditures of a hospital during a defined period. Global budgets are often tied to performance contracts that define a set of services and include preestablished annual targets (e.g., volume) and quality and other performance measures. As suggested above, global budgets complement DRGs by providing a disincentive to increase inpatient cases. DRGs, for their part, complement global budgets by providing information on case mix and costs, allowing for more precise budgeting.

Toward an Implementation Strategy

Several lessons have been learned from international experience with DRG implementation that can guide migration toward DRG in Brazil. Implementing DRG is a gradual process. It is

TABLE 4E.1
Comparison of the AIH and DRG Systems

Features	AIH	DRG
Objective	Replace fee for service with case-based charge system	Measure hospital resource allocation and costs and production
Principle	Group individual services for each patient according to the main medical procedure performed	Group patients according to main diagnosis
Basic classification criterion	Medical procedure	Main diagnosis (according to International Classification of Diseases, ICD)
Classification structure and coding	Classification of 2,300 procedures, grouped by medical specialty and subspecialty	Hierarchical classification with 23 major diagnostic categories and 600 DRGs (varies according to country)
Relation to cost and resource use	Original values loosely based on limited cost information	Grouping based on relative resource use (cost weighted)
Quality of diagnostic information	Variable (required, but weak, especially for secondary diagnosis; not basis for system)	Good (basis of the system)
Allows for severity or comorbidity	No	Yes; included in coding (in refined version)
Periodic reviews and updates	No major review	Several major reviews
Operation	Standard form, manual or computerized	Computer based
Distortions and fraud	"Procedure creep," low and distorted payment levels	"DRG creep"
Main control system	Bill auditing	Peer review
Country adoption	Brazil (1986)	United States (1970s–1983); Australia (1992); Germany (2003); Sweden and Portugal (late 1990s); Italy, Spain, Finland, United Kingdom (early 2000s)

Source: Authors' elaboration.

usually better managed if phased over a number of years. The remainder of this annex summarizes the application of lessons from DRG implementation to the Brazilian context.[70] The technical steps required for implementing a DRG system are summarized in box 4E.1.

- *Design.* Establish a working group at the Ministry of Health (MS) to coordinate the preparation of the new system and the transition process. This group will be responsible for preparing a framework and work plan to guide the design of the proposed system and its implementation. Particular attention should be paid to defining the objectives of the new system (e.g., increase efficiency, contain costs, or support case management) while recognizing the potential pitfalls and problems of the current system it seeks to reform. Build stakeholder support by portraying DRG as a way of remedying the well-known distortions of the AIH system and introducing a more transparent hospital payment system. The working group should consider assessing the lessons learned from other countries' experiences through an in-depth literature review and site visits.

Box 4E.1
Steps in Designing a DRG System

A DRG system classifies patients in groups that are clinically coherent (that is, they relate to the same anatomical system and disease group), economically homogeneous (they use a similar volume of resources and thus have similar costs), and statistically representative (they include a sufficiently large number of cases). Technically, implementation of a DRG system consists of three major steps:

1. *Determine the structure of case grouping.* This step implies creating major diagnostic categories; grouping cases as clinical or surgical, whether by treating these as two separate groups or by applying weights to cases according to the complexity of the procedure; and grouping cases according to age and other risk factors.
2. *Determine the cost distribution across International Classification of Diseases (ICD) codes.* The average cost per case is determined and then grouped and averaged within each ICD code, and outliers are removed to minimize distortions.
3. *Merge clinical and cost criteria to determine final case groups.* This involves creating case groups and calculating the average cost per case within these case groups.

Source: Cashin, Samyshkin, and O'Dougherty 2005.

- *Pilot-testing and roll-out.* Consider pilot-testing the transition to the new system in a small number of hospitals meeting basic requirements.[71] Introduce the new system gradually to ensure stability in financing and operations, as well as continuity in data collection.
- *Enabling organizational environment.* Facilitate DRG implementation by adopting performance-based contracting and strategic purchasing measures (within the context of global budgets)[72] and promoting organizational arrangements that ensure increased managerial autonomy in public hospitals, including the ability to allocate inputs and resources appropriately to achieve stated goals.
- *Capacity building.* Develop and implement a plan to strengthen regulation, oversight, and monitoring capacity of federal and state health authorities while providing technical support at the state or regional level to support transition and implementation at the local level. Any plan should include strengthening the purchasing and contract management capacity of states and municipalities, as well as providers' capacity for care and case management.
- *Information systems.* Strengthen the AIH case-based hospital information system, especially with respect to reliably recording primary and secondary diagnoses. Introduce a standardized cost accounting system that allows costing by case, not just by cost center.
- *Evaluation.* Plan for an impact evaluation, collecting baseline data in a sample of comparative hospitals with and without DRGs.

Notes

1. As described in chapter 6, public hospitals report that these are common problems.
2. Indirect administration generally refers to special organizational arrangements used in public hospitals, such as public foundations (chapter 5).

3. Until recently, AIH was the main payment mechanism used by the federal government to pay for inpatient care in public hospitals. It was replaced by federal grant transfers to subnational governments, which convert these funds to budgets to pay for hospital care.

4. The current AIH system was designed in several phases (see annex 4B).

5. The SUS uses a large number of payment mechanisms, mostly for primary and ambulatory care. Annex 4C contains a list of mechanisms.

6. Drugs and supplies are paid within the "hospital services" category.

7. Martins, Travassos, and Noronha (2001) found that because of underreporting of secondary diagnoses, a comorbidity index that the authors derived from AIH data was a poor predictor of the probability of hospital death and thus a poor indicator for risk adjustment.

8. Such problems are not limited to the SUS. Hsia et al. (1988), for instance, found that in the United States clinical information was incorrectly coded in 21 percent of the cases and that most of the errors were in the hospital's favor.

9. Auditing is supposed to check whether a patient bill includes unauthorized charges and whether the procedures performed are consistent with the diagnosis.

10. Because the AIH system is based on medical procedures rather than diagnostic groups, it is sensitive to technological change and therapeutic advances.

11. The AIH defines components by a different logic, based on two criteria: the receiver of payments, and separation of high-cost inputs for better cost control. The main components used in the AIH system are hospital services, professional (mostly physician) services, diagnostic services (tests), special (high-cost) procedures, general drugs and medical supplies, special (high-cost) drugs, and special materials. While some of these components relate to accounting line-item categories, other components, such as hospital and diagnostic services, include a variable mix of labor, supplies, and services that cannot be disentangled without considerable work. This discrepancy between accounting categories and AIH payment categories makes it difficult to estimate and control procedure costs consistently and thus reduces the usefulness of the AIH as a management information system.

12. There is no correlation between AIH procedures and International Classification of Diseases (ICD) codes.

13. For example, in recent years fee adjustments have either been flat, across-the-board increases or have favored complex and expensive procedures such as cardiac surgery and transplants. But as shown below, these are the most highly paid procedures in the AIH schedule and are less in need of price adjustment than some others. Annex 4D presents the main rate adjustments introduced in the AIH schedules in recent years.

14. The methodology used by the AMB is unknown, but anecdotal evidence suggests that the rates were based on consultations with its members. AMB (2005) presents the latest edition of a new schedule introduced in 2005.

15. In addition to copayments set by some health care plans, privately insured patients often have to pay out-of-pocket the difference between the insurance-paid amounts and the fees charged by the hospital. These patients also pay for diagnostic tests and for drugs not covered or only partially covered by their plans.

16. For reimbursement of privately insured patients treated in SUS facilities, the regulatory agency (ANS) has adopted a fee schedule, TUNEP, in which the rates are much higher than the AIH schedule applied to private hospitals under contract with the SUS and are also unrelated to the AMB schedule. The common feature of all these fee schedules is that they are based solely on negotiation between payers and providers without the benefit of reliable cost information.

17. These "packages" share some similarities with the AIH system but lag considerably in terms of accumulated experience and sophistication.

18. For comparison, the SUS reimburses R$7.55 for a specialized medical consultation.

19. This is the same survey used for the DEA and benchmarking analysis described in chapter 3. See annex 3D for sampling methodology.

20. By combining the classification of hospitals in the AMS survey by ownership and organizational arrangement, the main payment mechanism funding them was identified. For example, public facilities under direct administration are funded through the traditional line-item public budget.

The distribution of inpatient admissions by patient category and the mean estimated relative cost of an admission for each category of patient were then used to estimate the proportion of revenue deriving from each payment mechanism.

21. The assumption is that facilities catering to civil servants or the armed forces are funded through a mechanism similar to private insurance rather than the typical public budget.

22. The AIH covers only 34 percent of costs, if weighted by procedure frequency.

23. For this analysis, a technical classification of complexity was used rather than the MS categories of medium- or high-complexity and strategic procedures.

24. When the means are weighted by procedure frequency, the results hold, but with a reduction in the payment for high-complexity procedures to 8 percent above costs.

25. Several countries, including Germany, have dealt with this issue by reimbursing only for services produced with high-technology equipment purchased after obtaining approval.

26. Budgets for public facilities have three principal sources of financing: federal grant transfers to states and municipalities; special payments, included in the grant transfers, for high-cost tests, drugs, and materials; and state and municipal revenues. As mentioned, federal grant transfers to subnational governments have replaced direct AIH/SIA payments to most public hospitals. These transfers, which are based on AIH/SIA payments, are, however, complemented by budgetary resources from subnational governments. In short, because AIH/SIA rates are identical for public and private hospitals, SUS financing policies have favored public hospitals. This bias in favor of public providers is intended and is the outcome of an explicit policy favoring public provision since the introduction of the SUS reforms in the 1980s (see box 2.1).

27. On the crisis of nonprofit hospitals, see Comissão de Seguridade Social e Familia (2004).

28. Federação das Santas Casas e Hospitais Beneficentes do Estado de São Paulo (FEHOSP), "Panorama das Santas Casas e Hospitais Beneficentes," 2007 (press release). CREMESP estimates that the debt was R$1.5 billion in 2005 alone (CREMESP data).

29. Communication from official of the state health secretariat (not for attribution).

30. "A Crise dos hospitais"(editorial), *Estado de São Paulo*, December 30, 2004.

31. Secretaria Estadual de São Paulo, "Secretaria libera R$48 milhões extras para Santa Casas do Estado" (press release). http://portal.saude.so.gov.br (accessed May 14, 2007).

32. On nonprofit hospitals in the state of Paraná, see "Santas Casas em Crise," *Gazeta do Povo*, October 16, 2005.

33. www.cns.org.br./links/menup/noticiadosetor/clippings (accessed September 13, 2006).

34. It is common knowledge that physician-owners, board members, and directors of private facilities hold political office or are connected with officeholders in municipal and state governments.

35. The ratings were based on Brazilian hospital licensure standards.

36. Portaria 1721/GM, September 25, 2005.

37. IBGE (2003); $N = 428$. For sampling and DEA methods and a discussion of possible confounding variables, see annex 3D.

38. This grouping reflects the PPM accounting for at least 50 percent of revenues in the sampled hospitals.

39. For no hospital in the dataset was fee for service the main source of revenue. Furthermore, the number of hospitals under the global budget PPM group was insufficient for the analysis.

40. A case-mix index was computed from the costs of individual hospitals relative to the mean for each procedure and was used to adjust mean costs (see chapter 3).

41. Ratios of nearly 100 imply costs near the sample mean.

42. The results were compromised by the small number of facilities in some of these groups, and the facilities were classified by the main source of funding. Nonprofit hospitals derive revenues from a variety of PPMs.

43. Quality was measured by a quality index based on the hospital mortality rate adjusted for case mix, the ratio of nursing personnel per bed, and graduate nurses as a proportion of total nursing personnel. (See chapter 3 for a discussion of this index and annex 3D for the methodology.)

44. The measure of quality used here, like most other available measures, can capture only part of the full range of health service quality.

45. Although it is commonly assumed in Brazil that the proportion of nurses, and especially graduate nurses, to patients is an indicator of better quality, no systematic studies could be found to substantiate this hypothesis.

46. The relationship is regulated by Law 8080 and the Basis Operational Directives approved in 1996 (NOB/96). The convenio is informal because nonprofits are considered quasi-public entities. The SUS maintains more formal contracts with for-profit hospitals, but these contracts are also poorly managed or monitored.

47. The convenios date to the pre-SUS system operated by the Social Security Medical Institute (Instituto Nacional de Assistência Médica da Previdência Social, INAMPS). INAMPS issued contracts to private hospitals to provide the insured population with medical care. With the formation of the SUS and the decentralization of service provision, the contracts were not reissued, updated, or replaced. Thus, no SUS-funded private hospital is bound by a formal contract.

48. MS Decree (Portaria) 604/GM, April 24, 2001.

49. The draft regulation closely mirrors the regulation for contracting teaching hospitals, described later in this section. Some states are already implementing contracting instruments with nonprofit facilities in which performance is tied to a proportion of a global budget (São Paulo) or to investment financing (Minas Gerais). Minas Gerais state has recently negotiated and signed management contracts with a number of regional hospitals (SES-MG 2006).

50. The Lei Camata (São Paulo) and federal fiscal responsibility laws placed a 70 percent cap on government wage bills for public employees. No such limits were placed on "other personal services" (outsourcing). Outsourcing medical services is commonplace among for-profit facilities but not among nonprofits. Tax disadvantages create a disincentive for nonprofits and OSSs to hire in-house employees instead of outsourcing.

51. International experience suggests that public hospitals manage medical care outsourcing poorly. In general, outsourcing is an ad hoc and often opaque response to the symptom of excessive labor rigidities.

52. As described in greater detail in chapters 5 and 6, the OSS is an organizational and governance arrangement implemented in 16 new public hospitals. It entails autonomous decision-making authority by facility management, performance-based contracting and financing, contract enforcement, and a robust information environment.

53. A standardized cost accounting system has been implemented in all OSSs, in part because payments are based on a volume-cost calculus.

54. Teaching Hospitals Restructuring Program (Programa de Reestructuração dos Hospitais de Ensino); see Portarias 1702/1703 (August) and 2352 (October), 2004.

55. Of the 220 public teaching hospitals, 48 are federal, 108 are state, and 64 are municipal.

56. Therefore, unlike the case of the OSSs, the performance-based financing scheme is not linked to the entire budget.

57. For example, hospitals falling below 50 percent compliance with performance benchmarks will earn 50 percent of the value of the variable payment; those attaining scores between 51 and 75 percent will earn 75 percent of the value.

58. As described in chapter 6, most of the features of the OSS management contract and global budget were developed over a 10-year period, often through a process of trial and error.

59. Two possible exceptions are the states of São Paulo and Minas Gerais, both of which have established programs and systems to monitor contract performance. See SES-SP (2007); SES-MG (2006).

60. In São Paulo state, none of the teaching hospitals under contract receive the full variable transfer because of noncompliance with one or more indicators (communication from the state health planning secretariat, December 12, 2007).

61. More than 6,000 public payers (including each of the 5,500 municipalities) and 2,000 private payers are active in the health sector.

62. Such adjustment is important because the cost of care is heavily influenced by individual case severity and the mix of cases treated by a provider.

63. As described in chapters 5 and 6, São Paulo state is experimenting with performance-based global budgets in 16 new public hospitals.

64. See Zanetta (n.d.); Silver et al. (1992); Veras et al. (1990).

65. APR-DRGs (all patient refined DRGs) are a more elaborate version of basic DRGs: they are more representative of non-Medicare DRGs (basic DRGs were designed based on Medicare patients), and they incorporate the severity of illness so as to disaggregate the DRGs into subclasses.

66. The differences in approach to DRGs have, however, reduced the possibility of international comparison and the development of standard tools and methods.

67. DRGs rely on three key sources of information: hospital activity data, hospital cost data, and case mix. Specific information requirements include the hospital identification number, the patient identification number, patient sex, patient age, patient marital status, patient place of residence, date of admission, duration of stay, discharge status, main diagnosis, secondary and other diagnoses, procedures performed, source of admission, specialty, occupation, intensive care stay, linkage to resource data, case-mix group, day care indicator, and internal transfer (Wiley 2007).

68. These problems are already present in Brazil's AIH system.

69. Several authors (Veras et al. 1990; Veras and Martins 1994; Martins, Travassos, and Noronha 2001; Martins and Travassos 1998) have explored the commonalities between AIH and DRGs and the possibility of a migration toward DRG and have concluded that such migration is feasible.

70. This section draws on Schneider (2007) and Cashin, Samyshkin, and O'Dougherty (2005).

71. These basic requirements should include at least hospital bed size (medium to large facilities are best) and reliable patient data and cost information.

72. These issues are discussed in chapters 5 and 6.

5

Organizational Arrangements and Performance of Brazilian Hospitals

Incentives embedded in payment mechanisms influence provider behavior, but hospitals do not all react in the same way to similar financial incentives. Public hospitals respond differently from private hospitals, nonprofits from for-profits, and more independent facilities from less independent ones (Harding and Preker 2003; Bogue, Hall, and La Forgia 2007). Hospitals that are under competitive pressure or are held accountable for results behave differently from those that are not. How a hospital responds to incentives inherent in payment mechanisms, in a contract, or in regulations depends on its organizational form. Its degree of independence, accountability to both payers and public, and market exposure are key elements of its organizational arrangements that influence its behaviors and, ultimately, performance. The elements of organizational arrangement in Brazilian hospitals and their relation to performance are examined in this chapter.

Organizational arrangements are the least understood drivers of hospital performance and, from an analytical perspective, the most difficult to isolate. Although confounding variables preclude definitive statements on specific arrangements and their impact on performance, evidence is emerging, in Brazil as elsewhere, that certain arrangements yield better results than others. This is particularly true in the public hospital sector, where government is testing innovative models to improve the quality and efficiency of publicly financed public and private facilities and their clients' satisfaction with them.

A range of distinct hospital types has emerged in the past 50 years in Brazil, particularly in the public and nonprofit subsectors, and differences in their behaviors are apparent. Intuitively, it makes sense that hospitals with different degrees of independence and different mandates and goals will respond in different ways to a common set of incentives. This chapter attempts to identify differences among the types of hospital organization in Brazil that can be systematically linked to their performance. Where such a connection can be verified, recommendations are made for improving the performance of publicly funded hospitals by strengthening organizational arrangements.

Although direct management has dominated the public hospital sector in Brazil, alternative organizational arrangements have emerged in a few public facilities during the last 25 years in the form of private support foundations, public enterprises, social organizations, and other types of "autonomously managed" facilities. The array of models reflects dissatisfaction with the traditional direct administration modus operandi as practiced in Brazil. Together, the new models represent attempts to bypass or avoid restrictions and inflexibilities imposed by public sector rules involving human resource management and purchasing. The degree of autonomy varies considerably among these arrangements, and some types may be vulnerable to interest group capture. Recent innovations attempt to introduce more results-oriented accountability and incentive systems by combining autonomy with contracting and the introduction of alternative payment mechanisms.

Even in private facilities, especially nonprofit hospitals dependent on public financing, management and governance practices may not be conducive to good performance, and many facilities lack managerial independence. Some private facilities, however, are introducing more robust governance, contracting, and management models in order to improve performance and to compete in an increasingly challenging health care market. Unfortunately, only a subset of these experiences has been examined rigorously. The results of the relevant research are reported here.

Organizational Arrangements: Framework and Literature

Organizational arrangements consist of specific characteristics of the hospital environment that influence hospital behaviors and, in turn, performance. This chapter follows the framework developed by Harding and Preker (2003) and by Jakab et al. (2002). It consists of five dimensions: decision-making authority, particularly regarding input management (autonomy); exposure to market pressures in providing services to assorted purchasers (market exposure); retention of unspent earnings and responsibility for losses (residual claimant status); degree of directness of responsibility for performance (direct accountability); and specification of objectives and mission, as well as of revenues to cover service costs (social functions). These dimensions are considered characteristic of successful, market-oriented enterprises in a competitive environment.

Most of the work on organizational arrangements takes the form of prescriptions based on theory and country experiences. Together with payment mechanisms, these guidelines are seen to contribute to a performance-enhancing institutional environment in public hospitals. The Harding and Preker framework focuses on organizational structures that can contribute to an accountability environment or generate incentives for improved performance. Although Harding and Preker recognize that the components of organizational structure can vary considerably, they maintain that public hospitals in many developing countries perform poorly because of ill-defined and unclear objectives, weak or absent accountability or oversight structures, lack of autonomy and market exposure, political interference, and dearth of information. They advocate organizational reforms supporting autonomous decision making at the hospital level, pointing out that such reforms improve governance by promoting a strong performance orientation, by strengthening accountability structures, and by enhancing facility survival in the broader market environment. On the basis of the five analytical dimensions of the framework, and drawing on experiences with public hospital reform in developed and developing countries, Harding and Preker (2003) offer a typology and continuum of organizational arrangements, as follows:

- *Administrative unit.* The hospital is fully or nearly fully dependent on the hierarchical control of government authorities for most budgetary and input decisions. In effect, the facility is directly managed by its government owners. This form is commonplace in most public hospitals in developing countries, especially in Latin America.
- *Autonomous unit.* Facility managers enjoy greater decision-making authority in selling services, charging fees, and managing budgets, but facilities remain under public owner-

ship and are subject to public sector rules for procurement, labor, and contracting. Contracting may be partially managed by government administrative offices, in which case the facilities may be best described as semiautonomous units. Countries that organize some or all of their public hospitals this way include Argentina, Malaysia, Singapore, Tunisia, and the United Kingdom.

- *Fully autonomous unit.* Managers have full or nearly full decision rights over inputs, service mix, finance, and spending. They are accountable with respect to financial and service performance but are generally exempt from public sector rules.[1] Because such facilities are under public ownership, they must comply with legal mandates to attend to "public patients." Australia, Austria, Colombia, Estonia, Hong Kong (China), the Netherlands, New Zealand, Singapore, and Spain, among others, organize their public hospitals in this way.

- *Private unit.* This form encompasses nonprofit and for-profit facilities in which managers are not bound by public control (unless so specified in a contract with public payers). These facilities are fully exposed to market pressures with respect to finance and health performance. In theory, incentives are aligned so as to reward managers for earning revenues, monitoring and maintaining performance, and expanding or retaining market share. Countries with publicly funded hospitals organized in this way include Canada, Malaysia, Singapore, and the United States.

In Brazil examples of each of these organizational types exist and receive public financing. As is typical elsewhere as well, within-group variation is evident, particularly for the hybrid categories of semiautonomous and fully autonomous units. Organizational arrangements may not address all five dimensions of the framework, and considerable inconsistency in implementing new forms or changes has been observed in the international experience (Ham and Hawkins 2003). Some countries have focused on a subset of dimensions, leaving other dimensions untouched.[2] For example, the health social organization model introduced in public hospitals in the late 1990s in São Paulo state would receive high marks on autonomy, accountability, and social functions, but it represented a modest reform in terms of exposing the facilities to the market. In theory, consistency in implementing the full range of dimensions increases the potential for sustainable performance. Granting greater autonomy without the other dimensions, for example, may not result in improved performance.

In practice, introducing alternative organizational arrangements is a complex endeavor, and success may depend on factors outside the organizational environment, including political will, policy leadership, and availability of resources. Furthermore, organizational reform in hospitals rarely occurs alone; it is generally linked to parallel reforms in, for example, payment mechanisms, state modernization, and public-private partnerships. This has been the case in Brazil. These contextual factors constitute the confounding variables that challenge evaluators in isolating the impact of organizational structures on performance. Without such information, it is impossible to identify the policy lessons from successful (or failed) experiences.

Not everyone accepts this framework and typology. In a review of studies of "autonomization" reforms in public hospitals in developing countries, Castaño, Bitrán, and Giedion (2004) express pessimism as to whether these reforms improved hospital performance and claim that autonomous decision making remained limited. They cite several experiences with reforms that attempted to widen autonomy for facility management, as described next.[3]

Five cases examined by Govindaraj and Chawla (1996), in Ghana, India, Indonesia, Kenya, and Zimbabwe, showed little impact of greater autonomy on efficiency and quality. Equity appeared to be negatively affected in some cases, and autonomy did not result in improved accountability. Kamwanga et al. (2003), in their analysis of five semiautonomous hospitals in Zambia, reported no impact on performance, and the hospitals remained dependent on centralized, historical budgets. Eid (2003) found that in Lebanon boards established in corporatized hospitals had few decision-making rights and were often captured by facility managers. Board politicization resulted in loss of transparency and decision-making independence.

Other studies, however, suggest that autonomous organizational arrangements contribute to improved performance. Comparative research in Panama matching a public hospital operating under a fully autonomous arrangement with two hospitals under institutionally administered arrangements found that the former achieved significantly higher levels of production, efficiency, and quality (Bitrán, Má, and Gómez 2005). McPake et al. (2003) reported that the establishment of autonomous organizational and governance arrangements in five hospitals in Bogotá improved quality and efficiency. Parallel reforms in payment mechanisms and significant increases in overall system financing, however, make attribution of the results solely to autonomy difficult. Of the seven cases from developing economies reviewed by Preker and Harding (2003), four—Hong Kong (China), Malaysia, Singapore, and Tunisia—appeared to show improved quality and outputs, but the reforms also increased costs. In this chapter the performance of hospitals under autonomous organizational arrangements is compared with that of matched facilities directly managed by municipal and state governments.

Castaño, Bitrán, and Giedion (2004) identified some potential perverse effects of autonomatization.[4] For example, autonomous hospitals may have little incentive to deliver high-impact, but low-revenue, priority health services such as prenatal care and may focus instead on services such as tertiary care that attract wealthy or privately insured patients, especially if payment mechanisms favor these services. Consequently, free services or health care aligned with the health needs of the poor may be reduced. Autonomous hospitals also have an incentive to institute or raise user fees for public patients, to increase revenues.[5] If public budgets were cut, managers would be encouraged to seek alternative sources of revenue such as selling services or charging user fees, and this could have negative equity effects.

Another issue has to do with the regulatory environment. Autonomy, without proper governance, monitoring, regulation, and enforcement, could result in corruption, such as kickbacks between facility managers and input suppliers. Finally, autonomous facility management could make network integration more difficult, resulting in ineffective referral systems and lack of coordination with primary care providers. This chapter attempts to assess these issues within the Brazilian context for each of the arrangements examined here, to the extent that information is available.

Some of the suspected perverse effects suggested by Castaño, Bitrán, and Giedion are only marginally relevant in the Brazilian context, for two reasons. First, all publicly financed services are by law free to Unified Health System (Sistema Única de Saúde, SUS) patients in both public and private facilities, and there is little evidence of user fees or informal payments for SUS patients.[6] Second, direct public management, in which nearly all public facilities at each level of the delivery chain are owned and operated by government, dominates the public organizational landscape. There is little evidence that the direct administration model has achieved care coordination in Brazil (Mendes 2001). This is especially true of care that must be coordinated across municipal lines, between municipal- and state-managed services, and between publicly financed public and private facilities. In fact, a strong case can be made that networks, however defined, are dysfunctional or nonexistent throughout most of the country.[7] Therefore, at worst, enhancing facility autonomy would only reduce the potential power of an unused instrument, integrated public command. As mentioned in chapter 2, lack of coordination has more to do with the content and process of health decentralization, which delegates considerable authority over the organization and delivery of health to Brazil's 5,500 municipalities, than with organizational arrangements in public hospitals (Mendes 2005). Many Brazilians seek basic care in hospitals partly because publicly financed primary care is deficient or absent (Mendes 2002). In sum, there is strong evidence that health care in Brazil is already heavily centered on hospital-based delivery (CONASS 2005) and is not coordinated using existing direct administrative control instruments across facilities at different levels (primary care, diagnostics, hospitals).

Organizational Arrangements in Public Hospitals in Brazil

Brazil has struggled for 70 years to reform public administration, applying a series of strategies to combat clientelism and patronage employment.[8] Overall, advances have been irregular, with evidence of some successes as well as of back-pedaling on earlier reforms. While some sectors have displayed greater progress than others, a broad, systematic reform model for public administration has yet to emerge. Nonetheless, reforms have left their mark on the public sector in the form of small enclaves of good performance (Shepherd 2002). The outcome has been a mosaic of organizational arrangements in public institutions in nearly all sectors, including public hospitals. Given the superior results of some of these public hospital enclaves, the organizational building blocks for crafting a more comprehensive strategy to develop and expand high-performing public hospitals already exist in Brazil.

Brazil may present an exceptional case in the developing world because of its array of organizational arrangements in public and private hospitals. In a sense, the country can be considered a laboratory of natural experiments in such arrangements. Table 5.1 presents a breakdown of the total number of public and private hospitals according to major organizational model. Annexes 5A and 5B provide summary descriptions of each of the arrangements described in this chapter.

Three types of organizational arrangements are found in public facilities. *Direct administration* is the predominant arrangement (see table 5.1). Facilities in this category are essentially administrative units that are owned and operated by federal, state, or municipal government. Most do not manage a budget. *Indirect administration*, applied in about 2 percent of public facilities, refers to semiautonomous, parastatal organizations in which managers hold slightly greater decision-making authority with respect to some organizational functions such as procurement and budget execution. These facilities can best be described as hybrid organizations containing elements of both hierarchical control—typical of direct administration—and autonomy, typical of the third category, *autonomous organization*. Autonomous organizations, which make up less than 1 percent of public hospitals, have full decision-making authority over inputs, resource use, and production. Most were established in the 1990s.

TABLE 5.1
Organizational Arrangements in Public and Private Hospitals in Brazil, 2005

Classification	Type of organizational arrangement	Number	%
Publicly owned hospitals			
Direct administration	Federally, state, and municipally managed facilities	2,585	35
Indirect administration	Autonomous management units (*autarquias*)	62	} 2
	Public foundations (*fundaçoes públicas*)	75	
Autonomous administration	Autonomous social services (*serviços sociais autônomos*)	6	
	Public enterprises (*empresas públicas*)[a]	19	
	Private support foundations (*fundações de apoio*)	46[b]	} 1
	Social organizations (*organizações sociais*)	17	
Privately owned hospitals			
Nonprofit	Private foundations	107	
	Philanthropic and charitable associations and societies	1,700	} 25
	Cooperatives and employee unions	44	
For profit	Corporate or privately held	2,765	37
Total		7,426	100

Source: MS 2005; MS/Datasus.
a. Includes facilities classified as mixed economy enterprises *(empresas de economia mista).*
b. Estimated number of hospitals under direct and indirect administration that have affiliated support foundations.

Although developed in different periods, nearly all the indirect and autonomous forms were intended to circumvent the rigidities of direct administration and give managers flexibility and authority. Some forms have achieved (and sustained) this objective better than others. The complex legal and regulatory landscape, often compounded by multiple reforms in the public service apparatus and by systemic reforms such as decentralization, has contributed to the array of organizational forms, as well as to variations within specific forms. Annex 5B describes and compares each of these arrangements according to the dimensions of the Harding and Preker (2003) framework. Table 5.2 summarizes the comparison.

The current patchwork of organizational arrangements in the public hospital sector originated in three waves of reform:

- The administrative reform of 1967 (Law 200/1967), which established indirect administration arrangements.[9] As originally legislated, these arrangements entailed full managerial autonomy.
- The constitutional reforms of 1988, including subsequent legislation governing the civil service (Law 8112/1990), procurement (Law 8666/1993), and health system decentralization (Law 8080/1990). These reforms subjected all publicly owned and operated entities to the public labor, procurement, and financial regimes. In effect, they severely restricted the autonomy of public institutions under indirect administration.
- Administrative reforms implemented in the late 1990s (under the constitutional amendment of 1998) that led to the founding of autonomous organizational models such as social organizations.

TABLE 5.2

Comparison of Components of Organizational Arrangements in Brazilian Public Hospitals

Organizational component	Direct administration	Indirect administration	Autonomous administration			
			SSA	EP	FA	OSS
Autonomy (decision rights)	Very limited	Limited	High	High	High	High
Market exposure	Very limited	Limited	Moderate	High	High	Moderate
Accountability	Very limited	Very limited	Moderate	Moderate	Moderate	High
Residual claimant status	Very limited	Moderate	Moderate	Moderate	Moderate	High
Social functions	Implicit	Implicit	Implicit	Implicit	Explicit	Explicit

Source: Annex 5B.
Note: FA, private support foundation; SSA, autonomous social services; EP, public enterprise; OSS, health social organization, São Paulo state.

The Limits of Direct Administration

Direct administration refers to a set of structures, functions, and processes that dictate behaviors in public institutions owned and operated by government. Nearly all public hospitals, which are directly managed by line ministries or secretariats, apply this arrangement (see table 5.1). Hospitals under direct administration possess limited decision-making autonomy, are financed through historical line-item budgets, are generally not responsible for monitoring performance, manage in an environment in which accountability is diffuse and performance requirements are implicit, and have little exposure to markets. These characteristics are typical of government-operated facilities elsewhere (Preker and Harding 2003). All hospitals under this arrangement follow a single set of rules, as specified in federal framework legislation stipulating labor, procurement, and budgetary rules and procedures for the public sector.[10] This legislation, collectively known as public law or the public sector regime (*direito público*), predated but was considerably strengthened by the 1988 Constitution and the subsequent legislation.

The legal intricacy of the public sector regime, combined with the complexities of health decentralization, led most states and nearly all municipalities to centralize the implementation of labor, procurement, and budgetary processes in administrative and finance secretariats. For example, most subnational units have created central procurement and human resource units to handle these functions for line secretariats, and finance secretariats standardize most budgetary and financial management processes for all executing units.[11] Line secretariats and corresponding executing units such as hospitals simply implement budgets defined by higher-level authorities. In a number of states and municipalities, purchasing, recruitment, and budgetary management are performed outside the line secretariats, which may have only marginal advisory influence (World Bank 2007).

Decentralization in Brazil was a deep reform that was closely linked to the country's emergence from more than two decades of military dictatorship and the subsequent redemocratization. In the health sector the breadth and depth of decentralization have led some observers to refer to it as a "system shock" (Akhavan 2001: 8) because of the misalignment of (decentralized) responsibilities and existing managerial, technical, and fiduciary capacity at the municipal level.[12] In addition to mandating universal health coverage, the reform shifted full operational responsibility for the previously centralized health service delivery system to the municipalities.[13] Few municipalities were prepared for this responsibility or had prior experience in hospital management, and in nearly every instance the transfer of federal and state hospitals to state and municipal ownership and management has meant little or no change in the way facilities are governed and managed. Furthermore, most workers in decentralized facilities retained their federal status, making it difficult for municipalities to develop a human resource strategy for hospitals. Centralization in secretariats by local governments enabled greater consistency in the implementation of the laws but also introduced rigidities, particularly in recruitment, dismissal, salaries, definition of staff positions, and procurement practices (World Bank 2007), limiting the authority of health secretariats over these key functions.

The Rise and Fall of Indirect Administration

Between the late 1960s and the late 1980s organizational forms such as autonomous management units (*autarquias*) and public foundations (*fundações públicas*)—collectively known as indirect administration—emerged in Brazil, driven in part by the administrative reform of 1967. These reforms were originally enacted by a military government and were considered means of institutional control and clientelism by the military. The reforms, however, also sought to expand the scope of publicly financed services by establishing more agile institutions. They were applied to a subset of hospitals and other public health care institutions, and about 2 percent of all facilities (5 percent of public hospitals) now have indirect administration arrangements (see table 5.1). As originally designed, these arrangements granted autonomy to managers regarding budget management, hiring and firing practices, procurement, and supplier contracting. Managers could also retain leftover revenue (residual claims). Directors and other ranking personnel, however, were politically appointed. Under the extreme federal centralization in Brazil at the time, most of the indirect administration organizations were directly linked to the executive level and were run by the military government. These arrangements were criticized as sources of corruption and patronage practices.[14] Although this criticism was not necessarily directed at arrangements in the health sector, the general discontent with autonomous management units underlay changes in public administrative processes that were incorporated into the 1988 Constitution (Shepherd 2002).

Standardization of procurement, civil service, and budgeting reforms had the effect of imposing new rigidities on the indirect administration model. Although nearly all the formal organizational arrangements of indirect administration remained intact, the processes by which they operated changed drastically, compromising discretionary autonomy. The indirect administration models retained residual claimant status, continued to capture other than public financing, and maintained their status as autonomous budgetary units, but all procurement and personnel management were subject to government rules, as stipulated in the new laws.[15] As a result of the decentralization reforms, the previously autonomous facilities also came under the hierarchical control of local government regarding appointment of directors and supervision.[16]

In sum, the new procurement and civil service legislation significantly restricted autonomous decision making by indirect administration entities. Mendes et al. (2002) suggest that facilities under such arrangements are nearly indistinguishable from their direct administration counterparts.

The Emergence and Extension of Autonomous Organizations in Public Hospitals

Despite the reduced independence associated with constitutionally driven reforms, a few health institutions were able to secure and retain a high degree of autonomy through special legislation that responded to their prestigious, and often privileged, position in the sector and their strong political support. Other arrangements emerged or expanded partly in response to rigidities imposed by the 1988 Constitution and subsequent legislation. Collectively, these arrangements are referred to as autonomous administration in table 5.1 and annexes 5A and 5B. Although they account for less than 1 percent of public hospitals, they are receiving increased attention from policy makers at every level of government.

Pre–1988 Constitution

Two autonomous organizational models are found in some hospitals: public enterprises (*empresas públicas*, EPs) and autonomous social services (*serviços sociais autônomos*, SSAs).[17] Most of these institutions were established through special federal legislation in the 1960s and 1970s and enjoy high prestige and strong political support, especially the SSAs. Most are financed directly by the federal government through historical budgets or direct transfers. Public financing is the sole source of financing for some facilities, while others also sell services to the private sector. Despite calls to incorporate SSAs and EPs into the decentralized SUS system and the public labor and procurement regimes, these facilities have thus far maintained their autonomy, applying private sector regimes for labor, contracting, and procurement. Most are governed by a board of directors.

There is little documentation concerning the performance of SSAs and EPs, but they are no longer considered viable organizational models, and states and municipalities show no interest in enacting legislation establishing facilities under these prereform models. In any case, the administrative reforms of the 1990s that resulted in the creation of the social organization model (described below) created a disincentive for setting up SSAs and EPs.

Post–1988 Constitution

The 1990s brought the expansion and emergence of two autonomous organizational arrangements: private support foundations (*fundações de apoio*, FAs), resulting from initiatives within facilities, and social organizations (*organizações sociais*, OSs). Both were meant to bypass the restrictions of the public labor, contracting, and procurement regimes. Social organizations grew out of a second wave of administrative reforms led by the federal government. Although this model accounts for a small minority of organizational arrangements in public hospitals, it marked a major shift in organizational structure with respect to accountability, decision rights, market exposure, residual claimant status, and social functions.

Private Support Foundations

Although private support foundations existed in hospital facilities before the 1988 reforms, the number increased in the 1990s, reaching approximately 50 in 2005.[18] FAs are generally affiliated with highly specialized public teaching hospitals operating under direct administration.[19] As applied to hospitals, the FA is a parallel finance, governance, and management structure that is incorporated under the private regime for labor, procurement, contracting, and financial management. Establishing an FA requires neither special legislation nor broad political support. Rather, an FA is established through an agreement (*acordo*) with the federal, state, or municipal government that operates the facility or through a government statutory act (*acta*). The purpose of FAs is threefold: to capture additional revenue from private and, to a lesser extent, public sources to complement the government budget; to hire additional personnel and pay bonuses to civil servants; and to allow greater flexibility in the purchase of goods and materials.

Typically, FAs are founded by a group of professionals—most often, physicians—employed in a facility. The process is simple and consists of (1) establishing a board of governors (*conselho de curadores*) to appoint a director and formulate statutes and regulations; (2) obtaining approval of the foundation's constitution from the board of governors and the purveyor for foundations (*provedoria de fundações*) in the Attorney General's Office (Ministério Público); and (3) signing a partnership agreement (*termos de parceria*) that defines the terms of the relationship between the FA and the hospital. Once these steps are completed, the FA is granted tax-free status by the state or municipal government. The federal government's foundation comptroller is responsible for financial audits of FAs. The raison d'être of FAs is to support the public facility to which they are linked according to the partnership agreement and statutory act. FAs are required to be physically installed in the public facility for at least two years and to be fully self-financed.

In practice, FAs have raised additional revenues by selling services to private insurance plans and patients, securing donations, and obtaining public and private grants for medical research. With these revenues, they have hired additional personnel (under private contract law), provided bonus payments to staff, and purchased medical equipment. Some observers suggest that the FAs have helped retain prestigious specialists in public hospitals by financing bonuses, salary scale-ups, and medical research. FAs have also been agile in purchasing needed equipment that might have taken years to buy through public procurement channels. Box 5.1 describes how one foundation operates within a public hospital.

Detractors claim that FAs have created parallel management and stratified delivery systems within the hospital that favor paying patients, as well as FA founders, who invariably are physicians.[20] FA revenues and expenditures are generally small, compared with the facility's budget, and concentrate on services that are lucrative for the FA and its physician founders but do not necessarily improve access or quality for SUS patients.

The federal comptroller-general (*tribunal de contas*, TCU) has on several occasions challenged the raison d'être of the FAs (*O Globo*, July 26, 2006). Most recently, in an audit of five FA hospitals in Rio de Janeiro the TCU declared illegal the use of public funds to remunerate privately contracted medical personnel, as well as the provision of monetary benefits (e.g., bonuses) to civil servants. The TCU recommended that all personnel contracted under private law be replaced by civil servants through a public selection process. Some observers claim that FAs are "an illegality that has survived" (Kanamura 2006: 19) and that the model is no longer viable because of continuous legal challenges. Although more research is needed into the advantages and disadvantages of the FA model, the expansion of FAs over the last 15 years provides evidence that public facilities derive important benefits from them.

Social Organizations

The federal government's administrative reforms of the late 1990s introduced a new set of organizational arrangements, social organizations (OSs). This model was applied to a number

Box 5.1
Achieving Labor Flexibility within Public Direct Administration: The Pro-Heart Foundation

Founded in 1973, the National Cardiology Institute of Laranjeiras (INCL) in Rio de Janeiro is a national referral hospital for the treatment of cardiovascular disease. It is owned and operated by the federal government under a direct administration arrangement. In 1996 the INCL sponsored the establishment of the Pro-Heart Foundation (FUNDACOR), whose mission is to further the quality of cardiovascular disease training and treatment in Rio de Janeiro.

In 2004 FUNDACOR reported revenues of R$26.2 million and expenditures of R$21.3 million (51 percent of the INCL budget). Nearly 92 percent of the revenues came from the government—in the form of regular SUS (AIH) transfers, and additional transfers to treat patients on waiting lists in public facilities. Although the magnitude of FUNDACOR'S dependence on public financing is unusual, this arrangement can be found in other specialty hospitals with private support foundations (FAs). Sales to private insurers (health plans) accounted for 4.2 percent of revenues. This is a small share of income compared with that of nonprofit facilities and of other FAs, which derive 10 to 20 percent of their revenues from health plans (see the table below).

FUNDACOR Revenues and Expenditures, 2004

Revenue source (total revenue, R$26.2 million)	Percent
Private insurers	4.2
SUS (AIH)	21.7
SUS (special)	70.1
Other	4.0
Expenditures (total, R$21.3 million)	
Personnel	70.7
Materials and supplies	10.7
Information services	3.5
Diagnostic services	8.6
Other	6.5

Source: FUNDACOR data.
Note: AIH, Authorization for Hospitalization; SUS, Unified Health System.

More than 70 percent of expenditures goes to pay mostly professional personnel hired by FUNDACOR and to provide bonuses or salary upgrades for INCL professional and nonprofessional staff. In 2004 FUNDACOR provided bonuses or salary upgrades for 200 INCL professionals, or 40 percent of INCL professional staff. INCL and FUNDACOR representatives claim that FUNDACOR's production has increased steadily. For example, between 1998 (the first full year of FUNDACOR's operations) and 2003 the number of cardiac surgeries grew by 130 percent. Data from the pre-FUNDACOR period are, however, unavailable, and so the impact of FUNDACOR on this increase cannot be measured. Detractors assert that FAs cater to paying patients, but no substantiating evidence of such behavior was found for FUNDACOR. In 2002–4 SUS patients accounted for 94 of discharges, 97 of surgery cases, and 96 percent of outpatient consultations subsidized by FUNDACOR.

Source: Compiled by authors from documentation provided by FUNDACOR.

of hospitals operated by the São Paulo state government as part of a broad set of measures to reform the state apparatus (MARE 1996). Following "new public management" principles, the reform attempted to correct the structural inefficiencies in excessively "bureaucratic" Brazilian public administration and confer greater autonomy and accountability on public agencies and their managers.[21] The major features of the reform plan included:

- Strengthening decentralization of social services.
- Identifying and separating "exclusive" and "nonexclusive" functions of the state. (Social actions and services are considered nonexclusive state responsibilities and can therefore be transferred to the nonprofit sector.)
- Fostering increased autonomy and accountability for government agencies and their managers.
- Enhancing accountability by introducing mechanisms that orient the system toward results (rather than ex ante or input-focused controls), foster direct participation and control by beneficiaries and communities, and promote transparency in civil service and financial management.

The reform was incorporated into a 1998 constitutional amendment (Article 8) that modified Article 37 of the Constitution to enable the granting of full "managerial, financial and budgetary autonomy to indirect and direct administration entities." Autonomy was conditioned on the signing of contracts between managers and executive authorities that specified financing and expected performance. Significantly, the amendment also entitled any level of government to set remuneration, hiring and firing practices, position descriptions, and any other aspect related to human resource management. In short, the amendment provided constitutional support for introducing greater flexibility in public management and, to a certain extent, represented a "way out" (*saída*) of the contracting and human resource rigidities engendered by the Constitution and the relevant civil service laws.[22]

The constitutional amendment set the stage for the creation of social organizations as legal organizational arrangements for the provision of social services. Federal Law 9637 of 1998 established the legal framework for the OS as a nonprofit, private (nongovernmental) entity under private labor, procurement, and contracting law (*pessoa jurídica de direito privado*). Essentially, an OS is exempt from the confines of civil service and procurement rules.

Health Social Organizations in São Paulo State

On June 4, 1998, four months after the federal law creating social organizations was passed by Congress, São Paulo state enacted Law 846, establishing health social organizations (*organizações sociais de saúde*, OSSs).[23] OSSs were created as nonprofit social organizations "of public interest" (*utilidade pública*) that were incorporated under civil law (*direito privado*). Unlike facilities under direct and indirect administration, OSSs are not bound by public contracting, civil service, or procurement laws. The OSS is a legally independent organizational arrangement under the state law. No additional legislation is required to establish the arrangement in a specific facility.

Between 1998 and 2005 São Paulo state introduced OSSs in 16 new facilities. OSSs are general hospitals, averaging 200 beds per facility, that offer the four basic specialties: surgery, gynecology and obstetrics, internal medicine, and pediatrics. Most also provide psychiatric inpatient care, as well as "day hospital" and ambulatory surgery services. All maintain intensive care and neonatal units. Each facility offers emergency care, and two-thirds provide outpatient care for nonemergency patients; these hospitals are known as "open door" facilities. The remainder, "closed door" facilities, accept only referrals.[24] All are located in low-income neighborhoods in heavily urbanized municipalities on the periphery of the city of São Paulo.

Organizational Characteristics

The salient organizational features of the OSS model, as implemented in São Paulo, are outlined in box 5.2. Perhaps the most important innovation of this model is the granting of full managerial autonomy in decision making on inputs, managerial processes, and day-to-day operations of public facilities to private, nonprofit organizations in exchange for accountability for results that are specified in a performance contract and supported through a results-based financing mechanism. In turn, the state surrenders hierarchical control and direct management of tasks related to facility operations, human resources, and input procurement and assumes more arm's-length responsibilities related to contract management, negotiation, and performance monitoring. OSSs are not permitted to treat private patients or charge fees.

Box 5.2

Major Characteristics of Hospitals under Health Social Organization (OSS) Arrangements, São Paulo State, 2004

Legal framework
- OSS arrangement established under state law.
- Supported by federal framework law.
- OSS bound by civil law (*direito privado*).

Ownership
- Public: state government of São Paulo.

Responsible entities
- State government is financier but is legally responsible for property and service delivery system.
- Facility operations are the responsibility of a contracted private, nonprofit organization (EPNL), usually a university or philanthropic organization.

Selection of contractor
- Competitive tendering.

Financing
- Global budget allocated in monthly cash installments.
- Retention fund: 10 percent of financing retained against quarterly compliance with performance indicators.
- Capital financing and depreciation excluded from global budget.

(continued)

Box 5.2 *(continued)*

Accountability
- Trustees (EPNL governance board): operations and overall performance; compliance with state law and contractual terms.
- Payers/owners (state health secretariat): performance indicators and financial reporting requirements specified in contract.
- Regulators (state auditing agency): spending and management of public funds.
- Patients: no organized body, but contract mandates annual patient satisfaction survey.

Decision-making autonomy
- All inputs except capital investments.
- All managerial processes.
- All contracts with suppliers.
- Negotiation of performance targets with payer (state government).

Market exposure
- Not permitted to charge fees or to sell services to private patients or to insurance plans.
- Participate in pooled procurement schemes.
- May outsource clinical, diagnostic, and hotel services without government permission.

Residual claimant status
- Retain and invest "savings" in capital markets, but not to provide bonuses to managers, who receive fixed salaries.
- Unable to sell "shares" or seek outside investors.

Monitoring, information
- Robust information environment: quarterly reports on production, AIH, spending and costs.
- Standardized cost accounting systems implemented in all OSSs.

Results orientation
- Production targets and performance indicators specified in contract, linked to financing mechanism, and monitored by state health secretariat.

Social functions
- Legal and contractual mandate to serve SUS patients only; facilities located in poor neighborhoods.
- Services and activities and corresponding volume specified in contract.
- State government pays costs of specified production targets.

Source: São Paulo State Law 846; state OSS documentation.

Management Contract and Payment

The OSS model can be described as a type of contract management arrangement in which a legally incorporated private, nonprofit organization (*entidade privada não lucrativa*, EPNL) is contracted to direct and manage all functions and services of a publicly owned facility. The contractor is typically a university or philanthropic organization that already owns and operates hospital facilities and is selected through a semicompetitive process involving certification by the state.[25] Once certified—that is, authorized as an OSS—an EPNL can be contracted by the state to operate a facility through a five-year renewable management contract (*contrato de gestão*).[26] The EPNL is responsible for contracting all personnel and procuring all inputs (except capital inputs) to comply with production and quality targets specified in the management contract. It is not permitted to spend more than 70 percent of its budget on payroll.

OSSs are financed through a global budget negotiated between the state and the facility. Originally, the budget for each facility was determined through cost estimates based on historical spending patterns in other state (non-OSS) facilities. By 2001, however, the state had installed standardized cost accounting systems in each hospital. Currently, the costs generated by the systems are the basis for annual budget setting. Although the global budget represents a hard budget constraint, its allocation is divided into two parts, each tied to performance as specified in the management contract. The first part is linked to production targets; the second, to compliance with reporting requirements and quality indicators. Noncompliance with production targets, reporting requirements, or quality indicators can result in withholding or suspension of defined percentages of financing.

The state OSS law stipulates that the OSSs cannot collect fees or sell services to third parties. They can retain "leftover" revenues, but only for investment in health-related activities. Managers receive a fixed salary and are not permitted to receive bonus or incentive payments, but OSSs can pay performance bonuses to staff. EPNLs can obtain loans in the capital market to cover operating deficits but not to pay for capital improvements. Depreciation is not included in calculation of the global budget. Any capital investments are negotiated annually with the state government and are therefore dependent on the state capital budget and on political negotiations with state health authorities. In short, capital financing of the OSSs is similar to that for facilities directly administered by the state. The lack of financing for depreciation of plant and equipment is the major weakness of the model. As the facilities age, the OSSs are subject to the vagaries of state capital financing and may face delays in the upgrading of plant and equipment.

The state OSS law mandated the formation of governance boards in OSS-managed facilities (Law 846, Article 3). Consisting mainly of representatives of civil society, the boards are envisioned as the ultimate authority in the facility. This measure has yet to be implemented, and its nonfulfillment could challenge the long-term sustainability of the model. Although accountability is driven by the management contract and the performance-based financing mechanism, a case can be made that an independent governance structure with broad civil society participation—with responsibility for oversight of managerial practices, fiscal performance, planning and policy making, and accountability to individuals, communities, and governments—would enhance overall performance and community support.[27]

Comparative Review of Organizational Features in Public Hospitals

How do organizational models in public hospitals influence behaviors and performance? Drawing on facility surveys, this section reports on two comparative analyses of organizational arrangements in public hospitals. The first study compares patient mix and sources of financing, using a sample drawn from a 2002 national facility survey (IBGE 2003). The second analyzes organizational structures and behaviors of a small sample of facilities, following the models reviewed in the previous section.

Table 5.3, which draws on the first analysis, shows the estimated distribution of admissions by type of patient served according to the ultimate payer of services rendered (e.g., the SUS and health plans). The table also shows the proportion of financing derived from different sources or payment mechanisms.

All public hospitals cater mainly to SUS patients, but only facilities under direct administration depend heavily on traditional government budgets. A minority of these facilities, along with hospitals under indirect administration, attend to private patients as well as patients covered by private prepayment plans. These facilities have broadened their demand and consequently derive revenues from various sources, including health maintenance organizations (HMOs) and private, fee-for-service patients. To accomplish this, they have probably instituted private support foundations to permit contracting, billing, and collecting revenues from private payers. The facilities classified as autonomous administrative arrangements—mostly OSSs and autonomous social service organizations—cater exclusively to SUS patients. As mentioned, OSS-operated facilities receive a global budget and, by law, are allowed to provide services only to SUS patients.[28]

How do these arrangements compare in terms of creating a flexible organizational environment that fosters the conditions that allow "managers to manage"? These questions were the subject of the second analysis mentioned above, a groundbreaking study of organizational arrangements in Brazilian public hospitals by Mendes et al. (2002).

TABLE 5.3
Public Hospitals: Patient Mix and Sources of Financing, by Organizational Arrangement, 2002
(N = 284)

Organizational arrangement	Clients, by payer (% of admissions)		Main funding source by payment system (% of revenues)			
	SUS	Health plans	Government traditional budget	Government decentralized budget	Government (SUS) prospective payment	Private prepayment plans
Direct public administration	98	2	86	0	10	4
Indirect administration	90	10	0	56	28	16
Autonomous administration[a]	100	0	0	100	0	0

Source: Figure 4.1; Couttolenc et al. 2004.

Note: For each main analytical category ("Clients, by payer" and "Main funding source by payment system"), rows add to 100 percent.

Definitions of the main funding sources are as follows. *Traditional budget:* based on line-item allocation and used largely in the public sector under direct administration. *Decentralized budget* (including global budget and autonomous budgetary units): found within indirect and autonomous models; facilities with decentralized budgets generally have greater autonomy in the execution of the budget but may have to follow procurement and civil servant rules. *SUS prospective payment:* used by the SUS for paying hospital (AIH) and ambulatory (SIA) services to private and public hospitals. *Private prepayment health plans:* mainly HMO-type organizations; largely used in contracts between private (and public) plans and hospitals.

a. Includes social organizations and autonomous social services.

The researchers selected, through purposive sampling, 24 hospitals of similar size and complexity from every part of Brazil. One group, labeled "alternative," consisted of 10 facilities operating under indirect and autonomous models and 2 direct administration facilities with innovative organizational practices.[29] The researchers hypothesized that these facilities would have "flexible" structures which would enable more "strategic" and "autonomous" behaviors. The remaining 12 facilities, which operated under direct administration, were labeled "traditional." These displayed no evidence of innovative organizational practices and operated as administrative units of government. They were hypothesized to feature structures that responded to "hierarchical" control and would therefore display more "normative" behaviors (e.g., compliance with rules and reporting on these "compliance" behaviors). Based on a survey of facility managers and follow-up interviews, the research sought to determine how the hospitals differed within and across the two groups with respect to organizational structure (formal rules and processes) and organizational behaviors (application of rules and processes).

To investigate organizational structure, a survey was administered, consisting of a series of questions. The responses were used to construct a set of 25 variables grouped into six categories: professionalism and sustainability of managers (process of appointing senior management, management stability); decision-making authority over strategic issues (planning, budgeting, resource allocation, presence of hard budget constraint); accountability (accountability mechanisms related to owners, patients, and communities and information on performance and public disclosure); locus—in the facility or in the administrative hierarchy—of decisions regarding personnel (recruitment, dismissal, and remuneration); market exposure (ability to sell services, set prices, and tap nonbudgetary revenues); and competition (ability to compete with other providers and negotiate with suppliers). The researchers constructed four composite indicators based on these variables: accountability, decision making for strategic issues, decision making for personnel, and market exposure.

Based on the presence or absence of each element (variable), two sets of scores were generated to determine the degree to which the organization functioned either within a "hierarchical" rule set, in which most decisions and strategic issues were controlled by government officials and mandated by public service rules, or within a "flexible" or independent rule set, in which most decisions and strategic issues were determined by facility managers who had greater latitude to determine service and input mix and devise managerial practices. Thus, each hospital received both "hierarchy" and "flexibility" scores.[30] Not surprisingly, significant differences were found between the two groups of hospitals. Public hospitals featuring autonomous organizational structures were found to be significantly more flexible (or less hierarchical) than facilities under traditional structures (e.g., direct administration) for each of the four composite variables: accountability ($p < .014$), decision making for strategic issues ($p < .0001$), decision making related to personnel ($p < .0001$), and market exposure ($p < .0001$).

Figure 5.1 traces the flexibility and hierarchy scores received by each hospital in the sample. A clear separation was observed between the two groups of hospitals: alternative facilities had higher flexibility and lower hierarchy scores, while traditional hospitals displayed a nearly opposite correlation. Considerable dispersion was evident among hospitals with alternative organizational structures.[31] This is consistent with the previous discussion of variations

FIGURE 5.1
Hierarchy and Flexibility Scores for Organizational Structures,
Alternative and Traditional Hospitals, 2000
(*N* = 24)

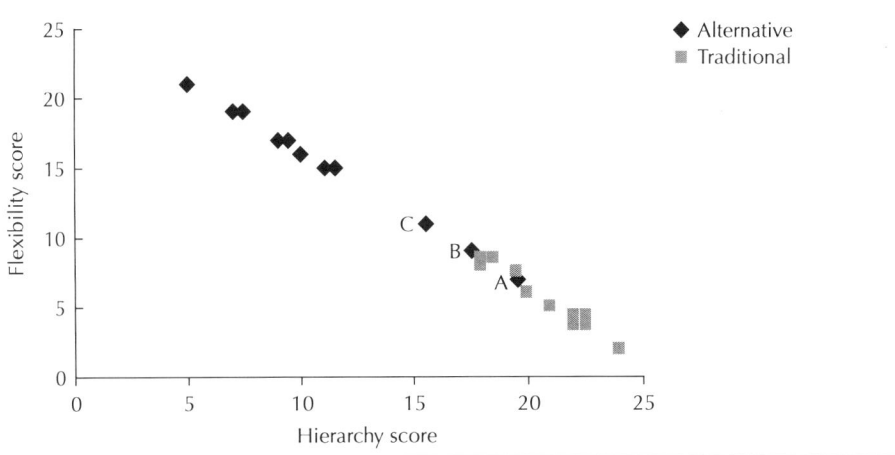

Source: Mendes et al. 2002.

among organizational arrangements in the indirect and autonomous categories. The alternative group consisted of a variety of organizations under direct, indirect, and autonomous administration. As discussed above, organizations under indirect administration are hybrids that contain the hierarchal elements of direct administration but also some elements of flexibility. By design, autonomous organizations have a high degree of flexibility and autonomy. Hospitals under direct administration are more homogeneous from a structural standpoint. This is expected because all are subject to a similar or nearly similar rule set.

Two direct administration facilities (A and B in figure 5.1) were originally hypothesized as "alternative" because they were known to have flexible human resource policies, including performance-pay schemes for professionals. The survey results, however, showed little evidence of flexibility on other structural dimensions or of innovative policies for other categories of personnel. These two facilities can therefore best be described as hierarchical organizations. A third facility (C in the figure) occupies a middle ground in structural rankings. The facility was one of several in a large complex that was managed by a state government and had established a private support foundation (FA). The foundation's insertion in the market, however, was minimal, deriving little revenue from nonpublic sources.

Private Sector Organizational Structures and Governance Arrangements

Nonprofit and for-profit hospitals constitute nearly two-thirds of all hospital facilities in Brazil. As explained in chapter 2, the SUS maintains service agreements with about 90 percent of the nonprofits, as well as half of their for-profit counterparts. About 56 percent of SUS hospital financing is directed to private hospitals. Table 5.4 shows that the SUS represents about 80 percent of the patient volume treated in nonprofits but less than half of their revenues.

TABLE 5.4

Private Hospitals: Patient Mix and Sources of Financing, by Organizational Arrangement and Ownership, 2002

(N = 304)

Ownership	Organizational arrangement	Clients, by payer (% of admissions)			Main funding source by payment system (% of revenues)				
		SUS	Health plans	Private	Government traditional budget	Government decentralized budget	Government (SUS) prospective payment	Private prepayment plans	Private fee for service
Private nonprofit	Philanthropic associations[a]	74	20	6	0	0	33	45	22
	Private foundations	85	10	5	0	0	48	29	23
Private for-profit	Corporate management	34	48	17	0	0	8	58	33

Source: Figure 4.1; Couttolenc et al 2004.

Note: For each main analytical category ("Clients, by payer" and "Main funding source by payment system"), rows add to 100 percent.

a. A small portion of this group (<2 percent) includes cooperatives and unions.

These facilities are increasingly seeking revenues from private health plans and private patients to compensate for shortfalls in SUS revenues.[32] In the case of for-profits, the SUS represents less than one-third of patient volume and is the source of less than 10 percent of their revenues. For-profits derive most of their income from contracts with private health plans. Fees collected from private, non-SUS patients are their second most important revenue source.

Little is known about organizational arrangements and management practices in the private sector, and what is known is limited to the nonprofits. Facilities operated by voluntary or charitable organizations are by far the largest category of nonprofits. There are about 1,700 such facilities, representing about 90 percent of nonprofit hospitals in Brazil, 37 percent of private hospitals, and 23 percent of all hospitals (see table 5.1).

Most nonprofit facilities are affiliated with a heterogeneous array of philanthropic and charitable associations (*associações filantrópicas e beneficentes*), including Masonic societies, charitable groups, and religious orders. A subset of this group has formed private foundations. Cooperatives or unions formed by professional organizations account for a small portion of the group.[33]

Philanthropic societies founded hospitals as well as other social assistance institutions such as orphanages, poorhouses, and schools. Although some facilities date to colonial times, most hospitals were founded in the early 20th century. About 30 percent of nonprofit hospitals are affiliated with religious organizations; most of the remainder belong to secular, "community-based" societies (17 percent) or civil societies (52 percent); see Barbosa et al. (2002). Nonprofit facilities are found throughout Brazil but are concentrated in the South and Southeast regions, usually in the interior. More than half of these facilities are located in municipalities in which they are the only source of hospital care.

Nonprofit hospitals operated by voluntary organizations became a well-established source of hospital care and professional training prior to the development of public systems. In fact, in some parts of Brazil, they were the only source of medical care. Over time, many of these organizations have shed other charitable work, such as running orphanages and poorhouses, to concentrate on furnishing hospital-based care and educating medical professionals.

The nonprofit hospital sector in Brazil is in transition. Most nonprofits were founded mainly as charitable institutions to deliver medical care, but an increasingly complex set of demands is forcing them to alter their mission, roles, and goals. A new environment has come about through an explosion in technology, education, and research, market diversification, irregular public funding, and changes in payment systems. To survive, nonprofits are being forced to change. Although many are still small "mom-and-pop" organizations, a growing number have embarked on modernization.

Mendes (1986) classifies the nonprofit hospital sector into two groups. The first is traditional, in the sense of maintaining the charitable mission established by the founding society or organization. These generally smaller, independent facilities are highly dependent on SUS financing. The second group is "entrepreneurial" and operates more like for-profit businesses. They are usually larger facilities and tap revenues from private insurers and patients. Some belong to nonprofit conglomerates that operate several facilities. Increasingly, these facilities are abandoning their charitable orientation and acting more like business enterprises, albeit nonprofit (e.g., they do not distribute revenues from operations to owners).

A recent survey provides evidence of the changing nature of philanthropic hospitals and their position in the health care market. In a sample of 530 nonprofit hospitals Giardi and Barros (2001) found that only 17 percent derived revenues exclusively from the SUS. Although still dependent on the SUS for a significant share of revenues, more than 80 percent reported income from contracts with private insurers, and 11 percent had established a facility-based prepayment plan.[34] Whether these facilities face market pressures or a hard budget constraint is an open question. For example, some states and municipalities assign government medical personnel to nonprofit facilities (Giardi and Barros 2001). Furthermore, as discussed in chapter 4, many nonprofit hospitals receive lump-sum subsidies, known as "public donations," when needed, in addition to the production-based Authorization for Hospitalization (Autorização de Internação Hospitalar, AIH) payments. This practice, although not uncommon, is difficult to quantify because the amounts, meant to keep the facility financially afloat, are usually politically negotiated between government and facility owners.[35]

Legal and Regulatory Framework

The 1988 Constitution established nonprofit organizations as legal entities and, unlike previous legal instruments, did not refer to such entities as philanthropic and charitable organizations. Importantly, the legal personality and private status (*direito privado*) of nonprofit institutions is protected by Article 5 of the Constitution. Nonprofit hospitals enjoy tax-free status if at least 60 percent of all services is provided to SUS patients.[36] All nonprofit facilities must secure (and update every three years) a certificate of nonprofit status (*certificado de filantropia*) from municipal, state, or federal social assistance councils.[37] The facility must present evidence of, among other things, the presence of elected governance executives,[38] nonremuneration of governance executives, continuous operation during the three previous years, annual publication of a financial statement; notarized registration of statutes, and use of income according to mission and statutes, as well as "results" for the previous three years and the annual minimal percentage of total care or infrastructure (usually beds) devoted to SUS patients. The last requirement is negotiated annually, case by case, with the government level that reimburses the facility.[39] In a 2002 census of nonprofit facilities, Barbosa et al. (2002) found that 15 percent did not possess a valid certificate.

Organizational Arrangements

Organizational arrangements in the private sector consist of private foundations, beneficiary associations, trade associations, and employee-operated cooperatives or unions (see table 5.1 and annex 5A).[40] This section focuses on those hospitals affiliated with philanthropic or charitable organizations (PCOs).[41] PCOs have a legally mandated governance structure of one or more statutory executives: board members (*conselheiros*), associates (*socials*), curators (*curadores*), or trustees (*instituidores*). These are part-time, pro bono positions. Each organization determines the role and responsibilities of its statutory executives with respect to facility management according to its by-laws (if any exist). The division of responsibilities between statutory executives and management is, however, established by law.

A few organizations have boards, made up of statutory executives, that meet regularly. In others, the statutory executives meet irregularly or informally to review the facility's financial performance. For a significant share of nonprofit hospitals, however, executives from the PCO exercise both governance and management functions (box 5.3). According to Barbosa et al. (2001, vol. 2: 61), the line between governance and management is often blurred:

> in various cases the separation between the [governing] entity and the hospital is neat and clear—especially in the case of larger entities and [multifacility] conglomerates, but in other cases the entity and hospital become confused—particularly in the case of small entities but also in large entities that operate a single hospital.

One way in which PCOs vary is in management, which some organizations take more seriously than others. According to Barbosa et al. (2002, vol. 3: 49), only 60 percent of the 1,414 nonprofit hospitals surveyed in 2001 had a formal management team. A philanthropic organization ran 34 percent, and about 3 percent outsourced management.[42] Smaller facilities are usually managed directly by the philanthropic society and larger facilities, by a management team.

Barbosa et al (2002) examined the type of executive responsible for facility management in samples of small and large facilities owned and operated by a single society, as well as (generally large) facilities belonging to a conglomerate, which may own and operate several facilities. Table 5.5 summarizes facility management responsibilities by executive position. Half of the small hospitals and a third of the large facilities did not have a facility-based executive manager. All but one of the 80 facilities belonging to conglomerates reported having a facility-based director. This is related to the fact that conglomerates' headquarters are usually located far from affiliates. In contrast, nearly all facilities reported having the *position* of medical director (not shown in the table), and two-thirds of those

---

Box 5.3
Governance and Management for Hospitals

Governance consists of an organization's structures and functions that set and enforce policies and exercise the ultimate authority for decisions made on behalf of the organization and its owners. The trustees, commissioners, or directors are ultimately responsible for the facility, including its assets and the quality of care. Important functions of hospital governance (based on models common among nonprofit hospitals in the United States and Europe) include defining and reviewing mission, role, and goals; providing financial stewardship; formulating future strategy; appointing and evaluating the chief executive officer (CEO); ensuring clinical efficiency and quality; and representing the hospital's stakeholder groups (Coile 1994). The trustees delegate authority to run the facility to a management team.

Management functions include defining business and medical strategies and drawing up plans to achieve the organization's goals and objectives; selecting, evaluating, hiring, and firing employees; formulating and analyzing annual budgets; setting service mix and prices; monitoring operations, including financial performance; overseeing use of physical and financial resources; and evaluating performance and outcomes and taking any necessary corrective actions (Rowland and Rowland 1984).

TABLE 5.5
Executives Responsible for Nonprofit Hospital Management, by Hospital Size and Type, 2002
(Percent)

Executive type	Individual facilities		Facilities operated by conglomerates (N = 80)[a]
	Small (N = 69)	Large (N = 15)	
Hospital-based executive	49	33	99
PCO statutory executive	22	33	0
PCO executive director and statutory executive	29	33	0
Total	100	100	100

Source: Barbosa et al. 2002.
Note: Small: mean = 67 beds. Large: mean = 576 beds. Conglomerates: mean = 136 beds. Columns may not sum to 100 percent because of rounding.
a. Eleven conglomerates with a total of 80 hospitals. Data were unavailable for one facility.

institutions reported having a general director. This apparent contradiction may have to do with the informality and merging of the governance and management functions. Many facilities simply reported the existence of these positions and did not distinguish among the executives who carried out functions related to the position. Barbosa et al. (2002, vol. 3: 74) explain:

> for the majority of the hospitals [in the sample], the statutory executives of the organization assume the position [of hospital director] together with the organization's executive director or hospital manager, or simply occupy the position of [hospital] general director without the position itself being explicitly instituted.

Table 5.6 shows that the decision-making authority of hospital management varies by function.[43] Although the hospital is free of the hierarchy of public control, the governing PCO retains decision-making authority over many functions in each of the three facility categories. Most facilities have discretionary authority in human resource management and procurement of drugs and medical supplies. About 60 percent report autonomy to open, close, or expand services; negotiate contracts with third-party payers (the SUS, private insurance plans); and contract out maintenance and hotel services. As expected, in most facilities the governing organization has authority over human resource policy, capital investments, and financial functions.

The degree of autonomy relates to facility size, as well as to the historical and centralized patterns of PCO management practices, including the above-described fusion and blending of managerial and governing functions (often in the same officer). Another factor is the part-time and voluntary nature of executive positions. For example, 22 percent of smaller hospitals and 33 percent of larger facilities are managed directly by the PCO statutory executive (table 5.5).[44] The degree of autonomy may be limited in these hospitals, partly because of the lack of separation between governance and management functions. Autonomy may also be constrained because of the part-time nature of both management and governance personnel.

TABLE 5.6

Nonprofit Hospital Executives Reporting Decision-Making Autonomy, by Function, Hospital Size, and Affiliation, 2002

(Percent)

| | Individual facilities | | Facilities operated by |
Function	Small (N = 61)	Large (N = 15)	conglomerates (N = 81)
Human resources			
Recruitment/hiring	80	73	77
Dismissal	77	73	83
Salary policy	40	47	52
Procurement			
Consumables	83	73	86
Equipment	67	67	59
Contracting out			
Maintenance	77	67	78
Hotel services	62	53	70
Capital improvements	46	53	42
Service mix			
Open new service	59	60	57
Expand existing service	62	67	62
Eliminate a service	59	60	57
Financial			
Budget approval	41	27	27
Borrowing	32	45	14
Financial investment	46	60	54
Negotiation—payer contracts			
SUS	57	60	58
Private insurers	62	67	65

Source: Barbosa et al. 2002.
Note: For definitions of facilities, see table 5.5.

As figure 5.2 shows, quite a few hospitals with facility-based executives report that these managers are volunteers and work part time. Smaller facilities are often managed directly by executives of the PCO or by part-time volunteer managers, while larger facilities usually have an autonomous, facility-based management team. As a general rule, most hospitals with full-time, paid executive managers have greater discretionary autonomy than those managed by part-time volunteers.

A significant share of nonprofit facilities has yet to modernize governance practices. In the current external environment, traditional practices are not conducive to organizational survival. In addition, the informality of decision making, combined with lack of separation of PCO-hospital governance and management practices, suggests diffuse accountability within the organization. This may hamper the execution of management functions and per-

FIGURE 5.2
**Percent of Full-Time and Volunteer Managing Executives of Nonprofit Hospitals,
by Facility Category, 2000**

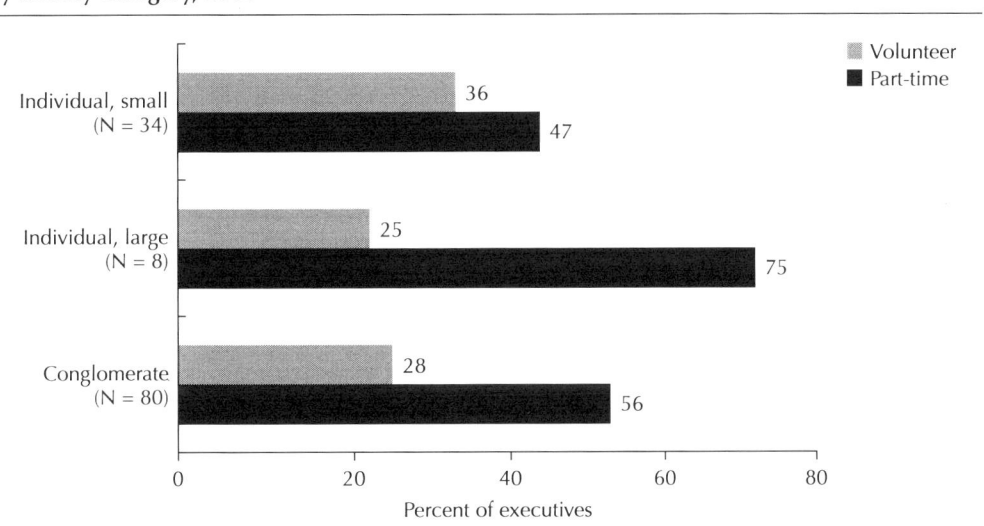

Source: Barbosa et al. 2002.

formance. Managerial practices in public and private hospitals are further discussed in the
next chapter.

Comparative Performance of Hospitals under Different Ownership and Organizational Arrangements

Organizational arrangements are important determinants of performance. Hospital behaviors do not respond to the external environment (e.g., payment mechanisms, public policies, legal and regulatory framework) in a vacuum. As seen earlier in this chapter, hospitals vary in their independence, decision-making authority, accountability mechanisms, and market exposure. The presence or absence of these elements influences behaviors and managerial practices and thus performance. The findings reported here show that sound organizational arrangements are associated with greater efficiency and that with the proper organizational arrangement and operational scale, public hospitals can be as efficient as their private counterparts, or more so. Furthermore, efficiency gains can be achieved without compromising quality.

This section presents the results of three analyses comparing facilities under direct administration with alternative or nontraditional organizational arrangements. Each analysis draws on different data sources.[45] The first is a comparison of the relative efficiency of private and public hospitals under various organizational arrangements, using the data envelopment analysis (DEA) described in chapter 3. The second is a comparative analysis of the performance of the sample of alternative and traditional hospitals discussed above.

The third compares efficiency and quality indicators for a sample of hospitals under the OSS arrangement in São Paulo state with those of a sample of direct administration hospitals from the same state.

Efficiency Analysis Based on a Facility Survey

This discussion synthesizes the findings of the DEA analysis on efficiency, disaggregated by organizational arrangement.[46] Table 5.7 shows total technical efficiency (TTE), internal technical efficiency (ITE), and scale efficiency (SE) scores, by organizational arrangement.[47] Because efficiency varies by hospital size, the table includes the DEA results for hospitals with more than 50 beds. As seen in chapter 3, the average TTE score was 0.42 for the 50+ bed sample (against a maximum efficiency score of 1.0), but 0.34 for the sample of smaller hospitals with only 25+ beds.[48]

Within the public sector, hospitals under autonomous and indirect organizational arrangements were found to be markedly more efficient, obtaining higher TTE scores than hospitals under direct administration. Among private facilities, for-profit facilities were slightly more efficient than nonprofit associations and foundations. Overall, public hospitals under autonomous administrative arrangements, mainly OSSs, were the most efficient group, followed by for-profits. Hospitals under the direct administration model were the least efficient for both the 25+ and 50+ bed samples, displaying TTE scores of 0.26 and 0.29, respectively.

Scale efficiency was a main driver of TTE, particularly for the 25+ bed sample. SE varied considerably among facilities in this sample, with public autonomous facilities displaying the highest SE scores and direct administration, the lowest. The small size of facilities under the direct administration arrangements contributed to the low TTE scores because most small

TABLE 5.7
DEA Scores by Ownership and Organizational Arrangement, Hospitals with More Than 25 and More Than 50 Beds, 2002

Ownership and organizational arrangement[a]	Hospitals with 25+ beds				Hospitals with 50+ beds			
	N	Mean TTE	Mean ITE	Mean SE	N	Mean TTE	Mean ITE	Mean SE
Public hospitals								
Direct administration	141	0.262	0.671	0.417	64	0.294	0.681	0.460
Indirect administration[b]	37	0.356	0.644	0.552	23	0.446	0.686	0.636
Autonomous administration[c]	18	0.398	0.626	0.688	14	0.470	0.670	0.716
Private hospitals								
Nonprofit foundations	53	0.385	0.668	0.562	22	0.449	0.834	0.535
Nonprofit associations	101	0.372	0.653	0.559	69	0.444	0.778	0.575
For-profit corporations	105	0.396	0.694	0.577	56	0.481	0.794	0.617

Source: Couttolenc et al. 2004.
a. Despite efforts to clean the data derived from the National Health Facility Survey (Assistência Médico-Sanitária, AMS) database, some of the groups are not fully homogeneous because of multiple interpretations of definitions of organizational arrangements.
b. Autarquias and public foundations.
c. Social organizations and autonomous social services.

facilities operate at very low capacity. In other words, the low volume of output results in significant unused capacity that in turn can respond to low demand. As expected, SE scores for each organizational arrangement of the 50+ bed sample are significantly higher than for the 25+ bed sample, with hospitals under autonomous administration and for-profits leading the way. ITE scores displayed little dispersion, particularly for the 25+ bed sample. Private, for-profit hospitals received the highest scores, followed by public hospitals under direct administration. For the 50+ bed sample, nonprofit foundations and for-profit facilities registered the highest ITE scores and hospitals under direct and autonomous administration, the lowest.[49]

Comparative Performance of Public Sector Organizational Arrangements

The second analysis is of the performance of alternative and traditional hospitals in the 2002 research reported in the preceding discussion.[50] Mendes and Costa (2005), following up on Mendes et al. (2002), classified as "traditional" those facilities that were rated "hierarchical" in their organizational structure and "normative" in their organizational behavior.[51] Facilities receiving high scores for "flexible" structures and rules and "strategic" organizational behavior were termed "alternative." The two groups were matched in terms of size, inputs, outputs, and complexity (case mix).[52]

The groups' performances were compared for a subset of quality and efficiency indicators. As shown in table 5.8, for all types of mortality rates, the alternative facilities were better performers. Significant differences were found in all rates except for cardiology. These

TABLE 5.8
Comparison of Selected Quality and Efficiency Indicators, Alternative and Traditional Facilities, 2003–4

Indicator	Alternative (N = 11)		Traditional (N = 11)	
	Mean	Range	Mean	Range
Quality				
Mortality (general)*	4.6	(3.4–5.7)	8.8	(5.8–11.7)
Mortality septicemia*	28.9	(22.7–35.0)	42.7	(35.1–50.2)
Mortality (cardiology)	10.5	(8.0–13.0)	13.8	(8.8–18.7)
Mortality (diabetes)*	5.3	(2.0–8.5)	12.5	(7.9–17.0)
Mortality (surgery)**	3.6	(2.6–4.5)	6.8	(4.6–9.0)
Mortality (>age 60)*	10.9	(8.6–13.3)	17.6	(13.2–21.9)
Efficiency				
Bed turnover rate	3.0	(2.2–3.8)	3.0	(1.4–4.7)
Occupation rate	68.3	(56–81)	75.5	(57–94)
ALOS	6.9	(5.8–8.1)	7.5	(5.7–9.4)
ALOS (> age 60)	8.7	(7.4–10.0)	8.8	(6.3–11.3)
ALOS (septicemia)	12.6	(10.5–14.7)	8.8	(3.1–14.4)
ALOS (cardiology)	9.3	(7.2–11.4)	9.9	(7.8–12.1)
ALOS (diabetes)	8.8	(6.8–10.8)	9.5	(6.5–12.5)

Source: Mendes and Costa 2005.
*$p < .05$. **$p < .01$ (Mann-Whitney test).

results suggest that the alternative facilities provide better-quality care. Regarding efficiency, although the alternative facilities demonstrated lower occupancy rates and lower average length of stay (ALOS), except for septicemia, the differences were not found to be significant. In general, the within-group variation for both quality and efficiency data was greater for traditional facilities.

Figures 5.3 and 5.4 display the percentage change for selected mortality and efficiency indicators between 1998 and 2003 for the sample of alternative and traditional facilities. For

FIGURE 5.3

Percent Change in Selected Mortality Rates, Alternative and Traditional Hospitals, 1998–2003 (*N* = 22)

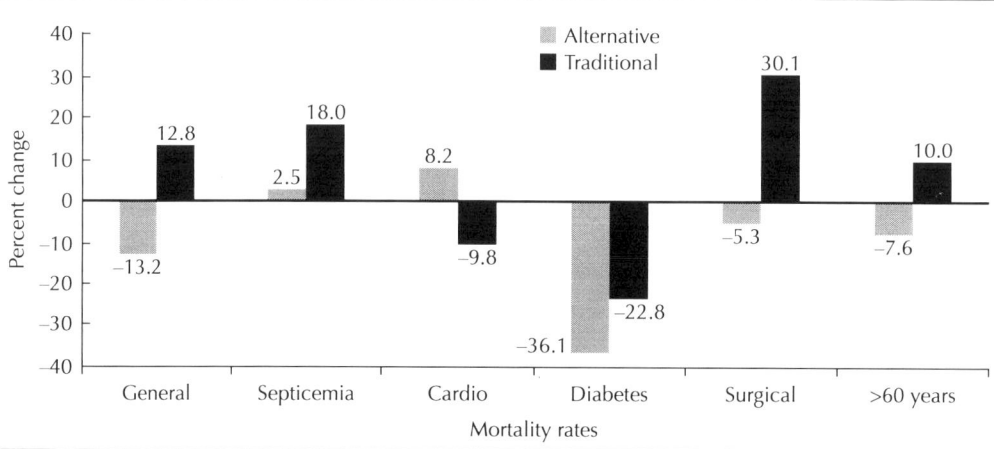

Source: Mendes and Costa 2005.

FIGURE 5.4

Percent Change in Selected Efficiency Indicators, Alternative and Traditional Hospitals, 1998–2003
(*N* = 22)

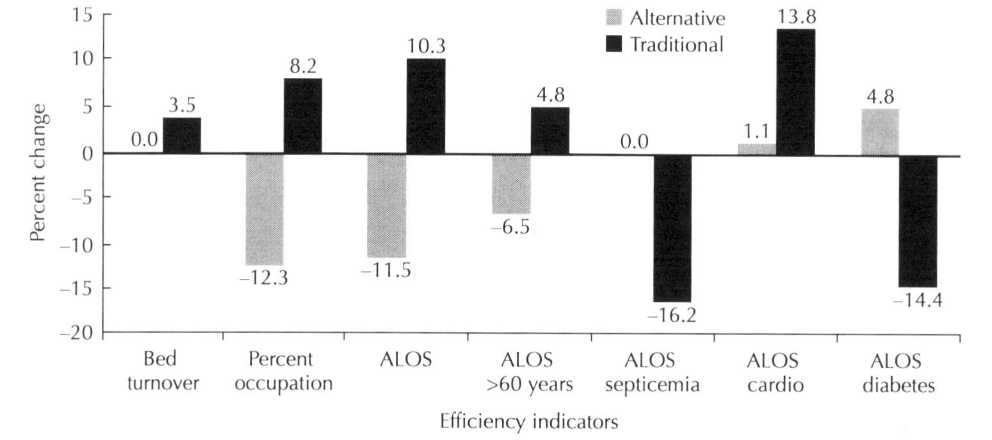

Source: Mendes and Costa 2005.

five of six mortality indicators in figure 5.3, the alternative facilities showed more favorable results: greater reductions in mortality, or increases at a lower rate than for the traditional counterparts. In four categories mortality rates actually increased in traditional hospitals. For only one category, cardiac arrest, did mortality increase for the alternative group while decreasing for the traditional facilities. Still, in 2003 the cardiovascular mortality rate was 13.8 in traditional facilities compared with 10.5 in the alternative group (not shown in figure). Although both groups made advances in reducing mortality from diabetes, the traditional group made greater gains.

Figure 5.4 shows that between 1998 and 2003 the alternative group registered decreases in occupancy rates, general ALOS, and ALOS over age 60 while showing no change in bed turnover. Over the same period the traditional facilities improved bed turnover and occupancy rates but also registered increases in general ALOS and ALOS over age 60. The traditional hospitals displayed impressive reductions in ALOS for septicemia and diabetes compared with increases or no change for the alternative group. Taken together, the alternative facilities displayed better gains for these efficiency indicators. The gains were achieved while improving quality (as measured by decreased mortality) over the same period.

Comparative Performance of OSS and Direct Administration Hospitals in São Paulo State

The performance of the OSSs can be measured in two ways: by degree of compliance with the terms of the management contract, and by comparison with other hospitals of similar size and complexity but operated under different organizational arrangements.[53]

The extent of contractual compliance is indicated by the results of the formal review of OSS performance by the state assessment commission, starting in 2002 (see table 5.9). On average, the OSSs exceeded aggregate production targets in both 2002 and 2004 except for outpatient services in 2002. In the same year, of the 12 OSS facilities, 7 reached or exceeded the targets for inpatient care; 8, for urgent care; and 6, for emergency care. Only five facilities met the target for outpatient consultants, but overall failure to achieve the aggregate target for 2002 was heavily influenced by the results for two facilities. In one of these, the state did not allocate a budget for outpatient care, and, consequently, all ambulatory care was delivered in the emergency room. The second case was a new hospital that encountered start-up delays. With these two facilities eliminated, on average the OSSs achieved the outpatient production targets in 2002. In 2004 nearly all facilities met or exceeded production targets, and the OSSs met the aggregate production target for each service. As for indicators linked to the variable component of the global budget, all facilities met targets related to information quality, care quality, and patient satisfaction in 2002 and 2004.

In 2003 São Paulo state compared 9 OSSs with 12 hospitals under direct administration organizational arrangements (5 hospitals directly managed by the state government and another 7 managed by the municipality of São Paulo). The results are presented in table 5.10. Although the hospitals were not matched for case mix, size, and spending, and the focus was mainly on financial performance, the results show that the OSSs deliver high-complexity services at lower cost.[54] The average AIH value for the OSSs—a proxy for complexity—is approximately 20 percent higher than values for the municipal and state facilities under direct administration, suggesting that the OSSs handle more complex, inpatient cases.

TABLE 5.9

Compliance with Production and Performance Targets Stipulated in OSS Management Contract, 2002 and 2004

(*N* = 12)

Production (fixed financing component)

	2002		2004	
Service	*Number meeting target[a]*	*% target reached[b]*	*Number meeting target[a]*	*% target reached[b]*
Inpatient	7	102	12	9.2
Outpatient	5	87	11	4.7
Emergency (walk-in)	8	105	10	9.1
Emergency (referrals)	6	108	11	6.4

Quality (variable financing component)

	Number of hospitals meeting target	
Assessment category[c]	*2002*	*2004*
Efficiency (ALOS)	All but 1[d]	All
Information quality	All	All
Quality of care	All	All
Patient satisfaction	All	All

Source: SES-SP 2006, 2003a.
a. Within allowable deviation bands.
b. Aggregate for all OSSs (N = 12).
c. See table 4.5 for definitions.
d. One facility did not meet the target for ALOS for normal births and consequently was penalized 2.5 percent of the variable budget.

TABLE 5.10

Comparison of Selected Hospitals under State and Municipal Direct Management with OSS-Managed Facilities, 2003

Indicator	*Municipal direct administration (N = 7)*	*State direct administration (N = 5)*	*OSS (N = 9)*
Average number of beds	254	200	211
Average number of annual discharges	6,684	9,636	11,904
Average number of discharges/bed	26.3	48.1	56.4
ALOS	6.5	5.3	5.5
Occupancy (%)	50.1	70.1	87.0
Average AIH (R$)	344	335	415
Average monthly spending, per facility (R$ millions)	N/A	2.90	2.75
Average monthly spending/discharge (R$)	N/A	3,603	2,774
Average monthly spending/bed (R$)	N/A	14,476	13,047

Source: State of São Paulo, CCSS and CGA database.
Note: N/A, not available.

The OSSs are also more productive as measured by discharges per bed, but their ALOS is slightly higher than in the state facilities under direct administration. Significantly, in per-facility and per-bed spending, the OSSs are the better deal, even though they provide more complex care. This raises the issue of quality; for example, are the OSSs cheaper because they maintain lower quality standards? As will be seen below, however, the OSSs display higher performance, based on selected quality indicators.

A second study rigorously matched 12 OSS facilities with 12 direct administration hospitals of similar complexity and compared performance data for 2003 and 2004. None of the hospitals in the sample were teaching facilities, and there was no significant difference between the two groups in the average number of beds, total spending, spending per bed, or number of professionals per bed.[55] The hospitals were also similar in terms of complexity.

The comparative performance results are presented in table 5.11. On the quality indicators, general and surgical mortality rates were lower in the OSSs, but the differences were only marginally significant ($p < .10$). Pediatric morality was slightly higher in the OSSs (2.8 vs. 2.6) but not significantly so. Three of the 12 OSSs are accredited, and several are working toward accreditation. None of the direct administration facilities have been accredited, nor are they seeking accreditation.

Turning to efficiency, the OSSs demonstrated significantly better performance on bed turnover rate (annual number of discharges per bed), bed substitution rate (average number of days a bed remains unoccupied between patients), bed occupancy, and ALOS. The OSSs use about one-third fewer physicians (full-time equivalent: $p < .05$) and one-third more nurses (full-time equivalent: $p < .10$) than the direct administration facilities. The substitution of nurses for physicians is consistent with international best practice and probably contributes to the lower expenditures described below.

The OSSs are significantly more productive as measured by general, surgical, and clinical discharges per bed. Given that average total expenditures are comparable for both groups of facility, the higher productivity drives lower unit costs. OSSs spend less per bed-day and per discharge, although only the latter was found significant. These production and spending results are consistent with the state-sponsored research described above.

For the entire sample of facilities, spending was highly correlated with production ($r = 0.66$), as measured by inpatient discharges. A regression analysis sought to determine the impact of additional spending on production for each category of hospital. Consistent with the efficiency results above, the findings showed that a 1 percent increase in spending would result in a 0.47 percent increase in inpatient discharges for OSS facilities, compared with a 0.22 percent increase for direct administration.

Although the two comparative studies are based on small samples, the results, taken together, suggest that the OSSs are more productive and efficient and provide higher-quality care than the comparison facilities.[56] In addition, they are a better bargain, as measured by value for money. The state-sponsored study also demonstrated that per-bed spending is lower, partly because of higher productivity but also because of a more appropriate personnel mix (e.g., nurse/physician ratios). The DEA analysis discussed earlier, which used a much larger sample of hospitals, also supports the superior efficiency findings observed in the OSSs. As practiced in São Paulo state, OSS is a robust alternative model for the organization and delivery of hospital care in public facilities. It should be noted, however, that the OSSs of São Paulo were implemented in new facilities and with strong political support.

TABLE 5.11

Comparison of Selected Quality and Efficiency Indicators, Hospitals under OSS and Direct Administration Arrangements, São Paulo State, 2003

Indicator	OSS hospitals (N = 12)		Direct administration hospitals (N = 12)[a]	
	Mean	Range	Mean	Range
Quality (mortality rate)				
General*	3.3	2.7–5.8	5.3	3.2–9.1
Surgical*	2.6	1.7–4.8	3.6	0.9–10.3
Clinical	11.6	9.5–14.0	12.0	10.7–14.1
Pediatric	2.8	1.7–4.2	2.6	1.1–4.9
Allocative efficiency (hours: full-time equivalent)[b]				
Physician**	143	95–273	203	90–339
Nurse	54	24–100	41	7–64
Auxiliary	234	78–385	257	89–391
Efficiency: descriptive statistics				
Bed turnover rate***	5.2	3.7–7.6	3.3	1.9–4.8
Bed substitution rate***	1.2	0.1–3.8	3.9	1.7–9.7
Bed occupancy rate**	81	52–99	63	38–76
ALOS**	4.2	3.8–5.6	5.4	4.1–8.1
ALOS surgery*	4.8	3.0–5.7	5.9	2.3–7.7
Technical efficiency (discharges/bed)				
General***	60	43–94	46	32–73
Surgical**	71	24–103	44	27–84
Clinical**	86	25–198	53	17–101
GYN/OB (N = 20)*	96	34–169	58	24–80
Annual spending (R$ thousands)				
Expenditures/bed	177	116–279	187	149–227
Expenditures/discharge**	2.9	2.3–3.9	4.3	2.9–7.0

Source: Costa and Mendes 2005.
a. For allocative efficiency and descriptive statistics, N = 10.
b. Full time equivalent = total hours/40 for nurses and total houses/20 for physicians.
*$p < .10$. **$p < .05$. ***$p < .01$.

Summary Assessment

Looking back over Brazil's organizational landscape during the past 25 years, the hospital sector can best be described as one in permanent transition, with its future direction still unclear. The first wave of "indirect" administrative reforms under the military regime granted considerable autonomy to hospital facilities, but these reforms were heavily criticized by subsequent democratic governments for enabling clientelistic patronage practices. Other observers suggest that the earlier reforms gave managers unfettered control over inputs and outputs, resulting in bloated payrolls and limited participation in the broader health system. The constitutional reforms of the late 1980s resulted in a policy shift manifested in back-pedaling on autonomous management under indirect administration and in the expansion of the hierarchical direct administration model.[57] Only a handful of public hospitals from the earlier period were able to maintain their decision-making authority. At the same time, the health system was being decentralized. Decentralization empowered governors and mayors, but decision-making rights were not transferred to the service delivery level. Decentralization did not involve organizational arrangements, governance, or management. Nearly all municipalities adopted the direct administration model, in part to facilitate compliance with procurement, financial management, and civil service legislation. Few had any experience or capacity in hospital management or in oversight of autonomous facilities.

The administrative reforms of the mid-1990s put autonomy back on the policy agenda with the passage of legislation promoting social organizations. Although the federal government appears unwilling to implement these reforms, partly for fear of the reaction of public employee unions, some states and, to a lesser extent, municipalities are taking the lead in exploring the social organization model and other autonomous alternatives to direct and indirect administration. Federal support for these efforts could catalyze and extend innovation nationwide. The social organization model is aligned with organizational reforms in public hospitals in Europe (see box 5.4 and annex 5E).

Box 5.4
Toward Greater Independence of Public Hospitals: Lessons from Europe

---

Direct hierarchical management of public hospitals remains a major organizational form in Brazil and in other countries of Latin America, but this is not the case elsewhere. Although the direct public management form was originally adapted from unitary public systems in European countries, particularly Spain and Portugal, today this arrangement is the least prominent model for public hospital organization in Europe. A variety of models has emerged. Many are hybrids, occupying a middle ground between semiautonomous and fully autonomous organizations. Some have significant decision-making authority over key managerial functions such as planning, budgeting, and human resource management. In other cases managerial autonomy has been increased by replacing line-item budgets with global budgets, and in still others public hospitals operate more like private organizations in which managers possess full decision-making authority but are responsible for the bottom line and are exposed to competitive pressures. In nearly all countries governments have introduced some form of purchasing arrangement in which performance targets are specified in contracts or intergovernmental covenants. In parallel with the introduction of organizational reforms and purchasing arrangements, countries have reformed hospital payment systems and placed increased emphasis on systematic measurement and comparative benchmarking of performance.

Annex 5E outlines organizational forms and their features in European public hospitals. Several countries have traditionally granted public hospitals wide decision-making authority over input and budget management. Austria, Belgium, and Germany are examples of countries in which public hospitals possess nearly full autonomy for input management, including hiring and firing of personnel, material purchasing, and budget management. But exposure to market pressures may be limited (e.g., hospitals may be unable to charge fees or make a profit). The Baltic states, Italy,

(continued)

Box 5.4 *(continued)*

Portugal, the Scandinavian countries, Spain, and the United Kingdom have gradually enlarged their hospitals' decision-making rights and responsibilities. These reforms have been accompanied by the introduction of purchasing arrangements that include the "internal" contracting of facilities to set explicit performance targets. In Spain several areas of the country are experimenting with alternative forms of public ownership such as foundations, consortiums, and public firms. The Baltic countries have restructured the previously state-owned hospitals into public enterprises that are able to contract with the government and with social insurance institutions. Finally, some of the newly independent states of Central and Eastern Europe still directly manage public hospitals, exerting direct hierarchical control over them, while others have transferred some decision-making authority for purchasing nonlabor inputs and for determining output mix. Traditionally, directors in public hospitals in the former Soviet Union wield considerable managerial power.

Implementing organizational reforms in public hospitals is a hugely complex task. As reviewed in this chapter, the OSS experience in São Paulo was facilitated by the fact that the reform was introduced only in new facilities. Introducing alternative organizational arrangements in existing facilities is much more difficult. In a review of European experience with more autonomous organizational structures, Maarse et al. (2005: 271) provide a cogent summary of the hospital reform process:

> In many countries, a strong reluctance to undertake large-scale reforms can be observed. The common pattern seems to be that governments move in incremental steps. Hospitals with budgetary structures have been converted to [more] autonomous hospitals [e.g., with control over non-labor inputs], which in turn have been transformed into [fully autonomous] models [e.g., with full control over all inputs, including labor]. Many governments, it appears, remain convinced that hospitals should keep their public status and that privatization will undermine the public goals of cost control, equity and affordability.

Source: Figueras, Robinson, and Jakubowski 2005; Preker and Langenbrunner 2005; Jakab et al. 2002; Ham and Hawkins 2003.

Is this second wave of organizational reforms sustainable? Although the government of Luiz Inácio Lula da Silva that came to power in 2003 has not supported the OSS organizational reforms initiated by the preceding government—now the political opposition—it has done little to stop them. In fact, given that all levels of government face high debt, tax burdens, and spending, financial authorities are increasingly seeking greater control of public expenditures. Recent pronouncements by finance and treasury officials make it clear that improving the "quality of public spending" is a major policy objective of the second Lula government (2007–11). The MS, for example, is considering a number of measures to contain rising costs, including reforming public hospitals along the lines of the OSS model.[58] It is, however, important to note that the sustainability of the São Paulo OSS model could be enhanced through implementation of facility-based governance structures, as mandated in the state law.

Public hospital reform is also an increasingly relevant topic at the subnational level. As noted in chapter 2, over the last 15 years municipalities and states have assumed a growing share of total public financing for health, while the federal government is financing a declining share. Hospitals represent the big spenders in subnational health systems, and states and municipalities are searching for ways to improve the quality of health spending, in part through hospital reform. Some states, such as Minas Gerais and Ceará, are adopting a public management reform program known as management shock (*choque de gestão*) that aims to curb cost escalation by putting tight controls on personnel and operating costs.[59] Both have recently introduced OSSs in new hospitals. Other states, including Amazonas and Rio de Janeiro, are considering OSS-type reforms to improve the efficiency and quality of public hospitals as part of a broader public management reform effort.

Organizational Arrangements and Performance in Public Hospitals

Organizational arrangements make a difference to hospital performance, as shown by the evidence presented in this chapter. This is especially true for public facilities. Public hospitals operating under autonomous organizational models display higher production, efficiency, and quality than facilities in which managers have little or no decision-making authority. They also appear to achieve greater gains in efficiency and quality over time than nonautonomous facilities. The worst-performing hospitals in Brazil are public hospitals under direct administration.

The most promising arrangement is that of the health social organizations (*organizações sociais de saúde*) implemented in São Paulo state. Their efficiency rivals that of for-profit, private hospitals. These high-performing public hospitals, founded under private law, receive state funds to provide services specified in a management contract. They do not follow public rules related to procurement, human resource management, financial management, or contracting. Managers have full autonomy regarding input management but are accountable to the state (and their boards) for providing specified service volumes, supplying financial and production data, and complying with quality benchmarks specified in the management contract. Accountability is reinforced through a financing system whereby a proportion of funding is tied to compliance with service volume targets and quality standards. Significantly, São Paulo state has in fact enforced contracts by withholding or denying payments to hospitals out of compliance with contractual provisions.

Hospitals with the independence and flexibility to manage inputs, set case mix, adjust capacity, reallocate resources, and perform other managerial functions are better performers than their counterparts without such independence. But independence alone may not be sufficient for improving performance; it must be accompanied by direct accountability mechanisms that lead managers to focus on results. Accountability mechanisms introduced in public facilities in Brazil include public performance-based contracting and financing, governance structures, contract management and monitoring, and market exposure.

The forms of autonomous hospitals reviewed here demonstrate that autonomy is difficult to define or categorize. For example, São Paulo hospitals under OSS arrangements do not have decision rights over setting fees, acquiring or selling capital assets, or selling services to third parties, but they do enjoy decision rights regarding labor, materials, service specification, outputs, and managerial processes. This suggests that autonomy is not an all-or-nothing attribute. Some decision rights may be more important than others in driving performance. Because hospital care is particularly labor-intensive, decision-making authority with respect to labor may be a key factor.[60]

Organizational Arrangements and Performance in Private Hospitals

The constitutional reforms protected the legal personality and private regime (*direito privado*) of nonprofit hospitals. In addition, the 1988 Constitution permits public financing of private facilities, and most nonprofits remain highly dependent on public financing. A not insignificant share of nonprofits is, however, out of compliance with legislation regarding governance and certification.

Private hospitals face a different set of problems than their public counterparts. The DEA scores indicate that nonprofits exhibit an intermediate level of efficiency between public direct administration hospitals and for-profit facilities. Their efficiency scores are similar to those of public facilities under indirect administration but below those under autonomous arrangements. Because information is lacking, no definitive statement can be made about the relation between the various organizational arrangements found among nonprofits (e.g., foundations, associations), but it appears that overlapping governance and management functions in nonprofit hospitals may compromise performance. Decision making among many nonprofits, particularly the smaller facilities, appears to be informal. Only larger hospitals have formal organizational structures, apply modern business practices, possess full-time management teams, and demonstrate separation between governance and management practices. Modernization of governance and managerial practices is a major challenge facing the nonprofit hospital subsector.

The experience of nonprofit hospitals in the United States provides some indication of the future direction of nonprofit facilities in Brazil (box 5.5). In a sense, nonprofit hospitals in Brazil hark back to a not-so-distant period in U.S. medicine in which nonprofit facilities were essentially physician workshops. In Brazil as in the United States, the formerly tight control by the trustees of umbrella charitable organizations has vanished and, arguably, has been passed on to physicians. A hypothesis worth exploring is that an undetermined number of nonprofit facilities in Brazil serve physician interests and are governed by physicians or their proxies. Management has not been a major concern, and this has impeded the professionalization of hospital managers, especially in smaller facilities—the vast majority of nonprofits. Local physician politicians with strong ties to nonprofits help small hospitals survive by securing government bailouts despite very low utilization (see the discussion of bailouts in chapter 4). Without competitive or performance-based contract pressures, this situation may continue into the foreseeable future.

Some Caveats

Except for the DEA analysis, most of the results discussed here draw on studies involving small samples. This is a consequence of the general lack of information available in direct administration hospitals, which requires researchers to conduct extended on-site visits to collect data. In some cases facilities were dropped from sample designs because even site visits did not yield enough information for comparative analysis. Direct administration systems in Brazil are information poor because managers are accountable for compliance with rules rather than for results.

Box 5.5
Managerial Modernization of Nonprofit Hospitals: Lessons from the United States

Like nonprofit facilities in Brazil in the late 1990s and early 2000s, nonprofit charitable hospitals in the United States faced an increasingly competitive environment in the 1970s and 1980s. The change was driven by new government payment policies that decreased reimbursement rates; the emergence of HMOs and other organizations intent on containing costs and therefore reducing demand for hospital care; changes in the legal and regulatory framework; and the growth of profit-making hospital chains. According to Starr (1982: 431–32), the emergence of for-profit chains contributed to the managerial modernization of U.S. hospitals. They introduced "standardized management practices, standardized accounting and other uniform services. These tendencies [were] as a rule less advanced in the nonprofit sector."

This environment eventually led to closings, takeovers by for-profit conglomerates, formation of nonprofit hospital systems, and mergers among nonprofit facilities. Of equal importance, nonprofits had to adapt business practices similar to those of for-profit corporations, modernizing their managerial and governance practices. To adapt to the incentives emerging from the external environment, the nonprofits had to strengthen their know-how in areas such as financial restructuring, cost accounting, clinical and nonclinical management, pricing, contract negotiation, process standardization, and measurement of data on efficiency and quality. Although the nonprofit sector has a long history of adapting to shifting external environments, Stevens (1989: 290) notes that nonprofit hospitals were no longer able "... to sit complacently, like medieval manor houses, on a rich and rightful social domain. The domain itself was being reconsidered."

As in the United States a couple of decades ago, charity as a founding principle of nonprofit hospitals is fast disappearing in Brazil and is being replaced by a business ethos. With the notion of business comes the notion of financial success, as well as the business practices required to achieve it. The informality of managerial and governance practices observed among philanthropic and charitable organizations in Brazil is unsuitable for the changing external environment.

Sources: Stevens 1989; Starr 1982.

The comparative analyses presented here examined the mean performance of groups of hospitals closely matched in size, inputs, and complexity. In fairness, a few direct administration facilities were found to be high performers, and some hospitals under autonomous arrangements were low performers. Further research using larger samples is needed to understand the relation between organizational arrangements and performance for these apparent outliers. Another major research gap concerns how governance and management practices affect performance in private hospitals.

Linkages between organizational arrangements, managerial behaviors, and performance, and particularly how the inherent incentive structure affects managerial practices and drives high performance, are explored in the next chapter.

Annex 5A

Organizational Arrangements in Public and Private Hospitals in Brazil: Summary

This annex reviews in a concise way the various organizational forms found in Brazil's hospital sector.

Direct Administration

Hospitals under direct administration are owned and operated by federal, state, and municipal governments. According to the Preker and Harding (2003) framework, they are "budgetary" organizations; they are generally financed through a direct budget allocation, often determined using historical criteria. Some facilities operating as independent budgetary units may also receive financing through the Authorization for Hospitalization (Autorização de Internação Hospitalar, AIH) reimbursement system. This is usually achieved through private support foundations in partnership with the facility (see below). Managers, who are political appointees, generally have little decision-making authority regarding human resources, investments, and contracting of auxiliary and hotel services. Human resource management and procurement must follow the rules stipulated in Laws 8122 and 8666; tasks in these categories may be embedded in the overall government apparatus and managed by administrative and finance secretariats. This is particularly true in states and municipalities. Personnel are government employees rather than hospital employees and are entitled to job stability. Pay scales are uniform for each category of worker—doctors, nurses, administrators, and so on. Monitoring is performed by government health authorities.

Indirect Administration

The array of arrangements offered by the indirect administration model confers more discretionary authority than the direct administration model, and organizations in this category can be classified as "autonomized." They enjoy nonprofit status if they provide social services. All were covered by Decree Law 200 of 1967 and were originally granted varying levels of autonomy, as discussed below. In most models, specific laws are necessary. The 1988 Constitution and the subsequent legislation subordinated these organizations to public labor, contracting, and procurement law, so that for these processes there is little difference between the direct and indirect models. Nevertheless, indirect administration organizations retain authority to tap nonfiscal financing, retain unspent revenues, and shift funds among budgetary areas. Directors are political appointees and answer hierarchically to the appointing government authority. Indirect administration organizations fall into several categories, as follows.

- *Autonomous management unit* (*autarquia*). This "decentralized administration" arrangement has been applied to organizations in a number of sectors, including hospitals and universities. Each autarquia is established through special legislation and is an independent budgetary unit with legal personality. Directors are political appointees. Governments control internal staffing decisions, which must abide by public labor legislation.

- *Autonomous management unit under special regime* (*autarquia de regime especial*). This arrangement, similar to the autarquia, has not yet been applied to hospitals. An advantage of this variant over the autarquia is that the managing director is appointed by the executive branch of government and confirmed by the legislature, affording some management stability across governments because replacing directors requires legislative approval. This form also enjoys residual claimant status.

- *Public foundation* (*fundação pública*). The public foundation is similar to the autarquia with respect to discretionary authority. These organizations were formerly common arrangements for indirect administration. They were founded through specific legislation and were subject to public labor and procurement rules. This type of arrangement is still common in the health sector; examples include the Hospital Foundation of Minas Gerais (FHEMIG) and parastatals such as the Oswaldo Cruz Foundation (FIOCRUZ) and the National Health Foundation (FUNASA). Facilities may retain budgetary savings as well as revenues from other sources, and procedures are currently similar to those of autarquias.

Autonomous Administration

Most autonomous administration arrangements have appeared during the last 15 years. Managers usually have considerable control over inputs, resource use, and production, compared with their counterparts under the direct and indirect models. All forms apply private labor and contracting law. In some, managers still respond hierarchically to government, but control is less direct. In at least one model, accountability for results is specified in performance contracts. These arrangements are best classified as corporatized organizations, although there are some differences between them and private organizations. Four types of autonomous administration are found among public hospitals, as follows:

- *Autonomous social services* (*serviços sociais autônomos, SSAs*). This form answers hierarchically to the executive branch of government. There are two major kinds of financing: budget transfers established through congressional law, and contributions from private insurers. The property is owned by the organization, which is governed by a board of trustees. These parastatal organizations are established through special legislation and enjoy great autonomy; they are not subordinated to a specific public authority except for financial reporting. SSAs are usually specialized organizations that direct their activities to specific beneficiaries. The most autonomous facilities under this form are a few public institutions that benefit from considerable prestige and political support. One such case in the health sector is the Rede Sarah Kubitschek, a network of inpatient and outpatient rehabilitation facilities that provides free specialized care.

- *Public firm (empresa pública)*. In some databases this arrangement is referred to as mixed economy enterprises (*empresas de economia mista*). Government is the major or sole holder of the organization's stock (voting capital), and management reports hierarchically to government. Private sector shareholders are residual claimants. This arrangement is uncommon in the social sectors. As in the case of autarquias and SSAs, each public enterprise requires special legislation and is an independent budgetary unit with legal personality. The arrangement offers no tax advantages over more traditional corporate forms. From a legal standpoint, this arrangement is best applied to an economic rather than a public service enterprise. It is an autonomous arrangement, and as a firm it can apply civil or private laws for labor, contracting, and procurement. This form has lost popularity since decentralization, but it has been applied to a few prestigious hospitals with strong political support, particularly in Rio Grande do Sul state.

* *Support foundations (fundações de apoio)*. Support foundations are private entities legally linked to public hospitals that typically operate under direct administration. Most highly specialized public teaching hospitals have adopted this arrangement. The foundations enable the facilities to circumvent public recruitment, staffing, remuneration, and procurement rules and to secure additional financing by selling services to the private sector (private insurers) or to other public entities. In some cases the foundations receive financing directly from government. The foundations generally focus on hiring additional personnel and paying bonuses to professional staff to complement government salaries. A general complaint is that they have been captured by medical professionals in order to "top off" salaries. Other criticisms include lack of transparency in financial management and the creation of a stratified delivery system within public facilities. Despite these concerns, the number of private foundations grew considerably in the 1990s.

* *Social organizations (organizações sociais, OSs)*. The OS is the most recent addition to the organizational landscape. Driven by the administrative reforms of the 1990s and established by the federal government in 1995, the arrangement consists of the contracting of nonprofit organizations to manage publicly owned hospitals. As practiced in São Paulo state, management contracts are competitively let. The winning organizations are issued a performance contract (with performance retainer) and a global budget. OSs apply private regimes for human resource management (Consolidação das Leis do Trabalho, CLT) and do not follow public procurement rules. Managers answer to a governance board of the nonprofit organization. OSs are dependent on government for investment financing, which is not included in the performance contract and the corresponding budget. A similar arrangement appeared in the late 1990s in the form of public interest social organizations (*organização de sociedade civil de interese público*, OSCIP) established in Law 9.790/99 under direct regulation by the Ministry of Justice.

Nonprofit Organizations

* *Philanthropic associations and charitable and benevolent societies*. These societies consist of hospitals affiliated with nonprofit, voluntary organizations that own and operate facilities. Most are highly dependent on Unified Health System (Sistema Único de Saúde, SUS) financing. Nonprofit organizations have a legally mandated governance structure with one or more statutory executives or trustees. These are part-time, pro bono positions. Each organization determines the role and responsibilities of its statutory executives with respect to facility management according to its by-laws. In a minority of cases

the organizations have boards that meet regularly and on which the statutory executives sit, and in other cases the statutory executives meet irregularly or informally to review the financial performance of the facility. In a significant share of nonprofit hospitals, voluntary organization executives carry out both governance and management functions.

- *Private foundations.* Little information is available on this organizational arrangement. All private foundations are maintained by private voluntary organizations or charitable societies. Anecdotal evidence suggests that there is little difference in governance and management practices between facilities under this model and the above-described associations. All foundations need to have governance boards. Foundations are regulated by the foundation purveyor (*provedoria das fundações*) in the Attorney General's Office (Ministério Público).

- *Professional associations.* These are mainly cooperatives of health professionals that own or manage hospitals. Under Brazilian law cooperatives are nonprofit, voluntary organizations. As is typical of cooperatives elsewhere, an assembly of members elects a board that constitutes the governance structure. In some cases board members exercise management functions. Relatively few cooperatives manage publicly financed facilities. More common are cooperatives that have public contracts to provide hotel and diagnostic services and, to a lesser extent, medical care. (Cooperatives also operate a number of private health maintenance organizations, or HMOs, and are then financed privately.) The publicly financed model is in jeopardy; the cooperatives' nonprofit tax status has been challenged in federal and state courts, and the Attorney General's Office is insisting that to receive public financing, a cooperative must win a public competition. Evidently, few are willing to compete. These organizations are regulated by the Justice Department.

- *Unions.* Health worker unions operate a small minority of facilities and also contract to provide specific services in public hospitals. Little is known about this model. Union-provided services are in rapid decline in the private sector because cooperative and privately managed health plans have become dominant. This model is regulated by the Labor Ministry.

For-Profit Organizations

- *Corporations.* The corporation is the most common arrangement in Brazilian hospitals. Corporations may be under limited or public ownership. The former are closely held enterprises; the latter issue equity shares to the public. Both distribute profits (residual claims). Little is known about governance arrangements and management practices in for-profit hospitals. Most large corporations maintain a governance structure such as a board of trustees. Such arrangements are rare for smaller firms with limited ownership.

Matrix: Features of Organizational Arrangements in Public Hospitals in Brazil

Organizational features	Direct administration	Indirect administration		Autonomous administration			
		Autonomous management unit	Public foundation	Autonomous social service	Public enterprise	Private support foundation (fundação de apoio)	Health social organization
AUTONOMY (decision-making rights) • Labor • Capital • Other inputs • Performance (targets) • Managerial processes	**Very limited** • Fully subject to hierarchical control. • Some managers can secure influence over personnel decisions because of ties to political authority. • Some states allow facility-based procurement in large facilities.	**Limited** • Possess decision-making authority regarding staff mix, service mix, budgetary management, and administrative processes. • Can set fees for non-SUS patients. • Subordinated to public administration rules for recruitment, salaries, and procurement. • Purchasing of supplies may be managed by state, municipal, or federal government. • No decision-making rights over assets or capital investments.		**High (full or nearly full autonomy)** • Possess decision-making authority regarding all inputs, including recruitment, dismissal, salaries and incentives, and material input purchases. • Able to define all internal managerial and supervisory processes, including setting financial and technical performance targets. • Evidence of managerial innovation (social organizations) • Set fees for non-SUS patients (except for social organizations). • Capital investment decisions dependent on government financing for all arrangements except private foundations and public enterprises. The latter organizations, however, rarely finance large investments.			

MARKET EXPOSURE	Very limited	Limited	Moderate	High	High	Moderate
• Revenues linked to productivity and performance • Access to capital • Negotiation with suppliers	• Funded through historical budgets. • Directors are political appointees. • Some revenues are indirectly tied to production through AIH payment system, but incentive is distorted by multiple payment systems.	• Financed mainly through historical budgets, but some revenues indirectly tied to production through AIH payment system. • Directors are political appointees. • Can sell services to private payers and other public institutions, but exposure to the market through sale of services is limited.	• Financed mainly through historical budgets but sell services to individuals, to private insurers, and to other public institutions. • Negotiate with input suppliers. • Most directors are political appointees. • Provide free services.	• Financed mainly through historical budgets but sell services to individuals, to private insurers, and to other public institutions. • Market exposure is evident, but contracted entities generally benefit from monopoly position in facility. • Negotiate with input suppliers. • Provide free services.	• Specialize in tapping resources from nonbudgetary sources, such as private prepayment plans (overall purpose) but can also receive budgetary allocations. • Negotiate with input suppliers. • Access nonpublic sources of capital.	• Financed mainly through global budget (from government), linked to production. (Portion of financing at risk.) • In most cases not permitted to sell services. • Negotiate with input suppliers. • Access private sources of capital. • Provide free services to SUS patients only.

(continued)

Organizational features	Direct administration	Indirect administration		Autonomous administration			
		Autonomous management unit	Public foundation	Autonomous social service	Public enterprise	Private support foundation (fundação de apoio)	Health social organization
ACCOUNTABILITY • To patients • To payers • To owners • To regulators	**Very limited** • Hierarchical supervision centers on financial, purchasing, and administrative processes. • Objectives and performance targets generally unspecified. • No results orientation. • Participation in irregular government programs to survey patient satisfaction.	**Very limited** (similar to direct administration model).		**Moderate** • Strong in-house supervision (management responds to board of trustees). • Results orientation (of private contracts) focuses on production but not necessarily quality. • Hierarchical supervision by government centers with respect to financial, purchasing, and administrative processes.	**Moderate** • Management accountable to board of trustees. • Results orientation (of private contracts) focuses on production but not necessarily on quality.	**Moderate** • Accountable to associated public hospital board and state attorney-generals' offices (*ministério público estadual*). • Focus on production. • Managers appointed and supervised by board, but supervision appears lax. • Results orientation may be specified in contracts with private payers.	**High** • Managers appointed and supervised by board of NGO, but accountability arrangement appears to be pro forma. • Strong results orientation through management contract and performance-based financing mechanism with government. • Focus on production, quality, and financial performance.

RESIDUAL CLAIMANT STATUS • Retention of "savings" • Responsibility for "losses"	**Very limited** • Unable to retain unspent budgetary revenue. • Losses can be shifted to government.	**Moderate** • Able to retain unspent budgetary revenue and "savings" from sale of services; losses can be shifted to government.		**Moderate** • Can retain unspent budgetary revenue and "savings" from sale of services, but losses can be shifted to government (except for support foundations).	**High** • Able to retain unspent budgetary revenue. • Losses cannot be automatically shifted to government.
SOCIAL FUNCTIONS • Responsibility to cover SUS patients • Unfunded mandates	**Implicit** • Mission often implicit: provide "free" (subsidized) care to SUS population. However, there is evidence of use of high-complexity care by high-income groups for procedures not covered by private insurers. • Unfunded or underfunded mandates common.	**Implicit** • Social functions stipulated in legislation creating the entity, but they are not distinguishable from those for direct administration.	**Implicit** • Provide subsidized care to entire population for general services. • Social functions stipulated in legislation creating the entity. • Unfunded or underfunded mandates common.	**Explicit** • Cross-subsidize care provided to poor through offsetting deficits and low salaries.	**Explicit** • Specified in performance contract. • Government subsidy based on real costs of care.

(continued)

		Indirect administration		Autonomous administration			
Organizational features	Direct administration	Autonomous management unit	Public foundation	Autonomous social service	Public enterprise	Private support foundation (fundação de apoio)	Health social organization
LEGAL AND REGULATORY FRAMEWORK	• Subject to public labor, contracting, and procurement laws.	• Each facility (or network) established as separate legal entity through special legislation. • Subject to public labor, contracting, and procurement laws.		• Each facility (or network) established as separate legal entity. • Private employment and contracting law. • Under political and legal pressure to follow public administrative regime for labor, procurement, and contracting.		• Created by statutory act and approved by federal Attorney-General's office (Ministério Público). • Not subject to public labor, contracting, and procurement law because funding is not governmental.	• Categorical arrangement established through government legislation. • Not subject to public labor, contracting, and procurement law.

SUMMARY ASSESSMENT

| ADVANTAGES | • Budgetary stability, particularly for personnel and investments. | • Budgetary stability, particularly for personnel and investments. • Retain residual claims and nonbudgetary revenues. • Potential for higher performance than direct administration, but variation is considerable. | | • Sustainable model (as long as political support continues). • Application of private labor and procurement regimes. | • Application of private labor and procurement regimes. • Budgetary stability and sustainable investments. | • Provides additional revenue to complement budgetary allocations. • Fosters retention of professional staff. • Fast track for professional recruitment and incentives. | • High performance in terms of quality, efficiency, and patient satisfaction. • Robust information environment. • Application of private labor and procurement regimes. |

DISADVANTAGES	• Subject to politicized decision making. • Low performance and high inefficiency because of incentive environment. • Absence of information. • Diffuse accountability.	• Nearly indistinguishable from direct administration. • Subject to politicized decision making. • Absence of information. • Diffuse accountability.	• Requires specific legislation. • Model dependent on one-time political support. • Unknown performance and weak accountability. • Not results oriented.	• Rarely used in hospitals. • Requires specific legislation. • Unknown performance and weak accountability. • Not results oriented.	• Evidence of capture by professional groups. • Absence of information. • Possible conflict of interest with mission of public hospital. • Bypasses instead of dealing with problems of direct administration. • In practice, model limited to new facilities. • Performance dependent on government capacity to manage contracts and monitor results.
ORGANIZATIONAL CLASSIFICATION	Budgetary organization	Semiautonomous ("autonomized") organization	Fully autonomous ("corporatized") organization	Hybrid organization (fully autonomous parallel organization)	Fully autonomous ("corporatized") organization

Note: AIH, Autorização de Internação Hospitalar (Authorization for Hospitalization); NGO, nongovernmental organization; SUS, Sistema Único de Saúde (Unified Health System).

Annex 5C
Methods for Analysis of Alternative and Traditional Hospitals

The discussion describes the characteristics of traditional and alternative hospitals examined in the Mendes and Costa (2005) study that was undertaken for this report. It then looks at the facilities' comparative performance.

Matching Alternative and Traditional Hospitals

Table 5C.1 shows that no significant differences were found between matching alternative and traditional hospitals with respect to average bed size, professional personnel per bed, physicians per bed, and nurses per bed. As expected, all traditional hospitals serve Unified Health System (Sistema Único de Saúde, SUS) patients exclusively, while seven of the non-traditional facilities serve a mix of SUS and privately insured patients.

Of the 13 traditional hospitals in the original sample, 12 were teaching facilities, whereas 7 of the 13 alternative hospitals were teaching facilities. This difference was found to be marginally significant ($p < .10$). Teaching hospitals generally receive more complex cases, suggesting that traditional hospitals treat more severe cases, but further testing suggests that this is only partially true. Several proxies for complexity were used: percentage of inpatients over age 60, Authorization for Hospitalization (Autorização de Internação Hospitalar, AIH) values, percentage of patients referred from other municipalities, and ratio of male to female inpatients. The percentage of inpatients over age 60 and the percentage of patients from other municipalities were not found to be significantly different between the two groups.[61] Although alternative facilities had higher average AIH values (general, surgical, and for inpatients over age 60), suggesting higher complexity, the difference between the two groups was insignificant. Traditional hospitals usually have a higher male to female ratio of inpatients than the alternative facilities, but the difference was insignificant. This suggests that alternative facilities may provide a higher proportion of maternal care, while traditional facilities may treat a higher proportion of trauma and chronic cases. In sum, the two groups are comparable in terms of complexity.

Comparative Performance of Alternative and Traditional Hospitals

The performance analysis was applied to 22 hospitals, 11 from each group. One alternative hospital was eliminated because it was an outlier. Another alternative facility and two traditional facilities were dropped because of lack of data.

The cost analysis was based on the AIH values adjusted for real procedure costs secured from a costing study performed in a separate sample of 24 hospitals (De Matos 2002). Figures 5C.1 and 5C.2 show that the two groups of facilities matched up well with respect to

TABLE 5C.1
Summary Input Indicators, Traditional and Alternative Hospitals, 2004

Indicator	Traditional (N = 11)		Alternative (N = 11)	
	Mean	Min–max range	Mean	Min–max range
Beds				
Total	304	131–579	349	70–1,005
Surgical	168	55–352	152	22–306
Clinical	107	49–209	159	33–584
Intensive care	30	0–67	38	20–412
Physicians				
Surgeons (number)	55	22–121	48	7–128
Surgeon-hours (FTE/week)	36	19–87	39	2–139
Surgeons/bed	0.2	0.1–0.4	0.1	0.1–0.2
Internists (number)	215	111–558	280	21–1,342
Internist-hours (FTE)	144	75–443	227	10–1,332
Internists/bed	0.7	0.3–1.7	0.8	0.1–1.8
Nurses				
Total (number)	55	1–94	94	6–457
Hours (FTE)	46	1–75	90	4–464
Nurses/bed	0.2	0.1–0.4	0.3	0.1–0.6
All professionals[a]				
Total (number)	619	53–1100	961	95–3,847
Professionals/bed	2.0	0.1–4.9	2.8	1.4–5.0
Equipment use index*[b]	91	46–100	97	85–100
Complexity (proxies)[c, d]				
Average adjusted cost AIH (R$)	1,557	925–2,016	1,623	971–2,252
Average AIH general (R$)	619	503–735	759	300–1,252
Average AIH >age 60 (R$)	670	554–786	970	317–1,578
Average AIH surgery (R$)	828	672–786	1,171	438–1,985
Patients >age 60 (%)	23	18–28	20	13–30
Patients from other municipalities (%)	31	26–35	36	15–25
Ratio, male/female inpatients	126	113–139	86	50–205

Source: Mendes and Costa 2005.
Note: FTE, full time equivalent.
a. Includes physicians, nurses, nurse auxiliaries, social workers, diagnostic technicians, and other professionals.
b. Index of percentage of existing equipment in use.
c. 2003 data.
d. Cost adjusted for the 60 percent most frequent procedures as previous PLANISA studies values for real costs.
* $p < .05$ (Mann-Whitney test).

adjusted costs and AIH values; the correlation between the two distributions for adjusted costs ($r = 0.987$, $p < .0001$) and AIH ($r = 0.987$, $p < .0001$).

Comparison of the performance of 6 alternative and 10 traditional teaching facilities (table 5C.2) shows that the alternative teaching facilities have a slightly more complex

FIGURE 5C.1
Adjusted Costs Based on AIH Values, 2003

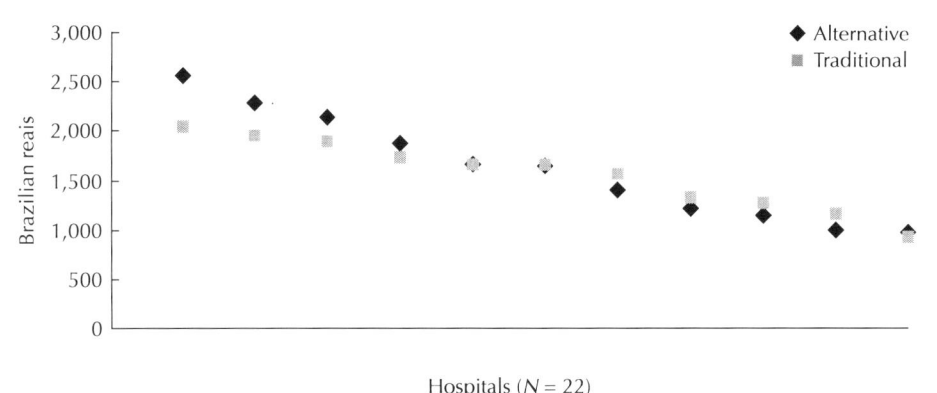

Source: Mendes and Costa 2005.

FIGURE C5.2
AIH Values, by Hospital Type, 2003

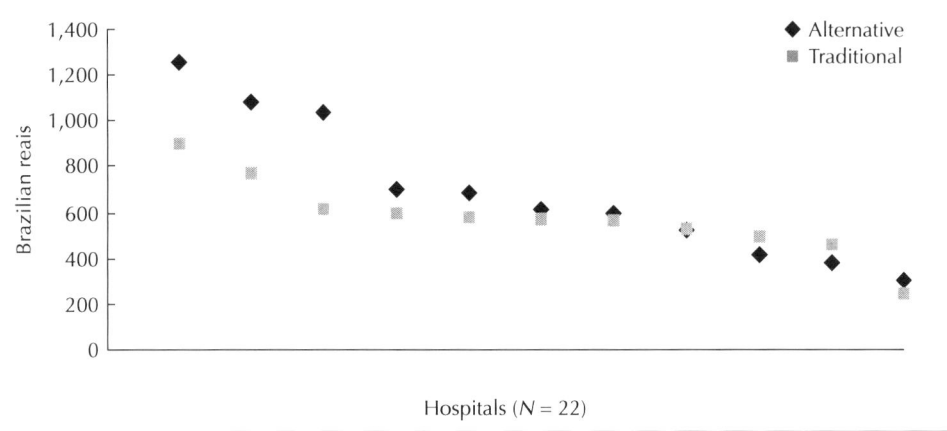

Source: Mendes and Costa 2005.

case load, measured by the proxy AIH value ($p < .10$), than their traditional counterparts. Alternative facilities also displayed significantly lower mortality rates ($p < .05$) and made greater use of available equipment. Although the alternative facilities were generally more efficient than the traditional teaching facilities, as measured by ALOS, the differences were not significant.

TABLE 5C.2
Comparison of Selected Quality and Efficiency Indicators, Alternative and Traditional Teaching Hospitals, 2003

Indicator	Alternative (N = 6)	Traditional (N = 10)
Complexity (AIH value, R$)[*]	864	607
Efficiency		
ALOS (days)	7.7	8.5
Occupation rate (percent)	68	75
Equipment use (percent)[**]	99	87
Nursing hours/bed	9.6	6.6
Professional hours/bed	96	68
Quality		
General mortality rate[**]	5.5	9.5

Source: Mendes and Costa 2005.
* $p < .10$ (Mann-Whitney test). ** $p < .05$.

Annex 5D
Methods for Comparative Analysis of OSS and Direct Administration Hospitals

Health social organization (OSS) and direct administration facilities were matched to avoid any significant differences between the groups in average bed size, total spending, spending per bed, discharges, physicians per bed, and complexity. No facility in the sample was a teaching hospital. Two direct administration facilities were eliminated from the sample because of data unavailability.

Direct administration facilities were found to have, on average, significantly more professionals and clinical beds. The facilities are of similar complexity, according to the proxy measure of Authorization for Hospitalization (Autorização de Internação Hospitalar, AIH), percentage of patients over age 60, and ratio of male to female inpatients.

TABLE 5D.1
Comparison of Selected Indicators, OSS and Direct Administration Hospitals, São Paulo State, 2003

Indicator	OSS hospitals (N = 12)		Direct administration hospitals (N = 10)	
	Mean	Min–max range	Mean	Min–max range
Beds				
Total	209	140–318	205	164–271
Surgical	63	26–106	75	36–202
Clinical[a]	49	20–81	92	56–180
Personnel (2004)				
Physicians (full time equivalent)*	143	94–276	203	90–339
Nurses (full time equivalent)	54	23–96	40	7–64
Expenditures (R$ thousands)				
Total spending	35,395	20,449–48,166	37,325	30,356–44,109
Spending/bed	177	116–279	187	149–228
Production				
Discharges (number)*	12,239	8,517–16,093	8,938	5,292–11,594
Complexity				
AIH general	419	320–525	420	294–597
AIH surgery	542	400–695	520	264–820
Patients >age 60 (%)	14	8.5–19	18	9–36
Ratio, male/female inpatients	76	45–132	59	45–75

Source: Costa and Mendes 2005.
*$p < .05$ (Mann-Whitney test).

Annex 5E
Matrix: Organizational Arrangements in European Hospitals

Country	Private or public ownership of hospitals	Decision-making rights of hospital managers	Recent changes
Albania	All hospitals public.	No autonomy with respect to skill mix, ward organization, or budget use.	Closure of small hospitals; conversion of 6 to 12 district hospitals to regional facilities.
Armenia	Mix of public and for-profit hospitals.	Considerable autonomy of managers to set prices, determine staff size, and negotiate contracts with staff.	Since 1993, incremental, increase in autonomy of hospitals.
Austria	In 1998, 49 private hospitals, 37 nonprofits, 142 public hospitals. Two-thirds of beds public.	Public hospitals have full autonomy in hiring, firing, skill mix, and ward organization but limited autonomy in budget use.	Introduction of performance financing.
Belgium	60 percent nonprofit private institutions; 40 percent facilities publicly owned by municipal welfare centers, provinces, state or intermunicipal associations	Public hospitals have full autonomy with respect to hiring, firing, skill mix, and ward organization but limited autonomy in budget use.	No information available.
Denmark	Most hospitals county-owned.	Autonomy with respect to hiring and firing, but limited autonomy to determine skill mix and utilize budgets.	In 2003 government issued plans to create autonomous hospitals.
Estonia	Most hospitals state-owned.	All public hospitals have been incorporated under private law as joint stock companies or foundations (known as trusts). Hospitals are managed by executive directors who are recruited competitively and have full decision-making rights.	Hospitals have merged into networks, resulting in reduction of number of facilities from 78 in 1998 to 19 in 2006.
Finland	Most hospitals publicly owned by federations of municipalities (i.e., hospital districts).	Decision-making rights limited; managers accountable to hospital districts; hospitals not allowed to make profit; assets owned by hospital districts.	Pilots under way to separate hospital districts from hospitals to introduce purchaser-provider split.

(continued)

Country	Private or public ownership of hospitals	Decision-making rights of hospital managers	Recent changes
France	25 percent public hospitals (1,000 out of 4,000); 33 percent nonprofit (1,400); 40 percent private for-profit (1,750).	In public hospitals, decision-making rights on staffing limited by national rules; most public hospital employees are civil servants with tenure. Director has no power to determine wages but has decision-making authority over other inputs.	Introduction of regional hospital agencies for planning and financial resource allocation for private and public hospitals. Introduction of strategic purchasing arrangements.
Germany	In 2000, of 2,030 general hospitals, around 790 publicly owned, 820 private nonprofit, 420 private for-profit.	Public hospitals have considerable decision-making rights regarding staff hiring and firing. Hospitals can run deficits and make profits. Investment costs are covered by the states (*Länder*); recurrent costs, by health insurance funds.	Countrywide diagnosis-related group (DRG) system introduced
Italy	About 60 percent of hospitals public (81 percent of beds).	By 2000, 98 autonomous hospital trusts established. Decision-making rights increased in hospital trusts. Managers empowered to define hospital's mission and objectives in three-year strategic plan.	Conversion of public hospitals to hospital trusts.
Netherlands	All hospitals private, not-for-profit.	Fully autonomous with regard to internal management, but major planning decisions must be approved by government.	Implementation of case-based hospital payment system.
Portugal	About 58 percent of hospitals public (78 percent of beds); remainder evenly divided between for-profit and nonprofit facilities.	Traditionally, public hospital managers have little budgetary flexibility or autonomy in investment and human resources.	In 2002 selective contracting was introduced with performance-based payment system. Hospitals are under reorganization with new classification system: public autonomous, public corporatized, and public corporate. The latter are private, but with the state as exclusive shareholder.
Slovenia	All hospitals public.	Most hospitals autonomous.	DRG payment system introduced.

Country	Private or public ownership of hospitals	Decision-making rights of hospital managers	Recent changes
Spain	About 42 percent hospitals public, 16 percent nonprofit, and 42 percent for-profit.	An array of autonomous arrangements has emerged in the last two decades throughout the country; forms include the foundation (*fundación*), consortium (*consorcio*), public firm (*sociedad mercantil pública,* or *entidad pública empresarial*), and autonomous organization (*organismo autónomo*).	Hospital reform is part of a broader systemic reform involving separation of purchasing and provision and application of performance-based contracting.
United Kingdom	Nearly all hospitals public.	Conversion of direct management hospitals into self-governing National Health Service hospital trusts. Each trust determines service mix, staffing structure, and size and employs own staff. Trusts own assets and can retain surpluses. Although autonomy is limited by civil service rules and hierarchical controls, trusts enjoy more decision-making rights than directly managed facilities.	Hospital reform is part of a broader reform to transform health authorities into buyers of services and hospitals into sellers.

Source: Adapted from Maarese et al. (2005); United Kingdom, Ham and Hawkins (2003); Spain, Martín Martín (2003).

Notes

1. Financial responsibility leads managers to be more focused on financial survival and hence on the income generated by service outputs.
2. In a review of country reform cases, Ham and Hawkins (2003) found considerable diversity in the breadth and depth of reforms along the five framework dimensions.
3. The organizational reforms listed were often accompanied by reforms in hospital payment mechanisms, as described in chapter 4.
4. Evidence supporting these effects was presented only in the case of user fees.
5. In some countries resource mobilization was a major driver of autonomy-enhancing reforms in public hospitals (Govindaraj and Chawla 1996).
6. The exception is for medicines and, to a lesser extent medical supplies, during stock-outs. This systemwide problem is evident at all levels of service delivery. In addition, there have been press reports of illegal, under-the-table payments for some procedures in publicly financed private hospitals, but such payments have not been systematically studied.
7. The city of Curitiba may be the exception (World Bank 2006a; Mendes 2005).
8. Nunes (1999) has characterized public administration in Brazil as clientelist, corporatist, (bureaucratically) insulated, and procedure centered.
9. The 1967 administrative reform, as originally designed, was part of a broader effort to decentralize the federal government. Decentralization was subsequently blocked by the military dictatorship and was not placed on the policy agenda until the return to democracy in the late 1980s.
10. State and municipal labor and procurement laws must be aligned with federal legislation.

11. The Constitution sought to fold all public institutions into a single public administration regime (*direito público*). Complementary civil service (1990) and public procurement (1993) legislation subjected most public organizations, including those under indirect administration, to the new procurement and civil service rule set. Presidential Decree 27 of 2000 also mandated that all public agencies were to follow a single set of budgeting rules and processes.

12. It is common for decentralization to reduce autonomy and make management problems worse, in part because of lack of institutional capacity at subnational levels (Jakab et al. 2002).

13. For example, by 1992 nearly 70 percent of all health care facilities were operated by municipalities, up from 22 percent in 1982. By 2004 municipalities operated nearly three-quarters of all public hospitals.

14. According to Shepherd (2002), 160 autonomous management units (*autarquias*) and public foundations were established, accounting for 58 percent of public employment. Most of these were public universities.

15. Under current practices, these indirect administration models can best be described as "decentralized" budgetary units in the sense that budgets are not centrally managed by government. Facility managers must follow standardized rules for procurement, human resource management, and financial management, often with considerable central (and ex ante) oversight.

16. Some observers suggest that centralizing processes enabled central control of patronage employment and opportunities for procurement-related corruption.

17. EPs are also referred to as mixed economy enterprises (*empresas de economia mista*). Although these models have different titles and are often classified separately in official databases, hospitals under public enterprise and mixed economy enterprise arrangements are essentially the same in both legal and organizational terms. Autonomous social services include, for example, the Sarah Kubitschek Hospital Network and the São João Batista Municipal Hospital. Both are legal entities founded (and protected) by special legislation.

18. In the past, and not necessarily related to the health sector, FAs have been used by politicians to direct public funds to "pork barrel" projects within their jurisdictions. They also have been used by corporations to finance philanthropic activities. FAs should not be confused with "public foundations." The 1988 Constitution eliminated the legal form of public foundation under private law and replaced it with the public foundation under public law. The new legal form offered few, if any, advantages over the direct administration arrangement, and in fact, an undetermined number of hospitals under the public foundation model were converted to direct administration after 1988.

19. High-profile examples of FAs include the Zerbini Foundation, which supports the Heart Institute of the Clinical Hospital of the University of São Paulo, and the Pro-Heart Foundation (Fundação Pró Coração, FUNDACOR) of the National Heart Institute of Laranjeiras in Rio de Janeiro (see box 5.1).

20. The FA arrangement can best be described as a collocation model, as is found in public hospitals in many developing and developed countries. Under this model, publicly employed professionals are permitted to earn additional income by providing services to private patients. Typically, the rationale is that this arrangement allows public facilities to retain scarce and highly skilled staff. In general, the model has not worked well in developing counties, resulting instead in stratified, two-tier care (La Forgia 1990) or hidden cross-subsidies from public to private services (Fiedler and La Forgia 2005). It can be described as an ad hoc, facility-based response to a labor problem that would be better dealt with systemically. For example, recognizing that the public service employment regime is not suitable for professionals working in public hospitals, European countries are increasing human resource flexibility (Figueras, Robinson, and Jakubowski 2005).

21. According to the architect of the reform, this new reform wave responded to the failure of previous "administrative" reforms to address institutional structures and was "designed to replace the existing mix of bureaucratic public administration and clientelist or patrimonialist practices in Brazil" (Bresser-Pereira 2003: 90). For the rationale behind social organizations, see Bresser-Pereira (1998: 235–50). Costa and Mendes (2005) suggest other motivations for the reform, including legal constraints on personnel spending under Law 82 of 1995 and the Fiscal Respon-

sibility Law (LRF), Law 101 of 2000. These restrictions drove governments to contract out service delivery to OSs and cooperatives. The LRF also sought to stimulate a new public management culture by mandating greater budgetary transparency, by planning revenues and expenditures, and by setting limits on public spending and debt. All levels of government were given percentage limits on personnel (civil service) spending but not on "other personnel expenditures," which could include spending for contracted services. This constraint gave local and municipal governments an incentive to look for alternatives to direct administration.

22. The debate over the constitutional amendment was heated and politically charged. The amendment itself left the final decision on how to move forward in the hands of federal, state, and municipal governments. In part as a consequence of the debate, complementary laws reforming civil service employment were never drafted. The OS law continues to face legal challenges based on the constitutional mandate that permits public financing of private providers of a "complementary" nature. This has been interpreted by some to mean that purchasing services from private providers is legal only in areas where there are no public providers. Because Congress has yet to enact legislation to implement the amendment, Vargas (2006) suggests that granting greater autonomy and applying contracts to public entities under direct and indirect administration will remain a paper reform only. As discussed in chapter 6, the failure to enact laws based on this amendment impedes conversion of direct administration hospitals to alternative and more autonomous arrangements.

23. Several states have enacted legislation to form OSSs, drawing on the federal framework law, but only São Paulo has fully implemented the OSS arrangement in public hospitals, as envisioned under the federal legislation. The states of Ceará and Minas Gerais were to introduce OSSs in public facilities in 2007.

24. In contrast, all public hospitals under direct administration are "open door" facilities. However, the state government is moving toward converting direct administration hospitals to "closed door" facilities in areas where municipal governments have high basic care coverage.

25. The relatively large supply of private, nonprofit organizations with hospital management experience in São Paulo favors the OSS model. The supply is considerably thinner elsewhere in Brazil, particularly in the North. Selection criteria require the bidders to have at least five years of experience in ownership and operation of health care units and to have a governance board (Law 846, ch. 1, sec. 1).

26. The term management contract (*contrato da gestao*) is specified in the state law. It should not be confused with internal contracting between government entities. The management contract is between a government purchaser, São Paulo state, and a private, nonprofit service provider (an OSS). Government contracting in health is described in chapter 4.

27. Currently, OSSs are formally accountable to EPNL governance structures, which generally include a board-like element. This arrangement, however, appears to be pro forma. EPNL boards are far removed from an OSS facility, and they oversee several entities, including universities, medical schools, other OSSs, or nonprofit facilities. Beyond reporting requirements, EPNL boards rarely question OSS hospital management or pressure managers to improve quality and efficiency. Bogue, Hall, and La Forgia (2007) found that public and private hospitals in Latin America with independent and facility-based governance boards reported higher performance levels than hospitals without boards.

28. Some autonomous social services sell services to HMOs and private patients, but these facilities were not part of the sample.

29. The sample consisted of 3 hospitals under autonomous organizational arrangements; 4 private support foundations linked to facilities under direct administration (OSSs); 1 public firm under a private labor regime; 1 indirect administration facility (autarquia); 1 public foundation; and 14 direct administration facilities. One of the direct administration facilities implemented an innovative performance payment scheme for physicians, and another contracted out medical and diagnostic services to professional cooperatives.

30. The maximum score was 26 on the flexibility and the hierarchy dimensions combined. In theory, a facility receiving a score of 26 for flexibility (and therefore 0 for hierarchy) was deemed to possess a fully flexible organizational structure according to the six organizational dimensions described in the text. Conversely, a facility receiving a score of 26 for hierarchy (and therefore 0 for flexibility) was considered to operate under full hierarchical control.

31. Flexibility scores were in a range of 7–21 for the alternative group and 2–8 for the traditional group. The ranges for hierarchy scores were 5–20 for the alternative group and 18–24 for the traditional facilities.

32. The divergence between patient volume and SUS-derived revenues is related to the below-cost payment mechanism. An undetermined number of nonprofit facilities receives irregular but significant lump-sum transfers from municipal governments to maintain operations

33. Of the estimated 1,851 nonprofit hospitals, 92 percent belong to philanthropic associations; 6 percent are private foundations, and 2 percent are cooperatives (see table 5.1).

34. The observed entrepreneurship of the nonprofit health sector has led to a sometimes heated debate on the role of these hospitals in the SUS. Some claim that the facilities provide stratified care and cater more to private, paying patients (covered by health plans or paying out-of-pocket). A 1999 government study found that the nonprofits' tax-free status "cost" the government $600 million in that year. The philanthropic organizations claim that because government pays below cost, they have to make up the difference by selling services to third parties (Giardi and Barros 2001).

35. The financial plight of nonprofit hospitals financed by the SUS is a constant theme raised by nonprofit trade associations. This issue has received attention in the press and from the Health Caucus in Congress.

36. Provision of less than 60 percent is permitted if approved by local SUS authorities (Law 9732/1998 [LOS]; Resolution CNAS 177/2000).

37. Under the Organic Social Assistance Law (POAS 1993); Decree 2536/1998; Decree 3504/2000.

38. These executives, known as "statutory executives," may or may not constitute a board.

39. Several agencies are involved in the regulation of nonprofit institutions. Federal, state, and municipal social assistance councils are responsible for issuing and renewing the nonprofit status certificate; the Ministry of Finance grants tax exemptions; and the federal MS or state and municipal health secretariats license facilities and pay for services provided to SUS patients.

40. This section draws heavily on the census by Barbosa et al. (2002), which covered 1,414 facilities, and their in-depth analysis of a random survey of 69 nonprofit hospitals.

41. Unfortunately, there is little information on organizational arrangements in hospitals operated by nonprofit foundations and for-profit societies and corporations.

42. No response was received from 191 facilities.

43. Barbosa et al. (2002) did not examine the relation between autonomy and specific organizational arrangements (e.g., private foundation, association, firm).

44. By law, this position is pro bono; not even an executive doubling as hospital manager is remunerated. About 80 percent of statutory executives work on a part-time basis.

45. More comprehensive analysis was impossible because of data limitations, particularly in hospitals under direct administration.

46. As explained in chapter 3, DEA estimates relative efficiency on the basis of the quantity of inputs used to produce one or more outputs. The DEA scores reported here are based on a random sample of 428 facilities with more than 25 beds drawn from the National Health Facility Survey (AMS) of 7,397 hospitals in 2002.

47. TTE consists of two parts: scale efficiency (SE) and internal efficiency (ITE). SE is directly related to facility size: efficiency increases as the volume of output increases because fixed costs are spread over larger quantities of output. IE is related to the production process and refers to obtaining maximum outputs for a given set of inputs. The DEA methods applied in this analysis are described in annex 3E.

48. This means that the typical facility was 34 percent as efficient as hospitals rated on the efficiency frontier. In other words, in comparison with the most efficient hospitals (which received a score of 1), the average facility produced about one-third the outputs for their level of inputs.

49. The ITE results, which are also affected by scale, deserve mention. Smaller facilities in Brazil tend to use fewer inputs and produce fewer inpatient stays but more emergency and outpatient visits. This makes them more efficient than large facilities with many inputs producing more inpatient stays. Furthermore, an increasing number of large facilities are limiting the volume of care provided in emergency rooms for nonemergency, on-demand services; the ER volume could lower ITE scores.

50. This follow-up research was commissioned by the World Bank and included two additional hospitals (one hospital under direct administration, the other under a contracting arrangement). The original sample contained 12 alternative and 12 traditional facilities. For the follow-up study, four facilities were dropped and two were added, for a total of 22. Of the four that were dropped, one alternative hospital was eliminated because it was an outlier in terms of complexity and could not be matched with any traditional facility, and one alternative and two traditional facilities were dropped because of insufficient data. The latter were replaced by two traditional facilities for the performance analysis. One alternative hospital was reclassified as traditional on the basis of the analysis of structures and behaviors described earlier.

51. This classification resulted in the placement of one facility that was under indirect administration arrangements (public foundations) in the traditional group.

52. See annex 5C for methods used to match and compare the two groups of facilities. The performance analysis was applied to 22 hospitals (11 from each group).

53. This discussion draws on three sources of information: yearly reports by the state assessment commission on compliance with performance targets specified in the management contract; a comparative evaluation performed by the state secretariat of health (SES-SP 2003a, 2003b); and a comparative evaluation commissioned for this volume (Costa and Mendes 2005).

54. The analyses were performed on the facilities for which data were readily available.

55. See annex 5D for a discussion of methods. Lack of available data for two direct administration hospitals led to those facilities being dropped for a subset of indicators.

56. The research was severely constrained by the general lack of information available in hospitals under direct administration. Even simple descriptive statistics were often unavailable, and considerable time and resources were expended in collecting data on site. Consequently, expanding the sample was not financially feasible within the research budget. In contrast, the OSSs exhibit a rich information environment, including data on standardized costs, production, productivity, and quality. This information is used by both facility and state managers to monitor performance.

57. In hindsight, a more circumspect policy would have been to reduce the payroll and intensify oversight instead of eliminating autonomy altogether by forcing adoption of the standardized public procurement and human resource management rules that emerged from the constitutional reforms of the late 1980s.

58. The proposed model, known as state foundations, is discussed in the next chapter.

59. The 2000 Fiscal Responsibility Law also set limits on personnel spending and other fiscal variables.

60. See, for example, Leonard, Masatu, and Vialou (2005); Das and Hammer (2005).

61. Inpatients from other municipalities are usually transferred from local facilities because of case severity.

6

Inside the Black Box:
Linking Organizational Arrangements, Managerial Behaviors, and Performance in Public and Private Hospitals

Hospitals are about getting quality services to people at an affordable cost. But hospitals are also labor-intensive, complex organizations. When patients receive timely, humane care and the treatment resolves their health conditions at a cost the health system can afford, the hospital can be considered a high performer. These patients are the "winners" of high performance. When patients lie for hours on a gurney in the corridor because of poor clinical management, suffer the ill effects of hospital-acquired infections, and do not receive timely treatment because of poorly maintained equipment, and the hospital constantly overspends its budget, the organization is a poor performer. Its patients are the "losers" of low performance. As seen in the previous chapter, hospitals under some organizational forms consistently display high performance, while hospitals under other forms consistently suffer from low performance. Why?

Managers commonly attribute organizational success or failure to managerial practices, but these practices do not occur in a vacuum. Managerial practices are organizational behaviors that respond to incentives inherent in the business and organizational environments. Chapter 5 dissected organizational forms and governance practices in Brazilian public and private hospitals, and the performance of hospitals under different organizational forms was found to vary significantly, particularly in the public sector. In this chapter managerial practices under different public sector organizational arrangements are examined. The following questions are addressed: How are managerial practices related to organizational arrangements, and how do they influence performance? Do nontraditional arrangements, such as those of autonomous administration, alter the incentive environment to enable or motivate high performance? Conversely, can managers in hospitals under traditional forms also innovate along the five organizational dimensions studied here—autonomy, accountability, market exposure, residual claimant status, and social functions—without first modifying organizational structures?

Managerial practices can be defined as "the set of formal and informal rules and procedures for selecting, deploying, and supervising resources in the most efficient way possible to achieve institutional objectives" (Over and Watanabe 2003: 122–23). Hospital management entails a wide range of clinical and nonclinical functions. Clinical areas include medical, nursing, and ancillary services. Nonclinical areas include personnel, materials, hotel services, finance, procurement, and public relations. There is abundant international literature, including guides, textbooks, and manuals, on structures, performance standards, work processes, information needs, controls, personnel qualifications, and financial implications for each of these areas, which are generally organized by departments within a hospital. This chapter does not delve into how these functions are carried out in Brazilian hospitals. Although descriptive information on this subject abounds, analytical work is sparse. Instead, the chapter focuses on broad management practices related to human resource management, procurement of materials, financial management, and contracting. Activities in these areas account for a large share of hospital expenditures and are important determinants of overall performance.

Management Practices in Public Hospitals

Drawing on the results of Mendes et al. (2002), chapter 5 compared organizational structures for a small sample of hospitals hypothesized as being "alternative" or "traditional." Alternative facilities were found to feature "flexible" organizational structures, while traditional hospitals responded to "hierarchical" rules and structures. This section reports on the results linking structures and managerial behaviors.

Organizational Structures and Managerial Behaviors

The researchers hypothesized that hospitals under hierarchical structures would display "normative" behaviors (e.g., compliance with an administrative rule set), while hospitals with more flexible structures would display "strategic" or autonomous behaviors and managerial practices. On the basis of a survey of managers in 24 hospitals (12 traditional and 12 alternative), the study attempted to determine how the hospitals differed within and across the two groups in terms of managerial behaviors (application of rules and processes) and whether structures, defined as flexible or hierarchical, were correlated with predicted behaviors.

The researchers examined evidence of behaviors and management practices across 34 variables related to organizational behaviors. These variables were categorized into 10 groups: strategic planning, budget management, investment management, performance and quality monitoring, human resource management, human resource policies, other administrative functions (information and equipment management), purchasing, patient relations, and market relations.[1] The maximum score on the groups was 37. The researchers also constructed four composite variables based on the 34 variables: demonstration of behaviors (e.g., application of processes and rules) related to accountability, decision making for strategic issues, decision making for personnel, and market exposure.

Each hospital was placed on a continuum based on the application of rules and functions in day-to-day management. Each facility received two scores: "strategic," and "normative" or "administrative." A *strategic* facility displayed evidence of practices for each of the above-mentioned 10 groups and did so autonomously. In other words, managers were actually managing—making decisions, exercising responsibility, and taking initiatives without prior higher-level approval on such matters as for example, hiring personnel, setting prices, determining service mix, selling services, accessing nonbudgetary revenues, and assessing patient satisfaction. A *normative* facility displayed evidence that functions and behaviors followed the hierarchy of governmental rules and controls, were the responsibility of government units external to the facility, or were not exercised.[2]

Hospitals were rated along both the strategic and normative dimensions. In theory, an individual facility could receive a maximum score of 37 for either dimension but not for both.

A facility receiving a strategic score of 37, and therefore a normative score of 0, was deemed to exhibit a strong strategic or managerial culture. Conversely, a facility with a normative score of 37, and therefore a strategic score of 0, was deemed to exhibit a strong administrative culture.

As in the analysis of organizational structures reported in chapter 5, significant differences, favoring the alternative facilities, were found between the two groups on the four composite variables derived from the 34 behavioral variables: accountability ($p < .0001$), decision making for strategic issues ($p < .0001$), decision making related to personnel ($p < .0001$), and market exposure ($p < .01$). Greater variation was found within both groups as to reported behaviors than was the case for structures.

The strategic and normative scores for each facility are plotted in figure 6.1. Three facilities originally hypothesized as being "alternative" (marked A, D, and F in the figure) received relatively high scores for normative behaviors. Facility A was under direct administration and contracted out most care services to physician and nursing cooperatives. Facility F was a nonprofit managed by a municipality that also contracted out all services to professional cooperatives. Both exhibited a normative pattern in all other behaviors and functions. Facility A also received high scores for hierarchy (see figure 5.1) and is best classified as "traditional." Facility D was a support foundation (*fundação de apoio*, FA) that displayed little integration into the market in terms of selling services to third parties. In contrast, one "traditional" facility (E in figure 6.1) that featured hierarchical structures and operated under the direct administration model received a high score for strategic and autonomous behaviors. This facility displayed innovations atypical of most hospitals in the traditional group, including strategic planning, programs to improve client satisfaction, expansion of the revenue base by selling services to private health plans,[3] special staff training programs, and incentive payment schemes. This was achieved despite hierarchical control in terms of organizational structure.

The case of this facility suggests that management can innovate under hierarchical organizational structures. In other words, change is possible in direct administration facilities, but the scope of such change may be limited by structural constraints imposed by hierarchical

FIGURE 6.1
Strategic and Normative Scores for Alternative and Traditional Hospital Behaviors, 2000
($N = 24$)

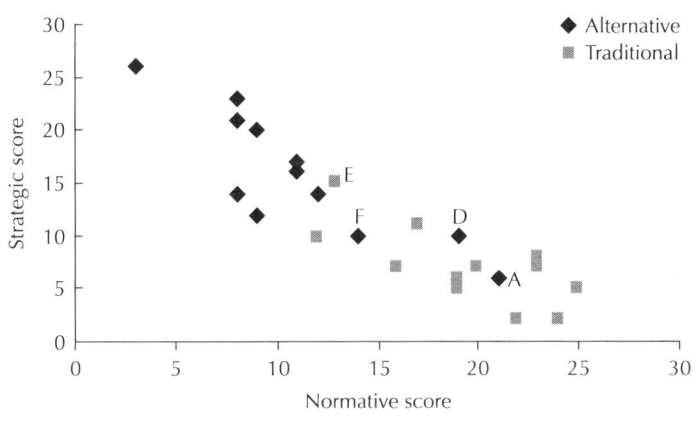

Source: Mendes et al. 2002.
Note: Letter designations for facilities are the same as those used in figures 5.1 and 6.2.

control. For example, none of the facilities under direct administration reported decision rights in human resource management, except for the payment of performance incentives.[4] Thus, organizational innovations are possible under direct and indirect administration and can serve as beacons of modest change for facilities operating under these models. Nevertheless, aggregate change remains elusive because of the structural constraints of hierarchical control imposed by the public sector regime. In contrast, one facility with an FA and two that contract out most services to cooperatives exhibited normative behaviors more aligned with direct administration. Apparently, possessing these arrangements does not lead to innovative managerial behaviors. As suggested in Chapter 5, FAs form parallel organizational structures within direct administration facilities, while cooperatives under contract with government are poorly monitored. More research is needed on how FAs and cooperatives impact hospital management and performance.

Structures are also strongly related to managerial behaviors. A high correlation ($r = 0.75$) was found between the scores on organizational structure reported in chapter 5 and the managerial behavior scores for the sample of alternative and traditional facilities, discussed above. Figure 6.2 plots the structural and behavioral scores for alternative and traditional facilities in the sample ($N = 24$). The higher the scores registered for structure (x-axis), the more flexible (and less hierarchical) is the organization. The higher the scores registered for behaviors (y-axis), the more strategic (and less normative) is the organization.

Hospitals displaying less flexible (more hierarchical) structures generally exhibited less strategic (more normative) behaviors. The opposite was also true: hospitals under flexible organizational structures exhibited strategic and autonomous behaviors. Nevertheless, some variation, especially in behavioral scores, was observed among both groups of hospitals. Four deviations from the pattern are worth noting.

FIGURE 6.2
Correlation between Flexibility and Strategic Scores, Alternative and Traditional Facilities, 2000
($N = 24$)

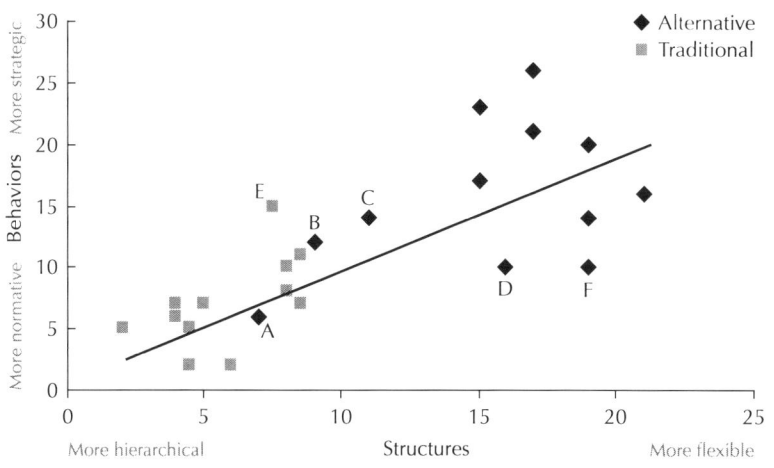

Source: Mendes et al. 2002.
Note: Letter designations for facilities are the same as those used in figures 5.1 and 6.1.

- Two alternative hospitals (B and C in figure 6.2) occupy a middle ground on both structure and behavior.
- One traditional hospital (E) that was rated hierarchical because of its structure displayed behaviors more in line with flexible organizations.
- One alternative hospital (A) scored low on both structure and behaviors and would be better classified as hierarchical and normative.[5]
- Two alternatives hospitals (D and F) demonstrated strong flexibility in terms of structure, but were more normative in terms of their behaviors. As mentioned above, one possessed an FA while the other contracted out medical services to professional cooperatives. These arrangements may not encourage strategic management practices in which managers make decisions independent of an hierarchically determined rule set.

Managerial Practices and Performance

Having established that organizational structures and behaviors are linked, the discussion turns to the typical managerial environment under the public sector regime. How are the facilities managed? Which behaviors can contribute to low performance? Are managerial roles and responsibilities clearly delineated? To answer these questions, analyses of procurement and human resource management in public facilities are discussed first. Because many functions are carried out in government units outside the facility, managerial capacity of state and municipal administrative units is then examined.[6] Annex 6A reviews the strengths and weaknesses of the legal and regulatory framework governing human resource, procurement, and financial management. These features are discussed briefly, next.

Complex Procurement Rules and Centralized Purchasing

About 20 percent of municipal facilities and 16 percent of state hospitals reported shortages of drugs and medical supplies. Nearly all managers of municipal hospitals and half the managers of state hospitals reported problems in maintaining adequate stocks of drugs and of medical and other supplies, as well as in accessing maintenance services (figure 6.3). The frequency of reported delays in the purchase and delivery of supplies in municipal facilities reached more than 80 percent for drugs and 60 percent for medical supplies. More than 40 percent of state facilities reported delays in purchase and delivery of drugs and 60 percent reported these problems for medical supplies.

Respondents cited problems in procurement processes—which are often managed by central secretariats in state and municipal governments—as the main reasons for the holdups, followed by poor inventory control[7] and delays by municipal managers in paying suppliers. In some cases the delays forced the temporary suspension of services. A recent procurement assessment found that excessive specificity of procurement rules led to a "constant stream of procurement disputes [that] results in delayed contracting and purchasing. The numerous administrative complaints and injunctions issued by courts of law may hold up the bidding by many months if not years" (World Bank 2004b: 2).

More than three-fourths of municipal hospital managers reported that most drug and medical supply purchasing was centralized in the secretariat of health or another municipal secretariat.[8] This contrasts with federal hospitals, which have autonomy to buy all drugs and medical supplies. State hospitals hold a middle position, with 70 percent possessing

FIGURE 6.3
Delays in Purchasing Supplies and Services, as Reported by Public Hospital Managers, by Subnational Level, 2003
(*N* = 24)

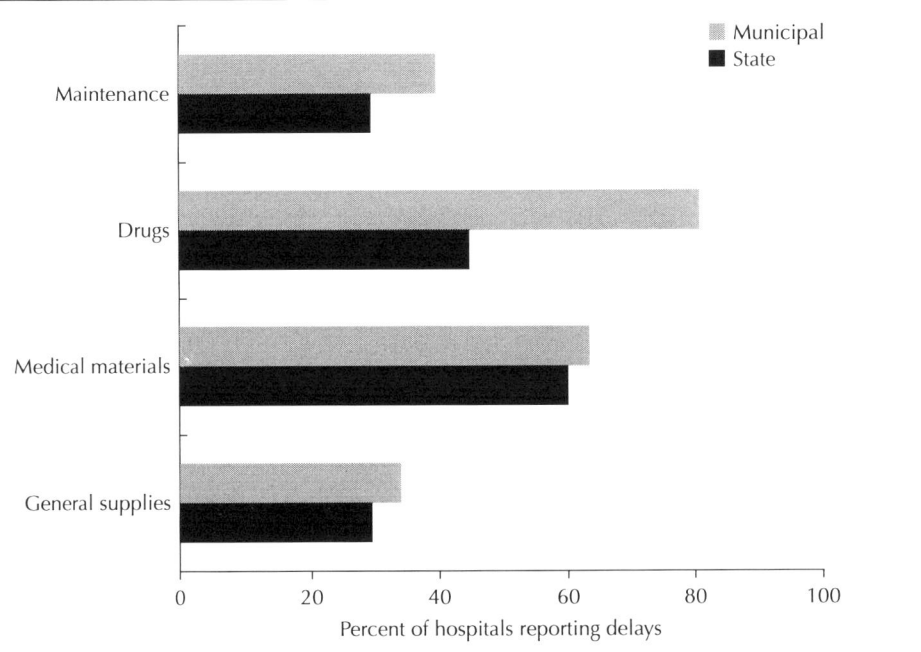

Source: World Bank 2007.

autonomy to purchase these items. Most facilities, however, make purchases through simpler and less competitive procurement procedures such as shopping (*tomada de preço*), direct purchases (*compra direta*), and requests for proposals (*carta convite*). This suggests that facilities generally have autonomy only for small purchases, usually in an emergency. Large purchases involving competitive bidding are managed elsewhere in government.

In terms of internal material management systems, about 60 percent of state hospitals and 30 percent of municipal facilities report not having intermediate stock control of drugs. Standardized formularies are absent in more than half the public facilities. Only about half the state hospitals have adopted a unit-dose system that could significantly reduce leakages.[9]

Centralized Human Resource Management and Rigid Civil Service Processes
Health care organizations are both labor-intensive and highly professionalized enterprises. The effective management of human resources—how an organization recruits, compensates, trains, rewards, and disciplines its staff—ultimately determines the practices and behaviors that contribute to performance. Staff behaviors, particularly those of professionals, are often driven by organizational forms and by the financial and nonfinancial incentives embedded in them.[10] Box 6.1 examines research on health worker behaviors under various organizational forms.

Box 6.1
Organizational Forms and Health Worker Behaviors

Recent research has shown that health workers behave differently under different organizational forms. Clinicians laboring in nonprofit hospitals in Tanzania provided care more in line with their technical capacity than did counterparts in public hospitals, when physician ability and facility characteristics were controlled for (Leonard et al. 2005). In the public hospitals, physicians provided care well below their capacity, resulting in routine misdiagnosis and incorrect treatment of patients. The authors concluded that incentives associated with organizational processes that were evident in the nonprofit hospitals and were absent in public hospitals—for example, managers' decision-making authority to recruit and dismiss staff, set salaries, and determine staff mix—were the determinants of higher-quality care. Similar research in India found that salaried public doctors do less than what they know and are less productive than private, fee-for-service doctors (Das and Hammer 2005). The researchers attributed the difference to salary-based employment combined with poor supervision and the lack of sanctions. In Uganda lack of autonomy of public hospitals to manage human resources contributed to less efficient use of staff when compared with nonprofit hospitals (Ssengooba et al. 2002).

   Physician absenteeism is another problem that plagues public facilities. Federighi and Pedrosa (2002) found that absenteeism ranged from less than 1 percent to 6 percent in a small sample of public hospitals in Brazil. In a survey of primary care facilities in five developing countries (Bangladesh, India, Indonesia, Peru, and Uganda), Chaudhury et al. (2006: 93) found that, on average, 35 percent of health workers were absent. Again, in nearly all cases, human resource decisions were made by the central government following rigid public rules. Few, if any, absentee workers were sanctioned. According to the authors, "Given the rarity of disciplinary actions for repeated absence, the mystery . . . may not be why absence from work is so high, but why anyone shows up at all."

In the survey results reported in World Bank (2007), nearly all municipal and state hospital managers identified human resource management as the top problem affecting facility performance. Figure 6.4 shows the responses from municipal and state hospital managers regarding personnel issues. Low productivity, work shirking, absenteeism, and mismatch between personnel skills and facility requirements are major problems, particularly in municipal facilities. Why is this the case?

Before proceeding, it is important to understand the broader context of human resource management across organizational arrangements. Annex 6B presents the summary features of labor regimes used to contract physicians. These features are generally similar to those for other categories of professionals such as nurses and technicians. Most physicians prefer part-time (20-hour) contracts, salaried remuneration, and an institutionalized employment link. Taken together, these preferences respond to instability in the labor market, provide access to benefits, and guarantee regular income (World Bank 2006a). Part-time employment allows professionals to secure work elsewhere or attend to patients privately, in part to compensate for low salaries or to meet income objectives. Multiemployment is the general rule for physicians in Brazil and is increasingly the case for other health professionals.

Although civil service (described below) is the dominant employment regime in public hospitals, it is not uncommon to find contracted professionals providing care in these facili-

FIGURE 6.4
Principal Personnel Problems Identified by Managers, State and Municipal Hospitals, 2003
($N = 29$)

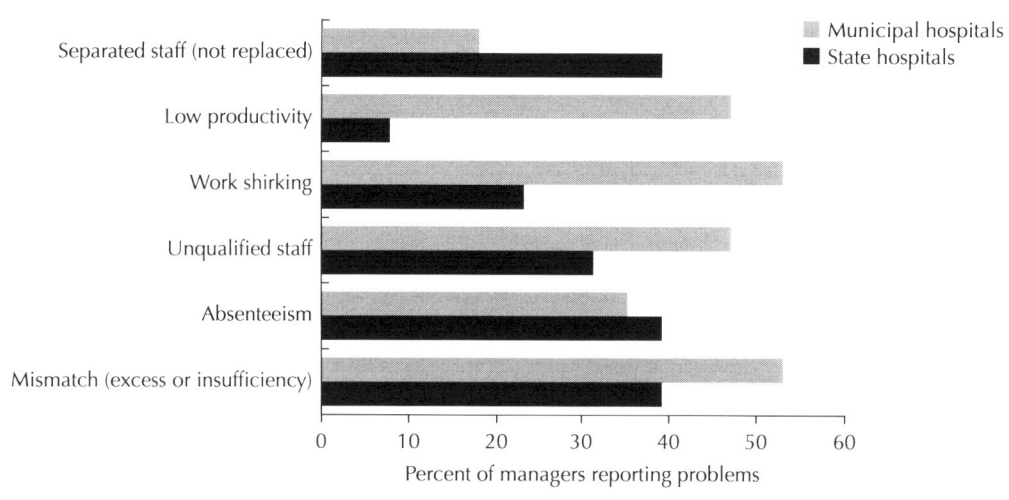

Source: World Bank 2007.

ties. These professionals may be contracted individually or through professional cooperatives (see chapter 4). They are generally paid part-time (20 hours) or full-time (40 hours) salaries that are determined by government, for individuals, or by the cooperatives, for cooperative-affiliated professionals.[11] Cooperatives, support foundations, social organizations, and other autonomous facilities follow the flexible private labor regime for salaried workers known as CLT (Consolidação das Leis do Trabalho; see annex 6B). Hiring processes, salaries, and staff mix are determined by the employer, usually hospital managers, according to facility needs or demand. Dismissal follows a legally determined "with-cause" or "without-cause" process. "With cause" follows a standardized process, according to CLT labor rules. "Without cause" is almost immediate (30-day notice) but the employer must make a severance payment allowance to the (former) employee. Benefits such as social security are required by law, but there is no guarantee of long-term employment.

As mentioned, most public hospital workers and professionals are civil servants. Facility managers have little influence over personnel recruitment, salary definition, or dismissal, partly because these processes follow civil service labor rules and are conducted by central-level human resource departments in the health or administrative secretariats of the state and municipal governments.[12] For example, recruitment invariably involves central-level selection of the highest-ranked individuals, based on scores on multiple-choice tests and review of curricula vitae, without the participation of facility managers. (The tests vary according to personnel category.) Candidates are not interviewed. Personnel within a specific staff category (e.g., nurse, nurse auxiliary, physician) receive the same rate of remuneration. Lifetime employment is guaranteed, after three years' probation. Dismissal processes are extremely complex and can take years. Many managers prefer not to initiate dismissal proceedings because of the time and personal costs involved. Managers state that these human resource practices result in the selection and retention of unqualified and low-performing staff who are not committed to the facility or public service. Civil servants receive pensions that are more generous than those under private sector regimes. Annex 6B contains a summary of the features of civil service (statutory) and private employment.

In the facility survey, managers reported an excess of some staff, usually low-skill, administrative, and support (e.g., cleaning, dietary) personnel, and a shortage of well-trained medical and managerial staff. More than 50 percent of municipal managers and nearly 40 percent of state managers cited such an imbalance. About 40 percent of state managers and 20 percent of their municipal counterparts reported a high number of workers on sick leave, with no substitutes.

Few managers are able to determine staff mix. Worse, the staffing of many public hospitals has not been updated in decades, even though services have been added, expanded, or eliminated. This has resulted in outdated job descriptions, or lack of positions to cover new technologies and services, and the retention of some staff with no functions. Revamping positions can take years, and staffing decisions are still subject to political influence. The presence of a significant proportion of staff ceded from or lent to other hospitals (usually due to political influence), refusal to deal with disciplinary problems, and failure to reallocate excess personnel to understaffed facilities impede effective and sustainable human resource management.

Finally, performance evaluation is a rarity, partly because of the difficulty of taking corrective action. For the most part, performance reviews center on personnel in the mandatory three-year probationary period. Despite the reportedly high levels of unqualified staff, managers have little influence over training. Few facility managers at the state and municipal levels generate or approve training programs.

Managerial Practices and Capacity in State and Municipal Bureaucracies

Since a large number of states and municipalities perform many managerial functions for public hospitals, particularly those under direct administration, this section focuses on managerial shortcomings at those higher administrative levels.[13] Public officials, usually located in municipal and state health secretariats, report deficiencies in planning, budgeting, and information management that contribute to large differences between spending targets, approved budgets, and executed budgets. Small municipalities and health facilities show low levels of budget execution. Inadequate funding is often identified as an important issue by subnational health authorities, but low capacity for budget execution and waste of available resources suggest that excessive formality and poor hospital oversight and supervision are major issues as well. The following are brief assessments of the planning, budgeting, and information environments.

- *Complex system but low planning capacity*. The planning process in the Unified Health System (Sistema Único de Saúde, SUS) is a complicated, formalistic process, mandating the preparation of an array of planning documents. The effectiveness of the process is questionable. First, municipalities report having insufficient or poorly qualified personnel to conduct robust planning exercises based on information analysis. Second, as discussed below, they often lack sufficient information for planning purposes. Third, the multiplicity of poorly formulated and unlinked planning instruments is a major problem and contributes to coordination failures among different phases of the process, as well as between activities and programs.[14] Fourth, planning in municipalities and smaller states is heavily driven by federal health programs and directives, with little initiative by local authorities. Plans are most often wish lists of objectives and targets, without corresponding strategies to guide implementation. Planning documents are produced because they are mandated, and once approved, they are usually forgotten and have little use as management and evaluation tools. Brazil has a long way to go to improve planning, particularly at the state and municipal levels—but this is the context in which most public hospitals operate.

- *Budgetary rigidities.* Rigid budget legislation and structure reduce budget flexibility. Where possible, state and municipal health secretariats bypass this rigidity by setting aggregate budgets and breaking down purchases and contracts into smaller amounts. Some municipal health secretariats have little decision-making authority regarding budgeting. Sizeable changes between initial allocation and final availability of funds reduce the utility of budgeting as a planning and management tool. Funds are not released, and payments are not made as planned, sometimes because of budget freezes. Delays and late payments are frequent, especially in releasing the first and last quarterly allocations. These factors and limited management capacity jeopardize executing units' ability to spend their budgets; it is not uncommon for facilities to be unable to spend all of a budget that had been deemed insufficient. Finally, the system for budget monitoring, control, and account rendering is well structured and formal but focuses mostly on compliance with established norms and financial control, with almost no concern for evaluation of results.

- *Coordination failures between planning, budgeting, and budget execution.* Budget preparation—which at the municipal level is generally the task of finance secretariats rather than health secretariats—follows a process that is often divorced from health planning, which is the responsibility of health secretariats. The structure of budgeting instruments is not aligned with the structure of planning instruments.[15] This impedes technical and financial performance and monitoring of health service delivery. In fact, there is little coherence among policies, plans, and budgets, although they are formally part of a single, integrated process. Budgeted funds at the local level are generally unrelated to demand or needs, for two reasons. First, funding responds to the availability of public revenue, with little concern for local plans, even when they exist. Second, facilities are allotted a defined level of service production, usually in the form of a spending ceiling that is independent of demand, the population's health problems, or costs. In general, the previous year's budget is the main source of information for subsequent planning and budgeting processes. Planning and budgeting often become a formalistic routine varying little from year to year, and this does not encourage good planning or management of service delivery. (Characteristics of a well-run system are outlined in box 6.2.)

- *Lack of information.* The overall institutional environment is devoid of information on inputs, performance, and costs, making it nearly impossible to link resource allocation to results. Impact evaluation is nonexistent. Monitoring centers on legally mandated financial controls and formalistic assessments. For example, budget monitoring and auditing focus on whether funds are spent according to legislation and budgetary rules, rather than on results. Similarly, rules governing federal transfers require states and municipalities to document spending of previous transfers (*prestação de contas*) and compliance with formal requirements such as establishment of a health council or approval of a health plan. Availability of disaggregated data on budget execution is limited, and this hampers tracking the actual application of budgeted resources. Information on costs is

Box 6.2
Characteristics of a Well-Run Planning and Budgeting System

A well-functioning budget process should be more than an accounting exercise to sustain routine activities of government organizations. It is through the budget process that the government's policy priorities are clarified, agreed on, and funded. Characteristics of a well-run planning and budgeting system include

- Availability of realistic revenue estimates and a projected resource envelope (e.g., based on macroeconomic projection) for the medium term, three to four years.
- A process by which policy priorities are compared and compete for limited funding. This implies availability of information required for deciding on tradeoffs.
- A clear statement of the government's policy priorities.
- Sectoral analysis of citizen demands and needs as a basis for each sector's policy priorities (preferably, with costing of each proposed intervention).
- Ability to estimate the medium-term fiscal implications of a given expenditure policy (e.g., recurrent cost implications of capital investment, such as staffing, materials, and equipment needed to run a newly built hospital).
- A transparent budget structure and regular reporting of budget execution to enable accountability and external control.

absent except in a few larger facilities. Many facilities have limited or no financial information whatsoever, partly because any such information that exists remains in central administrative and financial units. For example, figure 6.5 shows that in a sample of 49 (mostly large) hospitals, only 24 percent had cost information of any kind, and 26 percent had no financial information at all (World Bank 2007).

Management Practices in OSS and Direct Administration Hospitals in São Paulo State

Chapter 5 presented evidence that health social organizations (*organizações sociais de saúde*, OSSs) in São Paulo state demonstrate significantly higher performance, as measured by production,

FIGURE 6.5
Financial Information at Health Facilities, 2003
(*N* = 49)

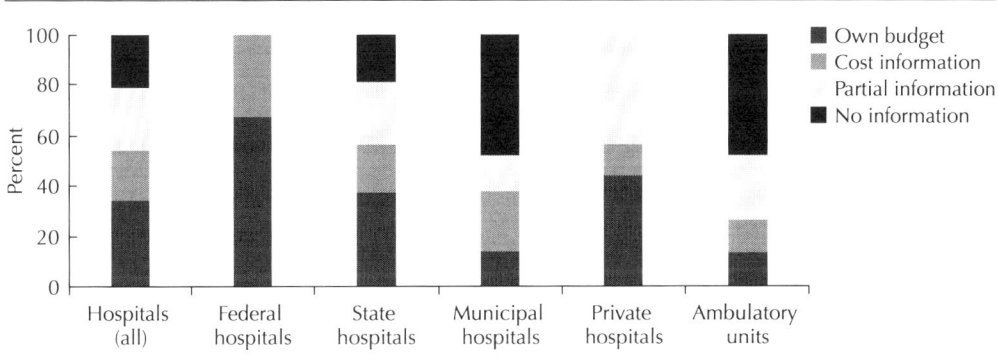

Source: World Bank 2007.

quality, and efficiency, than hospitals under more traditional organizational arrangements, such as direct administration. Why does the OSS organizational arrangement outperform other types? This question is the subject of an increasingly heated debate. Several reasons have been suggested. First, the newness of the facilities (none older than 1998) and the high visibility of the organizational arrangement may be contributing factors. Second, the OSSs are being constantly monitored by state authorities and receive frequent visits from local government authorities from elsewhere in Brazil. This "spotlight effect" may provide a strong incentive for sustained performance. Finally, most OSS facility directors have been in the job since their facilities opened, whereas direct administration facilities suffer from high rotation of ranking managerial staff.[16]

A number of OSSs have been in existence since 1998 and continue to demonstrate robust (and improving) performance, at least compared with other organizational arrangements. A more plausible reason for their continued good performance than those just cited has to do with the characteristics of the model (see box 5.2). Key elements include strong decision-making autonomy, specified accountability mechanisms (in the management contract), performance-based financing, and clarity of functions.[17] This, however, raises the question of how facility managers respond to the incentives inherent in the organizational arrangement. What is it about this organizational arrangement that leads to better performance?

Two recent studies have examined this topic. Ferreira (2004) compared five OSS facilities with five matched direct administration hospitals in São Paulo state to explore how the different models affected the behaviors of facility directors in managing human resources, outsourcing, finances, and procurement. The World Bank (2006a) assessed and compared human resource management in a small sample of OSS, direct administration, and private facilities.

Ferreira found notable differences in managerial behaviors. Box 6.3 presents salient conclusions and quotations from interviews with facility managers on processes and practices related to human resource management, financial management, contract management, and procurement.[18] Overall, the findings suggest that OSS managers respond to the incentive structure inherent in the organizational arrangement and demonstrate considerable autonomy, flexibility, and innovation in management processes. Facility managers make decisions concerning staff volume and mix and the recruitment, selection, sanctioning, and dismissal of personnel.[19]

None of the OSSs has developed a formal system for evaluating staff performance or tested a performance payment scheme. Nearly all in-house personnel are hired under private law. Although OSS budgets are set by state authorities in negotiations with facility management, all OSS managers reallocate funds among budgetary items to address financing shortfalls, cover emergency expenditures, and ensure compliance with production and performance targets specified in the management contract. Meeting the targets is particularly important because a portion of financing is tied to performance. Three facilities reported securing bank loans to cover short-term gaps in state financing. The failure to consider the financing of depreciation required to maintain plant and equipment originally allocated to the facilities is a major shortcoming of the OSS model.

Unlike their counterparts under direct administration, OSSs do not outsource hotel services, but they do outsource more medical and diagnostic services. OSS managers appear to be more strategic in selecting services to be outsourced. As nonprofit, private organizations they are not taxed on in-house services. Contracted firms and cooperatives, however, pay

Box 6.3
Managers' Assessment of Managerial Processes and Practices in Hospitals under Direct Administration and OSS Arrangements, São Paulo State, 2003

Direct administration (N = 5)	*OSS (N = 5)*

Human resource management

- Three managers considered human resources (HR) the most problematic area because they have little decision-making authority over HR processes, which are controlled centrally. One lamented that anything dealing with HR is "too complicated." (Two managers considered this area the least problematic because they "have nothing to do with it.") One manager mentioned that he has to constantly "negotiate with personnel" on completion of tasks and fulfillment of contracted hours.

- Absenteeism and work shirking are constant problems; personnel secure medical certificates to justify absenteeism and tardiness.

- All managers reported problems with insufficient numbers and poor quality of personnel. The number and type of positions (determined centrally) have not been revised since the facilities were inaugurated and do not match changing demand and technologies. Vacancies become available only through staff turnover. Some managers have initiated training programs, but even here central approval is required.

- Most personnel are hired through centrally administered public competition. Pay levels are set for each personnel category by the state. Managers have autonomy to hire temporary staff only.

- Low salaries are considered problematic, and some managers have implemented incentive pay schemes tied to production (state program).

- Disciplinary actions and firings are rare because the processes are hugely cumbersome and time consuming, rendering them ineffective. One manager maintained that dismissal of staff requires a transgression "so grave . . . that it is something out of this world."

- Instruments and processes for distinguishing between high and low performers are nonexistent. According to one manager, HR issues are engrained in the public administration apparatus: "The solution for the HR problems does not depend on hospital management. In fact, it does not even depend on the state health secretary."

- Only two managers considered HR problematic. In one case HR decisions are centralized in the nonprofit governing organization (*entidade privada não lucrativa,* EPNL), which the manager considered "out of touch with the reality of the hospital." A second manager mentioned the difficulty of molding a high-performance organizational culture among staff who considered the OSS a public facility. Staff "have to shed the public (servant) mentality . . . that they have the right to do anything but can't be obligated to perform [*tudo pode e nada deve*]." All managers (or their predecessors) have defined the volume and types of staff positions in their facilities. Changes must be approved by the EPNL.

- All managers reported that facility management recruited and selected all staff. Recruitment follows processes established by facility management or the EPNL. Recruitment problems relate to reluctance of personnel to travel to poor, distant neighborhoods.

- Low salaries were mentioned as a problem for nurses, but two OSSs are targeting recent graduates and providing supplemental training. No OSS has implemented a performance pay scheme. There is no evidence of instruments for evaluating performance.

- Most managers did not report problems with volume or quality of personnel. Two stated that more personnel were needed, but that budgetary limitations prevented additional hiring. Nearly all in-house personnel are hired under private contract law (CLT); some specialized personnel are hired through outsourcing to firms and cooperatives. Hospital managers determine pay levels on the basis of local labor market realities.

- All managers report using private law to dismiss staff, applying either with-cause or without-cause procedures. Most prefer the without-cause method, which is more rapid but more costly, as it entails payment of compensation.

(continued)

Box 6.3 *(continued)*

Financial and budgetary management

- The budget is set by the state with little input from facility management.

- Production targets are not specified, except to "maintain prior levels." No sanctions are incurred for not meeting these levels.

- Managers "administer" the budget and cannot reallocate funds among budgetary items. If equipment breaks down, requiring costly repairs, managers must seek additional financing or permission from state authorities to reallocate. This can take time, resulting in long service interruptions.

- The budget ceiling is set by the state with little input from facility management, but facility budgets are negotiated with the EPNL on the basis of production targets and costs.

- Production targets are specified in the management contract negotiated with the state on the basis of the budget envelope. A portion of the budget is at risk if production and quality targets are not met.

- All managers surveyed had full autonomy to "manage" the budget, reallocate it among line items, ensure compliance with production targets (or face loss of revenue), and make emergency purchases (e.g., for equipment repairs and parts). Some reported using their recurrent budget for capital purchases.

- Three managers reported securing bank loans to cover budget deficits because of delays in state allocation of the global budget.

Contract (outsourcing) management

- All facilities outsource hotel and maintenance services but not diagnostic or medical services.

- Managers do not negotiate prices or set contractual terms. The state sets standard prices for services for all contracts.

- All managers have adjusted contractors' prices (up to 25 percent), but only with central approval and if the necessary funds are available. Managers do not alter contractual terms without central approval.

- Only one manager reported cancellation of contracts.

- Little outsourcing of hotel services was reported, except in one facility, but maintenance and transport are mostly outsourced. Three facilities contract out medical services (anesthesia) and diagnostic services (laboratory, radiology, and hemodialysis).

- All managers negotiate prices and contractual terms. They also reported adjusting contractual price terms. In one case the governing institution performed these functions.

- All managers reported rescinding contracts for poor performance or noncompliance with contractual terms.

Procurement

- Periodic stock-outs were reported by four (of five) managers.

- Nearly all procurement is performed centrally; this is considered bureaucratic and slow. According to one respondent, "the timing (of central purchasing) has to be right, if not, you are left without stocks."

- Only one hospital reported possessing a standard formulary.

- All facilities have access to credit for emergency purchases up to R$8,000. Formal competitive bidding is not required for these purchases.

- All managers reported problems with the inventory infrastructure (physical space, ventilation, shelving)

- Stocks for three to six months are maintained because the state-operated procurement system makes large but irregular purchases.

- No stock-outs were reported.

- All OSSs carry out procurement according to internal rules published in the official state public record, *Diário Oficial do Estado*. In three facilities, facility managers execute all purchasing; in two, it is performed by the EPNLs. The latter is seen as advantageous because EPNLs participate in a pool procurement scheme with other facilities and secure lower prices.

- Emergency purchases are performed rapidly without restrictions (except for budget availability).

- Stocks for less than 45 days are maintained, thanks to the flexibility of the procurement system.

- No problems were reported with inventory control.

- All hospitals have developed a standard formulary.

Source: Ferreira 2004.

taxes on income, which would raise prices of contracted services and thus provide a disincentive for contracting.[20] Finally, procurement is performed by the facility or nonprofit entity (the EPNL) under contract with the state and follows OSS-developed internal rules published by the state. Managers report no problems or delays in procurement or inventory. All managers claim that they can make price adjustments to contracts, adjust terms, and rescind contracts.

In contrast, managers of facilities under direct administration act as administrators or processors of functions performed elsewhere in the state bureaucracy, and their autonomy with respect to human resource, financial, and procurement tasks is limited. Staff positions were defined when the facilities were inaugurated, which in many cases was decades ago, and can be adjusted only by state government—an irregular and infrequent process. Furthermore, recruitment occurs during periodic "mass *concursos*," when fiscal resources become available. Facility managers do not participate in the recruitment process related to the concurso. Invariably, they must hire the highest-rated individuals sent by the state government from the selection process.

Because nearly all OSS personnel are hired under CLT legislation, dismissal with or without cause after a probationary period is simple, compared with the procedure for dismissing a civil servant. Dismissal with cause calls for evidence of cause and a written warning, and if the transgression occurs again, the staff member may face a reduction in benefits. The staff member can contest any decision in labor courts, which generally favor the worker. Many OSS managers opt for dismissal without cause. This process is immediate, requiring just a single communication, but it can be financially costly because of severance and other compensation payments.

Under direct administration, lack of authority over staff leads to a complex managerial situation in which managers can do little but "negotiate" with staff to complete tasks, show up for work, arrive on time, and so on. This common practice throughout the public delivery system is known as the tradeoff, or favor exchange (*troca de favores*). Managers negotiate with professional staff the number of real work hours, which are always less than the contracted work hours. What this benefit essentially means is that working fewer than the contracted hours is condoned in most direct administration facilities as long as it is negotiated with managers.

As suggested above, sanctions and dismissals are rare in direct administration facilities, where managers must navigate a lengthy and complicated dismissal procedure that may take years, with high personal and time costs. Given most managers' short tenure, they prefer to avoid the process. In an OSS, work shirking and absenteeism are not tolerated. The threat of rapid sanctioning and, possibly, dismissal likely reinforces the incentive to perform.

Managers are unable to reallocate the few budgetary items under their command to meet increased or changing demand, or even to make an emergency repair. The slowness and irregularity of the state-managed procurement process contributes to stock-outs, while the typically large purchases are beyond the spatial means of facility stockrooms. All facilities under direct administration outsource hotel and maintenance services. Although the state sets prices and contractual terms, managers report making decisions to adjust these items. Contract management is generally performed by state administrative units.

From his observations of managerial behaviors of facilities under direct administration, Ferreira concluded that this organizational arrangement, at least as practiced in São Paulo state, was a "restrictive, "centralized," and "deficient" model that offered "few opportunities for innovation" (Ferreira 2004: 120). These public hospitals have difficulties in adapting to their changing environment, in part because of political interference in management and rigidities in civil service statutes that hamper the manager's ability to make necessary personnel changes. Ferreira cited human resource management as the most critical area. He concluded that civil service rules handicap managers who are attempting to develop and implement an effective human resource policy that would help improve performance in all facets of facility services and operations.[21]

In a recent interview with a director of an OSS hospital, the importance of the enabling environment created by that model was highlighted:

> I have become convinced that it is not possible to apply modern management techniques for human resource management and the agile purchasing of inputs without the [organizational] tools to do so . . . the OSS [model] is very agile, supplying the manager with the managerial means that are similar to private enterprise, and this is progress in terms of [public] administration . . . The great virtue [of the model] is the lack of [managerial] interference by the State Secretariat of Health, which makes the OSS accountable in terms of result indicators. (*Revista de Administração em Saúde* 6 [24]: 81)

The human resource issue was further analyzed in a recent in-depth study of personnel practices in seven facilities under direct administration, seven OSSs, four private facilities, and two public facilities with private support foundations (World Bank 2006a). The findings reported here focus on direct administration and OSS hospitals. The results confirmed the decision-making authority of OSS managers, and the lack of such autonomy for directors of direct administration facilities, concerning items such as wage bill control, personnel selection, and pay determination. Importantly, although the OSSs have significantly better information on production and efficiency, they do not systematically evaluate performance or implement a performance pay scheme. Direct administration facilities have implemented a state program, the Special Incentive Reward, for physicians, nurses, auxiliary nurses, and other professionals involved in care provision. In a finding similar to Ferreira's, the study concluded that the scheme is mostly ineffective because nearly all personnel receive a bonus.

Drawing on focus groups, interviews, and a staff survey, the study sought to test four human resource–related hypotheses to explain the observed higher performance of the OSSs when compared with direct administration facilities. The hypotheses were that (1) higher salaries in OSS hospitals permit managers to attract and retain higher quality personnel; (2) OSSs offer staff tailored bonus payments to improve performance; (3) OSSs provide superior supervision; or (4) OSSs offer better professional development and training opportunities.

All these hypothesis were rejected. The findings suggest, instead, that an important element of accountability contributes to performance: management's authority to recruit, select, and dismiss personnel. For example, directors advertised for physicians through informal networks within the São Paulo health care community to identify potential recruits. They interviewed all candidates and could check qualifications. Thus they were able to select those that best fit the organization's mission and management style. Nursing positions were announced in public advertisements, but again, selection followed a formal interview process.[22] In contrast, and similar to Ferreira's (2004) findings discussed earlier, hospitals under direct administration must follow civil service rules that require managers to select the candidates scoring highest on a multiple-choice, standardized test and a review of curricula vitae by state human resource administrators. Candidates are not interviewed, and whether the selected candidate is suited for the organization is not considered.

As mentioned above, flexible working hours appear to be an integral part of the incentive structure of the personnel systems ingrained in the public service regime. Health professionals typically hold multiple jobs to meet income goals and mitigate the risk of loss of any single job (CREMESP 2002). Most physicians are hired for 20-hour work weeks, and most nurses work 30 hours. Health professionals seek employment or continued employment in direct administration facilities because of the flexible hours and lifetime tenure.

This practice is purposely permitted because public salaries are considered low. There is little evidence, however, that salaries in direct administration are lower than those paid in the OSSs, where negotiable working hours are prohibited. In fact, interviews with staff who had worked in both types of facilities suggest that the salary differences are not significant, yet OSSs extract considerably more production from their medical staff (World Bank 2006a).

Some managers under direct administration have introduced state-sponsored incentive pay schemes to raise production. Such incentive schemes have not been evaluated, but their impact may be minimal. Bonuses are generally applied to an entire category of staff (e.g., physicians and nurses), with little differentiation among individuals. None of the OSSs offered performance bonuses, nor was there any evidence that OSSs offer more opportunities for training or professional development than their direct administration counterparts.

Finally, the research suggests that many professionals consider the OSSs superior and increasingly prestigious work settings (World Bank 2006a). This perception, along with the newness of the infrastructure and the "spotlight" effect of the innovation, may contribute to higher production. But in fact, the overall incentive regime—autonomous authority to manage human resources and apply CLT procedures, accountability for production targets within a hard budget constraint as specified in the management contract, and performance-linked financing—drives managers to strategically recruit staff with the "right fit" and to dismiss them rapidly when performance problems arise. In a sense, professionals must align their individual incentives with institutional incentives or go elsewhere.

Managerial Autonomy and Organizational Arrangements

Autonomy is considered a principal determinant of managerial behaviors because it "lets managers manage." It is seen as the key driver of performance, partly because it provides managers with flexibility in purchasing and allocating all inputs. But autonomy is not an "absolute state" (Castaño, Bitrán, and Giedion 2004: 3). As international experience has shown, autonomy is tricky to validate: it varies across organizational models, as well as across managerial dimensions for any given model (Preker and Harding 2003). Formal arrangements may not result in real decision-making authority. It is important to understand the real allocations of decision making that determine behaviors.

As noted, organizational structures and managerial behaviors have been found to be correlated. The OSS case study showed that, in comparison with their direct administration counterparts, OSS facilities apply modern and more effective managerial practices to human resource, purchasing, and financial management. Strong decision-making authority appears to be an essential contributing factor.

The link between autonomy and managerial practices is explored here through a typological analysis. Table 6.1 presents the available evidence on the range of decision-making autonomy for major managerial dimensions across organizational forms found in Brazilian hospitals.[23]

Managers of facilities under direct and indirect administration arrangements exercise restricted decision rights. If a hospital is an independent budgetary unit, as are federal hospitals and most facilities under indirect administration, managers have some latitude in budgetary management.[24] Under direct and indirect administration, most subnational governments do not permit managers to operate incentive payment schemes, even if funding is available.

TABLE 6.1
Managerial Autonomy in Public Sector Organizational Arrangements
(key: N, none or very limited; R, restricted; F, full or nearly full)

Managerial dimensions	Direct administration	Indirect administration	Autonomous administration		
			FA	SSA	OSS
Human resources					
Recruitment and dismissal	N	N	F	F	F
Promotion	N	N	F	F	F
Remuneration	N	R	F	F	F
Staffing mix	N	R	F	F	F
Promotion	N	N	F	F	F
Service mix					
Open or close services	N	R	N	F	R
Procurement					
Consumables	R[a]	R	F	F	F
Equipment	N	N	F	F	F
Price negotiation	N	N	F	F	F
Contracting (outsourcing)					
Definition	N	N	F	F	F
Negotiation	N	N	F	F	F
Contract management	R[b]	R[b]	F	F	F
Budget and finance					
Budget formation	N[c]	R	R	F	F
Budget modification	N[c]	R	R	F	F
Accounting system	N	N	R	F	F
Capital					
Plant	N	N	N	F	N
Equipment upgrading	N	N	R	F	N
Organizational					
Definition of structure	N	R	F	F	F

Source: Authors' elaboration.
Note: FA, private support foundation; SSA, autonomous social services; OSS, health social organization.
a. Federal facilities conduct their own purchasing. Most municipal facilities do not. In most cases procurement by facilities is limited to small purchases. Some states, such as São Paulo, permit larger facilities to purchase all drugs and supplies.
b. Facilities may have some authority to expand or eliminate contracting of nonmedical services, but this is usually done in coordination with government authorities.
c. Federally operated facilities, as well as a minority of state and municipal facilities, are independent budgetary units and therefore have limited autonomy in budgetary management.

Managers of facilities under indirect administration also have restricted decision-making autonomy in defining services and staffing mix. Their decision rights over recruitment and dismissal of staff are limited; as in direct administration, those managers must follow the public sector labor and procurement regimes.

The autonomous administration models displayed in table 6.1 allow considerably more autonomy, but restrictions also apply. All the models grant full or nearly full autonomy for decisions involving human resources, purchasing, and outsourcing. Only autonomous social services (*serviços sociais autônomos*, SSAs) enjoy across-the-board decision-making autonomy. This model, however, is rare in hospitals and is dependent on specific federal legislation. As has been seen, the OSSs grant managers extensive decision rights, and managers exercise those rights, demonstrating autonomous decision-making behaviors and practices along an array of managerial dimensions. Capital investments in OSSs are, however, dependent on and managed by government. OSSs can create, eliminate, and expand services without government approval, but they are not permitted to sell services to private patients or insurers.[25]

Contracting and Contract Management

As reviewed in chapters 4 and 5, the management contract is a key element of the OSS accountability arrangement that drives the model's higher performance results. The OSS contracts specify production targets, quality benchmarks, the implementation of medical record systems, financial reporting requirements, and quality improvement processes. Annual financial audits are performed by the state comptroller-general

São Paulo state faced a steep learning curve regarding arm's-length contract management. It was not an easy transition, considering the direct administration culture that permeated all aspects of health management within the state health secretariat before the OSS policy. Learning to influence hospital behaviors through contracting, specifically through contract negotiations and management, did not occur overnight.[26] For example, the original contract (in 1998) did not include variable financing linked to performance, nor was it very precise in the specification of outputs. In 2001 the state began to withhold 10 percent of the OSS quarterly budget allocation, to be disbursed on the basis of performance indicators. Not until 2001 did the state secretariat of health form a service contract coordinating unit to monitor and manage the OSS contracts. The secretariat also mandated the installation of information and cost accounting systems to provide the state with data needed for robust service specification, monitoring, and budget formulation. Given the potential for conflicts of interest, OSS legislation mandated the creation of an independent assessment commission, which was finally formed in 2001. Each quarter, the commission, consisting of representatives of the state executive and legislative branches and of civil society, assesses OSS performance and contract compliance and makes payment recommendations based on compliance with production targets and quality indicators.

The state's growing contract management capacity is another element of the accountability arrangement. The state has demonstrated both willingness and capacity to enforce contractual terms, withholding part of the variable budget in a number of instances and canceling an OSS contract. In 2002 one facility failed to meet targets for average length of stay (ALOS), and a portion of the variable budget was withheld. Another facility lost part of the variable financing because of deficient accounting practices. In 2004 two hospitals' variable payments were reduced, one for noncompliance with information quality targets and the other for failure to meet quality of care targets. In 2007 the state did not renew an OSS contract (with an EPLN), partly because of low performance.

Brazil's Experience with Hospital Conversion: Overcoming Human Resource and Financial Obstacles

Converting hospitals under direct administration to more autonomous organizational arrangements is an important issue for Brazil and has been raised by state and municipal authorities. A number of state and municipal officials are interested in conversion but do not have the institutional capacity and technical know-how to guide change. They also fear political fallout (from employee unions and their supporters) and perceive little federal support for more autonomous organizational arrangements (box 6.4). Some states and municipalities are considering legislation to facilitate facility conversion. Thus, there is evidence that

---

Box 6.4
The Politics of OS Implementation in the Health Sector

Social organizations were seen as the centerpiece organizational arrangement for performing social activities and services wholly or partially funded by the government. As described in this chapter, in the health sector a few states moved to introduce OSs in *new* hospitals, but only a handful of *existing* hospital has been converted to this form. There are several reasons for this.

First, conversion would require civil servants to shed their rights and protection under civil service law and enter into a private labor regime (CLT) that could offer higher salaries but would not guarantee lifelong employment. Public employees have little incentive to switch, and the political cost of forcing a transfer would be prohibitively high. Second, because OSs hire all staff through the private labor regime, local governments would lose control of an important opportunity for patronage. Finally, debate on OSs has been intense and often ideologically driven. Public health employee unions, as well as some professional associations, consider social organizations a form of privatization linked to the "neoliberal" administrative reforms associated with the government of Fernando Henrique Cardoso (1996–2002). These opposed groups are politically aligned with President Lula's Workers Party (Partido dos Trabalhadores, PT), which gained power in 2003 and enacted a policy of strengthening the direct administration model and expanding civil service employment.[a]

Importantly, on March 10, 2005, the National Health Council issued its Deliberation 1, which declared the OSS arrangement a form of outsourcing (*terceirização*) that was unconstitutional and unaligned with "SUS principles." The decree mandated the elimination of OSSs and gave states and municipalities 12 months to enact the appropriate measures. Although the decree has little legal authority and the claim of unconstitutionality can be challenged, the action sent local governments a clear message of opposition to expansion of social organizations by the Ministry of Health. Nevertheless, the second Lula government (2007–11) appears to have shifted its position and supports legislation creating an OS-like organizational arrangement in public hospitals, as described in this chapter.

a. This policy is driven in part by the party's strong political base among public sector employee unions. For example, in 2004 the federal government attempted to eliminate the hiring of long-term consultants under private contracts (CLT, temporary, and other forms) in federal ministries and mandated that any federal workers occupying these positions be civil servants. Some ministries and departments within ministries were restaffed through public competitive selection *(concurso público);* others are still waiting for approval to launch the selection process.

a new generation of reforms may emerge, this one seeking to transform public hospitals into alternative organizational forms.

Only a few health facilities under direct administration in Brazil have been converted to an alternative arrangement. This section reports on two current experiences in São Paulo state, with a large state emergency and ambulatory care center and a municipal hospital that were converted to OSSs.[27] Because these are recent initiatives and data from the preconversion period are sparse, the findings reported here are preliminary and should be interpreted with caution; none have been evaluated. These experiences, however, do provide indirect evidence of the potential for efficiency and quality gains, as well as the impediments related to thorny personnel management and finance issues involved in conversion. It is important to bear in mind that the OSS-managed hospitals described earlier involved new facilities and thus avoided some of the issues described here.

Case 1: Luzia de Pinho Melo Emergency and Ambulatory Care Center

In late 2004 São Paulo state completed construction of a new 270-bed inpatient facility that was annexed to an existing emergency care center with 50 observation beds and a specialty ambulatory care unit. All of the center's 690 staff were state civil servants.[28] Most professional staff had contracts for 20-hour work weeks. The new hospital was inaugurated under OSS management with a global budget and management contract. The original idea was for the OSS to manage only the hospital, while the emergency center would remain under direct administration. This arrangement, however, was short-lived, in part because of differences in accountability arrangements and management styles between the two models.

Several months after the hospital's inauguration, the OSS assumed management of the emergency and ambulatory care center. The center's personnel were offered the option of remaining at the facility but abiding by OSS personnel rules, including compliance with the number of contracted hours, or going to a position in another, state-operated facility. More than 60 percent chose to leave within the first year of OSS management, and most obtained positions in facilities under direct administration elsewhere in the state. Forty-five percent of the physicians (129 of 290) and 84 percent of nurses and nurse auxiliaries (185 of 220) sought positions in other facilities or quit, claiming "incompatible work hours" or "inability to adapt" to the OSS work regime.

This experience suggests an employee preference to negotiate real working hours (and work schedules) at direct administration facilities and not be subject to the more demanding work rules of the OSS. As noted, this practice enables multiple job holding, which is common among medical professionals in São Paulo. For example, many nurses had arranged "12–36" work schedules in which they worked a 12-hour shift and then received 36 hours off. The OSS demanded six-hour daily shifts to enable more continuous patient care and stronger ties to the facility. Most of the nurses left because they worked other jobs during their off periods. It was also common knowledge that an undetermined number of physicians worked for less than their contracted hours.

The OSS found creative ways to gain the commitment of civil servants who remained. For example, the OSS bypassed civil service rules and gave promotions and raises to 36 staff members who, unofficially, were qualified for and occupied managerial positions but had not been promoted because of lack of vacancies in government employment registers or rigidities in public sector rules. In effect, these staff members were not receiving remuneration commensurate with their qualifications or the jobs they were performing.[29] Recognizing this discrepancy, the OSS granted these workers contracts under the CLT to work additional hours with commensurate remuneration for jobs for which they were qualified, and which they were doing. The OSS also provided additional benefits such as uniforms, a monthly food subsidy (*cesta básica*), and life insurance for all workers, as well as educational scholarships (*bolsas de estudos*) for some.

The OSS assumed management of a facility in disarray. The center's stockrooms and pharmacies were disorganized, with out-of-date medicines. Equipment maintenance was lax, and sanitary conditions were substandard. The OSS invested in upgrading equipment and plant and in training staff. It renegotiated cleaning and janitorial contracts, thus reducing prices paid by 40 percent while benchmarking performance. It standardized processes for managing patient flows (e.g., triage in the emergency center, intrafacility referrals), staff scheduling, visitor access, requisitions and billing, central supplies, inventory, laboratory, pharmacy, food service, and laundry. It introduced information systems to track prescriptions, pharmaceutical distribution, billing, and payments. Finally, it expanded auxiliary and specialty care offered at the emergency center, adding 12 specialties and 3 diagnostic services: tomography, mammography, and echoencephalography.

Most of these improvements were funded through the global budget negotiated with the state for the newly constructed hospital. During the second year of operation the budget for the center was incorporated into the hospital's global budget.[30] Significantly, the facility did not retain the monetary value of the salaries of transferred staff; any additional hires to replace transferred staff were financed through the global budget. Efficiency gains derived from the renegotiation of supply and service contracts were invested in facility upgrading and service expansion. Some of the equipment purchases had been made by the state government prior to conversion, but the OSS completed installation of the equipment and initiated service expansion.

The available data suggest significant gains in production and productivity. Between 2004 (before conversion) and 2006, the annual number of emergency consultations at the center increased 50 percent. Clearly, the increase in production resulted in part from the addition of new specialty services such as neurosurgery. Still, the emergency unit (now the hospital's emergency room) currently operates with a smaller staff than before conversion, suggesting productivity gains. For example, in 2007 the emergency unit employed 272 physicians, nurses, and nurse auxiliaries, a decrease of 8 percent from 296 in 2004. The total number of staff—medical personnel, receptionists, technicians, registrars, and so on—was reduced slightly, from 319 to 316. The improvement in plant and equipment, the introduction of standardized processes for materials and pharmaceutical management and for the ordering of patient flows, and the continuous presence of physicians and nurses point to quality gains. In 2006 the hospital and emergency center were accredited by the National Accreditation Organization (Organização Nacional de Acreditação, ONA).[31]

Case 2: São José dos Campos Municipal Hospital

In 2006 São Jose dos Campos, a large city with 600,000 inhabitants just north of the city of São Paulo, asked an OSS to take over management of a 275-bed hospital operated directly by the municipality. In 2005 the hospital's R$84.6 million (US$35 million) budget consumed about half of the municipal health budget.[32] In July 2006 the OSS assumed management of the facility under a global budget and management contract aligned closely with the OSS model implemented by São Paulo state.

This facility had 900 workers prior to conversion. Upon conversion, 200 staff, including 102 nurses, requested and obtained transfers to other facilities in the municipal network. As in case 1, discussed above, most preferred to negotiate their work schedules at facilities under direct administration rather than abide by the stricter work rules imposed by the OSS. Importantly, the municipality welcomed these transfers because it enabled the health secretariat to fill human resource gaps elsewhere in the service delivery system. The OSS hired 809 part-time employees under private labor law, including 139 physicians, 58 graduate nurses, and 213 auxiliary nurses, to fill critical human resource needs throughout the hospital and to staff new and expanded services.

Like the OSS managing the center in case 1, the OSS invested in new plant and equipment and information systems, in the amount of about US$1.3 million. It also arranged for nearly 10,000 hours of training to upgrade staff skills, established standardized processes for clinical and nonclinical management and pharmaceutical management, and introduced a triage system in the emergency room. The hospital initiated new outpatient specialty services (neurology and endocrinology) and expanded services in cardiology, otorhinolaryngology, and physical and occupational therapy. Unlike the preconversion situation, inpatient, intensive care, and emergency services now operate with the continuous presence of a full contingent of nursing staff. Several outpatient units extended working hours from 8 to 12 hours.

Preliminary data from the 10 months after conversion (August 2006 to May 2007) suggest production and efficiency gains when compared with the corresponding 10 months before conversion, August 2005 to May 2006 (table 6.2).[33] The volume of ambulatory visits, inpatient discharges, and surgeries increased markedly. Emergency visits declined as a result of the

TABLE 6.2
Municipal Hospital São José dos Campos: Comparison of Available Production, Efficiency, and Quality Indicators Before and After Conversion

Indicator	Before conversion (10 months, August 2005–May 2006)	After conversion (10 months, August 2006–May 2007)	Percent change
Ambulatory visits	37,715	45,115	19.6
Emergency visits	211,804.0	205,555.0	−3.0
Inpatient discharges	12,536[a]	15,160[b]	20.9
Surgeries	5,029	5,658	12.5
ALOS (days)	4.5	4.3	−0.04
Bed turnover rate[c]	5.0	5.9	18.0
Neonatal mortality rate[d]	8.5[e]	5.5[f]	−35.0

Source: Statistical registers, Hospital São José dos Campos.
a. Nine months, August 2005–April 2006.
b. Nine months, August 2006–April 2007.
c. Average number of discharges per bed per month.
d. Infant deaths during first 28 days of life per 1,000 births.
e. 2005.
f. January–June 2007.

implementation of a triage system that reduced the number of unnecessary visits. The increase in bed turnover rate and the slight reduction in ALOS indicate efficiency improvements. The reduction in neonatal mortality suggests significant quality enhancement. According to hospital officials, these reductions were achieved through improved clinical management, including the hiring of a neonatal specialist, the establishment of a committee to review infant and maternal deaths and recommend procedures for avoiding future deaths, and the application of protocols in obstetric and neonatal units.[34] It is worth repeating that these improvements in performance, together with quality upgrades and training, were achieved mainly through efficiency gains rather than budgetary increases.[35]

The management contract was the source of all investment and recurrent financing. The contract specified a budget of R$81.3 million (US$ 37.3 million) for the 12-month period from August 2006 to July 2007.[36] This amount was essentially the same as the budget for the previous 12 months.[37] In other words, the OSS managed the facility within the same financial envelope as its predecessor, the municipality, did under direct administration.[38]

Within the budgetary envelope, the OSS financed mainly facility upgrading, quality improvement, and service expansion, drawing on three sources. First, the OSS retained the monetary value of the 200 transferred staff (evidently, the municipality possessed budgeted vacancies elsewhere in the delivery system to enable absorption of these workers). Second, the OSS achieved efficiency gains by renegotiating contracts with suppliers and service providers. For example, after diagnosing the workloads of personnel hired through service contractors (e.g., security), the OSS demanded and secured reductions in the value of these contracts by eliminating redundant staff.[39] The main source of finance, however, was windfall savings derived from the elimination of nearly all overtime pay. Before conversion, about 700 workers received overtime pay, amounting to 25 percent of the facility's personnel budget.[40] The dramatic reduction in overtime yielded savings of approximately US$525,000 a month, and most of this was used to hire new staff.

Lessons from the Case Studies

What lessons can be taken from these conversion experiences?[41] The first lesson involves the critical area of human resource management. In part to avoid legal challenges, upon conversion civil servants were assured of their employment link to government, as well as maintenance of their salaries and benefits. They were also given the options of remaining at the OSS-managed facility or transferring to another government facility. The transferred staff was replaced in part with personnel contracted by an OSS under the private labor regime. The cases reveal civil servants' reluctance to accept work rules such as those demanded by the OSSs; if given a choice, many would seek relocation to direct administration facilities. Experience suggests that between 20 and 50 percent of staff will seek transfers, but the percentage may be higher among physicians and nurses. Unless subnational governments have a large unmet need for personnel elsewhere in their delivery systems and can underwrite additional budgetary outlays, most can ill afford to continue to pay salaries for civil servants placed elsewhere in the system while assuming the additional cost of new hires in the converted facility. Also, given the difficulty of dismissing civil servants for poor performance, the OSS has an informal understanding with the local government in each facility to transfer inept, unreliable, and low-performing staff to facilities elsewhere in the system. This may be ideal for securing institutional commitment of staff and improving the performance of the converted facility, but it offers few advantages to the facilities receiving these unwanted workers. The experience a decade earlier with the Health Care Plan (Plano de Atendimento à Saúde, PAS) was that civil servants who were relocated to other facilities had insufficient work, contributing to higher costs with little or no impact on service production.[42] This demonstrates that in any system, there is a limit to available vacancies for placing disgruntled civil servants.

Civil servants are reluctant to relinquish their public employment ties. Some favor the security of life-long employment. Most have many years of service and have built up a nest egg for retirement in the public social security system, which offers benefits superior to those in most private systems. Under these conditions, civil servants have had little interest in resigning from the public service and taking private sector contracts (CLTs).

Another limitation relates to the supply of nurses and physicians. São Paulo state has a large supply of medical professionals, but other regions in Brazil would be hard-pressed to find replacements to staff in converted facilities because of the scarcity of supply.

Once a converted facility secures a critical mass of staff, whether civil servants or CLT employees who want to be there and to abide by the OSS-mandated work rules, an enabling environment for human resource management has been established that is conducive to improving performance. As practiced in São Paulo, the conversion model related to human resources is limited by the availability of budgeted personnel vacancies elsewhere in the health system for absorbing transferred workers and by the overall market supply of personnel to replace the departed workers in the converted facility. Furthermore, few civil servants would be willing to convert to the private labor regime. Given these restrictions, subsequent conversions may occur much more slowly (and display less immediate results) because civil servants would be only gradually replaced with CLT-contracted personnel through attrition. Issuing CLT contracts to civil servants to work additional hours (as was done by the OSS in case 1) can generate staff commitment to the facility and improve accountability for performance.

As is discussed in the next section, international experience suggests that conversion would be facilitated and possibly accelerated through legislation that creates autonomous institutional structures and flexible employment regimes for health workers. Box 6.5 reviews issues and opportunities in Brazil's legal framework supporting autonomous management and alternative labor practices related to hospital conversion.

A second lesson involves the potential for efficiency and quality gains that in turn can defray the costs of conversion. In both cases, government did not have to significantly increase budgetary or investment outlays for these facilities because of the savings realized by reducing overtime pay, renegotiating and managing supplier and service contracts, eliminating duplicate personnel, and standardizing processes related to material and clinical management, patient flows, and diagnostic services. In effect, these savings underwrote the costs of hiring replacement staff, extending service hours, introducing new services, and investing in improving quality structures and processes. The limited evidence suggests that the converted facilities obtained greater value for money, demonstrating major productivity and quality gains without significant increases in payroll or overall spending levels. Nevertheless, more research is needed on balancing the savings generated by improved resource management with the costs of transferring and maintaining disgruntled employees elsewhere in the system.

Third, interviews with staff suggest that conversion implies a "cultural shock" with respect to hospital management and work processes. It entails transforming a management style that is employee-centered and focused on complying with norms and rules to one that is

Box 6.5
Hospital Conversion in Brazil: Legal Constraints and Opportunities

A 1998 constitutional amendment (Article 8, modifying Article 37) mandated the extension of "financial, budgetary, and managerial autonomy" to hospitals under direct and indirect administration and authorized the drafting of a law to determine personnel remuneration, as well as contracting terms and processes. In principle, the amendment established the legal foundation for converting public hospitals to more autonomous forms and for dealing with the touchy issue of personnel conversion. Congress has yet to begin drafting the legislation.

Federal social organization (OS) legislation was not specific to the health sector or to hospitals. The original intent of the drafters was to transform the management of museums, research institutes, social institutions, and other parastatal agencies to OSs. The law contains a disincentive for public personnel—the main input in public hospitals—to transfer to the private regime. OS legislation (Article 14) prohibits civil servants from retaining any benefits (e.g., career paths) and rights (e.g., lifetime employment) from the public regime once they are incorporated into a (private) regime under the OS. As was also the case in Colombia, Portugal, and Spain, the authors of the OS law thought that civil servants would be gradually replaced through attrition by personnel contracted under private law (Bresser-Pereira 1998: 246). The law does not permit civil servants remaining in the converted hospital to receive any additional remuneration or benefits paid by the OS beyond those specified in the public regime. Consequently, employees of a to-be-converted facility would likely seek relocation, in part because flexible hours would be eliminated and therefore more work would be demanded without additional compensation.

In the case of São Jose dos Campos Municipal Hospital, discussed in the text, the OSS issued CLT contracts to civil servants who held coordinator positions or performed tasks for which they were fully qualified but were unrecognized by the civil service. It also issued private contracts to public employees to work during hours outside their public contract. According to the OSS, such an arrangement is legal because it involves a separate contract rather than additional remuneration or bonuses and does not interfere with public contract hours or responsibilities.

Personnel conversion has also occurred in nonhealth public agencies converted to OSs, for example, several parastatal agencies.[a] Some public servants voluntarily resigned from the civil service and accepted private contracts. These experiences require evaluation to flesh out the nuances of labor practices.

Source: Authors' elaboration.

a. These agencies included the Riquette Pinto Education Communication Association (Associação de Comunicação Educativa Riquette Pinto, ACERP), the Mamirauá Sustainable Development Institute (Instituto de Desenvolvimento Sustentável Mamirauá, IDSM), and the National Basic and Applied Mathematics Institute (Instituto Nacional de Matemática Pura e Aplicada, IMPA).

patient-centered and involved with fulfilling contractual obligations related to performance. It also requires application of modern clinical and nonclinical management practices. Conversion demands accountability for processes and results where there had been none. Not all personnel or managers who have spent years laboring in direct administration facilities can make this transition. In each of the cases discussed, employee resistance was often manifested in the press and through local politicians. There is constant pressure, particularly from professionals transferred to other posts, to return to the status quo ante. Although conversion is still a work in progress, this resistance has been overcome through strong and continuous support from state and municipal governments and from civil society organizations allied with the OSS, such as universities and nonprofit hospitals. But the experiences also suggest that conversion means investing in staff: upgrading skills, improving working conditions, providing access to new knowledge and technologies, improving remuneration, creating opportunities for promotion, and linking pay levels to responsibilities. Rigidities in the public sector labor regime, combined with lack of decision-making authority, limit managers' ability to apply innovative labor practices.

Finally, conversion involves winning over the clients and the community. Reduction in waiting lists, quality improvements, service expansion, and extension of hours helped gain community support for the converted facilities. It is best if these benefits are observable in the short term.

International Experience with Hospital Conversion

International experience suggests that conversion is a long-term, incremental process fraught with political challenges. Although no rigorous evaluations have been published on the effects of conversion on performance, preliminary assessments in several countries suggest that efficiency and productivity gains have been achieved, with no decrease in quality or patient satisfaction.[43] Conversion, however, does not occur in a vacuum. Experience demonstrates that it should be part of a broader hospital reform package oriented toward rationalizing supply and improving efficiency and quality. Important features of such a package include reforming payment mechanisms, separating finance from provision, reducing excess infrastructure and consolidating overlapping services, introducing autonomous organizational structures, and modifying human resource management practices. This section summarizes experiences in six countries that have converted public hospitals: Austria, Australia, Colombia, Estonia, Portugal, and Spain. The discussion focuses on three key categorical elements of the process: formulation of a master plan, modification of the legal and regulatory framework, and regulations affecting human resource management.

Legal and Regulatory Framework

Legislation sets the stage for the gradual transformation of public hospital governance and management. In all countries a legal framework was approved that converted public facilities into private, nonprofit entities (e.g., foundations, trusts, associations, joint-stock companies) under private law. A master plan prepared the way for drafting key legislation. Alternative organizational arrangements established in Austria, Colombia, Estonia, and Spain are reviewed below.

Austria
Starting in the late 1990s, municipal hospitals, with their assets, were transferred to state-level hospital holding companies incorporated under private corporate law in each of Austria's nine states.[44] Although the facilities are publicly owned, they are operated privately through the nonprofit holding companies. The state government remains the main owner of the holding company and maintains contractual arrangements with it. This model had the added advantage of placing most facilities in a multihospital network under a single

command and management structure (the holding company). This assisted horizontal integration of facilities within each state and led to efficiency gains through reduction of underutilized infrastructure, merging of specialty and hospital services, and centralization of support and diagnostic functions such as information technology and laboratory services.[45] The organizational reforms were accompanied by the introduction of a diagnosis-related group (DRG) payment mechanism for hospitals. Cost containment results have been impressive; once the reforms were in place, annual cost increases were more than halved (Fidler et al. 2007: 332).

Colombia

Law 100 of 1993 ushered in a wave of far-reaching reforms that transformed the Colombian health system. A key feature of the reform was the conversion of government- or social security–managed hospitals to autonomous organizations known as state social enterprises (*empresas sociales del estado*, ESEs) governed by private law. By 2004 nearly all secondary and tertiary hospitals had been converted to ESEs. Hospital managers enjoy decision-making rights with respect to supplies, case mix, managerial processes, and capital investments, but they do not enjoy residual claimant status, and, as explained below, they possess limited decision-making authority in managing human resources. Decisions regarding the use of surplus funds rest with government. Management is overseen by governance boards consisting of representatives of government, employees, and users. Under the reform, ESEs compete for contracts from insurers and HMOs but receive direct subsidies from government to provide the uninsured population with services. Consistent with the ESE reform, government is restructuring the public hospitals to improve the efficiency and quality of care and enable the hospitals to compete in the provider market. Restructuring involves reducing labor costs and supplier debts, introducing modern management techniques, and applying performance-based financing vis-à-vis government and insurers. Toro et al. (2007) found that the 179 restructured hospitals demonstrated higher production and productivity and lower production costs than control facilities; operating deficits were also significantly reduced.

Estonia

A national law of 2001 converted public hospitals into private foundations or joint-stock companies. In each instance, hospitals were granted independent legal status with financial and managerial autonomy, but assets remained public. Nearly all the facilities operate under private law for management of inputs, including human resources. The extent of residual claimant status and access to markets varies. In several cases legislation mandated the formation of facility governance boards that are accountable for financial and operational performance. Because government is the main owner or founder of the foundations and joint-stock companies, it is strongly represented on the boards. Consonant with a master plan for hospital investments, a number of facilities were merged under the newly formed organizational arrangements. Some foundations thus manage multifacility networks of hospitals, ambulatory units, and diagnostic centers. These changes resulted in improved efficiency through facility closures, reduction in underutilized bed capacity, consolidation of redundant services, and improved clinical management. Data on three regional networks demonstrate significant reduction in beds and length of stay, together with increases in bed occupancy and number of discharges per bed, as a result of the reforms (Fidler et al. 2007).

Spain

Since the early 1990s, several of the independent subnational governments have initiated reforms of their public hospital systems, establishing an array of alternative autonomous arrangements. These efforts were part of a broader reform involving the separation of purchasing and provision and the application of performance-based contracting. Several organizational types were legally created: the foundation (*fundación*), consortium (*consorcio*), public firm (*sociedad mercantil pública*, or *entidad pública empresarial*), and autonomous organization (*organismo autónomo*). Depending on the legal and regulatory framework, which was often specific to the subnational government as well as to the individual facility, these new arrangements were applied to conventional public facilities that had previously operated as budgetary arms of government. Under the new arrangements, hospitals received funding through global budgets and other mechanisms specified in contracts with public purchases. These organizational arrangements have yet to be evaluated.

Human Resource Management

Regulations governing labor practices can facilitate or restrict the ability of an organization to manage its workforce effectively. Legislation that restricts flexibility in human resource management at the organizational level is being challenged in public systems throughout the world. A number of European countries, for example, are gradually replacing rigid, "procedurally tortuous" macroregulatory modalities of human resource management with more flexible, targeted, microregulatory forms (Dubois, McKee, and Nolte 2006).[46] These regulatory instruments demand greater accountability and improved performance of health care organizations. Organizations are gradually being granted greater decision-making authority through incremental transformation from traditional bureaucratic and centralized control to more localized arrangements. Making personnel management for nascent autonomous institutions more flexible was part of hospital reform legislation in several countries.

In many countries, as in Brazil, the main impediments to facility conversion are rigid civil service rules and centralized (and often politicized) decision making in human resource management.[47] Diverse human resource solutions are evident among countries that have converted or are converting their public hospitals. In Colombia, Portugal, and Spain transitional models emerged based on legislation or on explicit and implicit policies. In these countries, conversion is a long-term endeavor that hinges on attrition of civil servants and their replacement by staff under private contracting arrangements. In other cases, such as Austria and Estonia, legislation mandated revocation of civil servant status and rapid incorporation under private law.[48]

Portugal

Staff could choose to remain under the public regime or switch to a private contract. Most senior staff have opted to remain civil servants, but new personnel are hired through private contracts. Thus, staff conversion will take place gradually, through attrition, while hospitals operate with personnel under both private and public regimes. The government is preparing career paths for the new staff members.

Spain

Hospitals were granted the right to manage human resources under private law. In all cases, facilities retained the civil service regime, partly as a result of pressure from public employee unions. Nevertheless, a transitional model emerged in a number of subnational governments. As in Portugal, the civil servant status and salary schedules of existing employees were respected, but these employees were given a choice between remaining civil servants or being recontracted under a private labor regime. This, like Brazil's *direito privado*, gave managers greater flexibility in nearly all facets of human resource management. Incentive schemes were set up to encourage personnel to migrate to the private labor regime, but personnel at some facilities were given a chance to change their minds even after choosing the private option: they could take a leave of absence and return to the civil service regime within three years. In most cases new hires were contracted through the private regime. In some facilities physicians and other professional staff were given special incentives to motivate "exclusive dedication" to the facility, full time, thus facilitating the establishment of a core professional staff.

Colombia

ESEs are subject to certain restrictions that constrain their decision-making authority in managing human resources. Governance boards and facility managers must follow cumbersome civil service rules regarding human resource management, which severely limit their ability to set salaries and to evaluate, dismiss, promote, or transfer employees. Collective bargaining agreements governing certain types of employees further curtail ESE decision-making authority. In light of the strong presence of government officials on the ESE boards, a case can be made that personnel decisions remain in the hands of government. Because of the political sensitivity of the issue, the government does not have an explicit policy on human resource management under ESE arrangements. Nevertheless, since individual ESEs can hire new staff under private labor law, one implicit policy already being implemented by most facilities entails the gradual replacement of civil servants by personnel contracted through third parties, outsourcing, and individual contracts—all under private labor law. As civil servants retire or seek transfers to other facilities, they are replaced by personnel contracted through one of those mechanisms. An estimated 20 percent of personnel is now employed through these arrangements, expanding facilities' flexibility in human resource management.

Austria and Estonia

Legislation in Austria mandated the transfer of hospital employees to the private, nonprofit, multihospital holding companies, but they remained employed under public law. Some special rights, such as flexible working hours and protection from layoffs and transfers, were abolished, and public employment law was modified to enable the companies to manage personnel under a regime essentially similar to private law. Thus, employees became accountable to the management of the holding company, which possesses decision rights to hire, dismiss, and transfer staff. Compensation continues to follow state employment law. Unlike the transitional models described above, Austrian authorities considered it important to have all employees contracted under a single but flexible labor regime.

In Estonia civil service rights were revoked for all medical personnel, and they were incorporated into a private labor regime. There, it was important for government planners to grant hospital managers full employer rights.

Managerial Practices in the Private Nonprofit Sector

This section examines the formality of management functions, as well as the soundness of management practices in SUS-funded, nonprofit hospitals. It draws heavily on the results of a survey by Barbosa et al. (2002).[49] The discussion focuses on the composition of the management team, management practices, and overall ratings of management competence.

Management Team

Between one-third and one-half of hospital managers work part time, and more than half are volunteers, as was seen in chapter 5. The informality of hospital management spills over to other positions. Table 6.3 shows the percentage of facilities that have formal positions for essential general and specialized hospital management functions. (The existence of a formal position, however, does not mean it has been filled.) Most smaller facilities (mean: 75 beds) report the absence of such positions for financial, human resource, general services, materials, and information managers. Since many of these facilities provide a limited volume of inpatient care, functions may be assumed by the facility's medical director or by executives of the philanthropic and charity organizations (PCOs). Nevertheless, between 20 and 30 percent of these facilities lack positions for medical, nursing, and general directors, suggesting that these are the responsibility of PCO executives. The extent to which these functions are covered by a PCO-based management team is unknown. Clear lines of authority and responsibility seem to be, at best, incipient in smaller nonprofit facilities, given that both

TABLE 6.3
Formal Management Positions in Private Nonprofit Hospitals, by Major Function and Hospital Category, 2001

(percent)

Position or function	Small (N = 64)	Large (N = 15)	Conglomerates (N = 81)	Non-SUS (N = 10)
Medical director	81	93	64	100
Nursing director	78	93	67	100
General director	67	73	81	90
Financial director	41	73	N/A	90
Human resources administrator	33	60	N/A	100
Materials manager	32	53	N/A	90
General services manager	29	60	N/A	70
Information manager	29	93	N/A	90
Planner[a]	12	27	N/A	40

Source: Barbosa et al. 2002.
Note: N/A, Information not reported or not available.
a. Includes contracting of consulting services.

governance and management functions are often centered in one or two PCO volunteer and part-time executives and that there are no formal, specialty managerial positions.

Most large facilities report having formal positions for general, medical, and nursing directors, but many lack positions for human resource, general services, and materials management. Considering the size of these facilities (more than 599 beds), the volume of services would probably require a more formal arrangement encompassing full-time, specialized personnel. Nearly all non-SUS hospitals reported having a full contingent of general and specialized managerial positions.[50] A case can be made that their market position drives these organizations to develop a modern and specialized management structure at the facility level.[51]

Management Practices

Table 6.4 shows the prevalence of specific management practices and instruments for each category of nonprofit hospital. In line with managerial patterns discussed above, most of the smaller facilities have not put in place essential managerial practices and tools related to finance, human resources, materials, and maintenance. More than half of them apparently do not possess a formal organizational structure, as evidenced by the absence of an organization chart.[52] Nearly all small facilities lack electronic information systems to support clinical and nonclinical management. Modern management techniques are more evident in larger facilities, and again the non-SUS-financed hospitals are more advanced with respect to the formal implementation of essential business practices. Human resource performance evaluation is common among most facilities, but promotion systems are generally lacking.

Few small hospitals sponsor training opportunities for the staff or feature employee incentive schemes, whether monetary or in-kind. This shortcoming (not shown in the table) could contribute to the high staff turnover—more than 20 percent annually—reported by a fourth of the smaller hospitals. Larger facilities, with more robust human resource systems, report lower staff turnover rates.

A formal business plan is conspicuously absent in a significant share of independent, SUS-financed facilities, suggesting that many hospitals lack medium- or long-term business and health care strategies. Systematic monitoring, internal auditing, and performance review appear to be the weakest functions across all hospitals except non–SUS financed facilities. This is perhaps the most troubling finding: few hospitals are concerned about performance. Data are neither collected nor analyzed, impeding the identification of problems and development of corrective measures. The lack of focus on performance compromises an organization's capacity to provide minimal standards of quality care or to survive in an increasingly complex and demanding environment. This environment is characterized by changes in public policies, modifications in payment systems, technological change, rising costs, increasing competition, changing labor force characteristics, and rising community expectations—all of which require modern and robust governance and management practices.

Management Ratings

On the basis of survey responses to about 70 questions on governance, organizational structures, and management practices of nonprofit hospitals, Barbosa et al. (2002) crafted a management modernity index. The index ranked, on a scale of 0 to 10, six essential management

TABLE 6.4

Formal Managerial Instruments and Practices in Nonprofit Hospitals, by Category, 2002

(percent)

Managerial instruments and practices	Small (N = 69)	Large (N = 15)[a]	Conglomerates (N = 81)	Non-SUS (N = 10)
Organization chart	44	93	82	90
Performance review[b]	30	N/A	N/A	80
Monitoring system[c]	26	47	31	80
Market analysis	26	67	33	60
Formal plan	26	47	68	60
Human resources				
Salary schedule	51	80	48	90
Job specifications	12	27	7	50
Performance evaluation[d]	41	60	64	90
Promotion system	9	33	12	40
Auditing				
Independent	30	85	N/A	100
Internal	21	54	N/A	40
Financial				
Annual budget	36	60	74	80
Budget review	29	53	57	80
Statement of cash flow	32	69	N/A	90
Accounts payable/receivable	83	88	N/A	100
Depreciation fund	30	77	N/A	100
Hospital cost system	35	34	N/A	80
Materials				
Annual inventory	30	58	N/A	70
Use of ABC method[e]	23	67	52	N/A
Product standardization[f]	38	80	63	N/A
Equipment maintenance				
Preventive	54	100	85	N/A
Maintenance records	30	93	57	N/A

Source: Barbosa et al. 2002.

Note: N/A, information not reported or not available.

a. For auditing and financial (nonbudgetary), N = 26.

b. Per service, function, or global (formal).

c. Including use of targets and indicators.

d. Systematic and formalized.

e. Activity-based costing (a common stock-management technique in which materials are prioritized according to expenditures).

f. Medical materials only.

dimensions: planning and executive management; economic and financial management; human resources; logistics (materials); technical services (medical care); and information technologies. The researchers classified as "incipient" (inferior) facilities that scored less than 5 and as "in development," those that scored between 5 and 9. Facilities receiving the top score of 10 were classified as "advanced." The index was applied to 63 small and 13 large SUS-financed facilities and 10 non-SUS hospitals (figure 6.6).

For small facilities, the average score was 3.4. Most (82 percent) of their management structures and processes were classified as "incipient." Only 11 of the facilities (17 percent) received a rating of 5 or better. Small facilities scored particularly low on functions related to financial management (2.6) and information management (2.9). They did best on technical services (4.6).

Turning to large facilities, the average score was 6.1, but 5 of the 13 were rated "incipient," and the remainder (8) fell into the "in development category." Although several facilities received tallies of 10 for specific managerial dimensions, no large hospital received a 10 on all dimensions. The largest hospitals—those with more than 600 beds—scored the highest. This subgroup (not shown in the figure) scored best on information technology, technical services, and logistics but lagged in human resources and financial management.

Finally, the non-SUS-financed hospitals tallied the highest marks, displaying an average rating of 7.2. Nearly all (9 of 10) were in the "in development" category. Only one hospital in this group, a small, 50-bed facility, was rated as "incipient." As in the case of the large SUS-financed facilities, a number of hospitals in the non-SUS group received perfect scores on several management dimensions, but none received 10 on all dimensions. The group scored highest, on average, for information technology, technical services, logistics and materials management, and executive management and planning. Most scores were more than double those received by smaller, SUS-financed facilities.

FIGURE 6.6
Management Development Scores of Nonprofit Hospitals, by Category, 2001

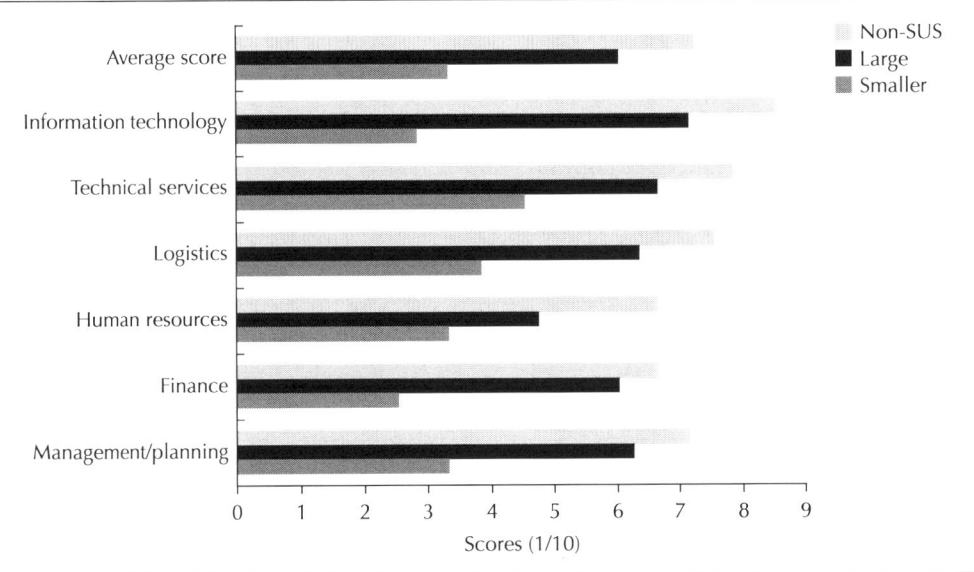

Source: Barbosa et al. 2002.
Note: Maximum score = 10.

Summary Assessment and Recommendations

Drawing on the performance results reported in chapter 5, this chapter has explored what is known about organizational structures and incentive environments affecting managerial practices in order to see what contributes to performance in public facilities. A strong relation is evident between organizational arrangements and managerial behaviors. Public hospitals with flexible organizational arrangements related to decision-making authority over inputs, accountability mechanisms (contracts, public disclosure, and information on performance), market exposure, and explicit definition of functions exhibit managerial practices in line with the incentive environment. These practices include strategic planning, introduction of programs to measure and improve client satisfaction, expansion of the revenue base by selling services to third parties, use of incentive payment schemes, and application of private rules for hiring and firing personnel. In contrast, facilities under hierarchical structural arrangements, usually of the direct administration model, demonstrate normative behaviors—administering processes, rules, and controls mandated by higher levels of government.

The chief problems related to the governance and managerial environments of traditional hospitals and the government bureaucracies to which they respond were also reviewed: complex procurement rules and unwieldy centralized purchasing; centralized human resource management subject to rigid civil service rules; lack of information for planning and monitoring; and disjuncture between planning and budgeting. Given the restrictions of civil service rules and the excessive centralization of human resource and procurement decision making, coupled with poor information, most managers of public facilities lack the means to improve performance.

Alternative facilities were found to be better performers than their traditional or direct administration counterparts, as was shown in chapter 5. Not all facilities, however, fit this schematic. For example, two hospitals under flexible organizational structures displayed normative behaviors more in line with conventional, direct administration facilities, and one hospital under a hierarchical structure showed behaviors more like the alternative group. Further research is needed to distill the relationship between structures and behaviors in these facilities.

Although autonomy appears to improve performance in public hospitals, the relation between autonomy and performance appears to work less well in private nonprofit hospitals. Without contracts to fulfill or competition, there is little pressure to perform. Management practices in nonprofit facilities are far from optimal, especially in small facilities—the vast majority of SUS-financed private hospitals. Management instruments—for example formal budget, salary schedule, and job specifications—and such processes as monitoring, inventory control, and maintenance, are absent in a disturbingly large number of facilities. Many small and medium-size hospitals appear to be unmanaged or informally managed, suggesting inefficiency and low quality.[53] All these facilities depend heavily on SUS transfers for their economic survival.[54] Part of the problem rests with the SUS's contracting mechanism and its passive approach to contracting.

Why OSSs Work

As implemented by the São Paulo state government, the OSSs, which involve the separation of purchasing from provision, represent the most robust example of an alternative organizational arrangement in Brazilian public hospitals. The chapter examined why OSSs exhibit superior performance. OSS managers respond to the incentive environment inherent in this organizational arrangement by applying private law to human resource management, particularly in hiring and firing practices; developing and implementing effective procurement processes and procedures; displaying accountability through compliance with contractual conditions; outsourcing services when it makes economic sense to do so; and managing and reallocating resources to meet production targets. Of equal importance, the state shows a willingness to enforce contractual terms by reducing or denying payments, or canceling contracts altogether.

The elements of the OSS model merit policy makers' attention. The findings suggest that an accountability arrangement is at work here that includes five essential characteristics: autonomy, flexible human resource management, strategic purchasing, contract enforcement, and a robust information environment. Together, they constitute the basics of a strategy for reforming the Brazilian hospital sector.

Autonomous Authority

Autonomy, although probably insufficient to sustain high performance by itself, appears to be the critical feature of the organizational models. Autonomy allows hospital management flexibility. Without autonomy, it is difficult for managers to be accountable to system objectives or incentives—whether specified in contracts, norms, or regulations or rooted in payment mechanisms. Without authority, managers cannot assume financial responsibility for the bottom line, expand capacity, alter input and service mix, incorporate new technologies, or improve quality and patient satisfaction. Government maintains excessive hierarchical control over most public hospitals in Brazil, so that they function as budgetary arms with little decision-making authority. Hospital managers are administrators of decisions made elsewhere in government; they have limited flexibility to fulfill their roles as leaders and authority figures. Facility managers' lack of authority to manage their staff, combined with their relatively short tenure, contributes to a phenomenon best described as "managing the unmanageable."

Flexible Human Resource Management

Although autonomy creates the enabling conditions for successful human resource management, the results reported here suggest that not all managers under autonomous organizational structures put in place effective human resource practices. OSS directors did, however, use their authority to apply private law to identify and recruit qualified professional personnel with the right organizational "fit." They recruited staff through informal networks and public advertisement, and all candidates were interviewed. No manager used the public competitive merit process (concurso), in which the state bureaucracy, without any interviews, selects the "winners" on the basis of a review of curricula vitae and high scores on a multiple-choice test. Under such a system, facility managers have little flexibility or discretion.

OSS managers also appear willing to fire nonperforming personnel, applying the without-cause modality that enables rapid separation but requires compensatory payments. Dismissal under public law is a protracted process that few managers are willing to undertake. Furthermore, unlike their direct administration counterparts, OSS managers are not bound to a rigid number of authorized posts (*padrão de lotação*) that are infrequently updated. They add, transfer, or cut personnel to respond to changing technologies and demand.

Finally, the OSS experience contradicts a commonly accepted axiom among civil service professionals in public hospitals—the need for a tradeoff, or favor exchange, under which professionals gain maximum flexibility in terms of real working hours in exchange for a low salary. The OSSs do not pay professional staff significantly higher salaries than traditional public facilities, but they are able to secure significantly better performance.

Strategic Purchasing

The concept of strategic purchasing has recently entered the policy agenda in Brazil, but only in a handful of states. Strategic purchasing implies "more discriminating and prudent" contracting (Robinson, Jabubowski, and Figueras 2005a: 7). It involves selective identification of providers, specification of outputs and outcomes, linking of financing to performance, and robust contract management and enforcement by the purchaser. Strategic purchasing means replacing passive government payment agents with "intelligent purchasing agents" who seek to maximize performance (Preker 2005: 38).

São Paulo state was the first government entity to move systematically from an integrated command-and-control public model with passive contracting of private providers to one that involves active purchasing with specific performance targets set by the state. Importantly, these targets are linked to financing. As applied in the OSS-managed facilities, the state has substituted contractual relationships for hierarchical control. The OSSs are directed to provide care in low-income urban areas in São Paulo state where people's access to hospital services has been difficult. Through pro-poor targeting, most OSS-managed facilities were built in urban *favelas* (slums). According to the management contract, OSSs are not permitted to provide services to the privately insured or to charge fees, mainly because of the universal nature of the SUS. Access is unrestricted, and the extent to which higher-income patients use these free facilities is unknown. Given their locations, however, it is unlikely that they are frequented by the well-off.[55]

The state selected OSSs from among institutions with considerable experience in hospital services. Most were universities and charitable organizations that already owned and operated hospitals and possessed the institutional capacity and governance structure to enter into a contractual relationship with the state and deliver the agreed-on services. Unlike the situation elsewhere in Brazil, the supply of eligible organizations is relatively developed in São Paulo.

The type and volume of services, as well as the resources allocated, are specified in a management contract negotiated between state authorities and the OSS. At the onset, there was no specific priority-setting methodology, resulting in midyear adjustments. With time and the introduction of information systems, data on unit costs, production, treatments, and disease incidence have become the main inputs for negotiating annual contractual terms. The contracts constitute the basis for a prospective global budget payment mechanism. Average unit costs of specified outputs and negotiated volume targets are currently the basis for determining the global budget.[56] Significantly, the state has linked financing to performance by tying a proportion of financing to production, patient satisfaction, and quality indicators. Managers are expected to stay within the budget and still meet the performance targets. The state has not increased the budget of any OSSs in deficit, and several OSSs have secured loans in the private sector to cover funding shortfalls.

Contract Monitoring and Enforcement

Provider autonomy requires strong accountability mechanisms. As has been seen, the SUS has been a passive payer of services through the convenio instrument. The purchasing-based framework described above requires vigorous contract monitoring and management by the purchaser. Without monitoring and contract enforcement, accountability does not materialize. The state's contract management capacity has been built up over time, and a change in the health secretariat's public service culture from a "hands-on" to a more "hands-off" approach was needed. The state had to learn to be proactive but not to micromanage. In other words, "hands off" does not mean "do what you can and want to."

Several procedures and mechanisms have been put in place to facilitate monitoring. First, OSS spending ledgers are audited by the state court of accounts (*tribunal de contas*). Second, OSSs are required to provide monthly statistical, production and cost reports to the state health secretariat. Third, performance is monitored by a service contract coordinating unit. This unit also manages the performance-based payment system and determines whether full or partial payments will be allocated. Fourth, purchaser-contractor monitoring sessions are held regularly to review progress vis-à-vis the contract. Finally, the state has set up an independent assessment commission that meets annually to review contract compliance and overall OSS performance.

Contracts are meaningless if the purchaser will not or cannot enforce the contractual provisions. The state has enforced these provisions by withholding payments from facilities that fail to fulfill reporting requirements and performance targets. Failure to comply with contractual terms resulted in the cancellation (and rebidding) of one OSS contract. Unlike the situation in the early years of the OSS initiative, the state does not provide additional resources beyond the negotiated global budget to an OSS facing a deficit.[57]

The capacity to monitor and enforce contracts took several years to develop and is still a work in progress. The local context was conducive to building this capacity. The São Paulo area contains a number of universities and consulting firms with considerable technical and managerial know-how and experience on which the state has drawn to develop monitoring and information management capacity. This is not necessarily the case elsewhere in Brazil. Finally, the state has encouraged evaluation of the OSS experience, allowing researchers and students ready access to information and staff.

Robust Information Environment

The ultimate success of any contracting process depends on the availability and use of information to make decisions on contractor performance and to track progress in the context of broader policies, plans, and objectives. More specifically, how a contract is managed depends on the information that comes from the provider for contract monitoring purposes. A purchaser needs timely information on progress, technical performance, and costs to permit decisions on corrective action, if needed.

Over time, São Paulo state established an enabling information environment to facilitate OSS monitoring and evaluation. The state mandated the installation of standardized cost accounting and other automated information systems in all OSSs to provide managers (and the purchaser) with disaggregated data on service production and costs.[58] OSSs are required to generate and provide data on activities, volume, and quality. Some data are reported monthly; other information is reported quarterly and annually. The state measures performance against targets for each OSS and compares performance across OSSs.[59] The reporting requirements facilitate regular feedback on progress and identification of potential problems. For example, state managers prepare comparative ledgers that are shared with the OSSs. Managers can thus see how their performance compares with that of other OSSs for a common set of production and quality indicators. The secretariat of health publishes the annual financial statements in the official state record, *Diário Nacional do Estado*, And the results of the annual contract compliance assessment performed by the independent assessment commission are presented to the State Assembly and made available for public review.

Conversion of Public Hospitals: The Next Step?

Brazil has made only limited efforts to convert health facilities under direct administration to alternative organizational forms such as OSSs. The OSSs in São Paulo and other states were implemented in new hospitals and therefore avoided a number of difficult personnel, legal, and financial issues related to the conversion of existing public facilities. Ambiguity and disincentives in the legal and regulatory framework, which may reflect fear of political fallout from employee unions and their political supporters, has resulted in a regulatory hornet's nest for states and municipalities seeking conversion of their public hospitals. Most state and municipal authorities, although privately interested in converting public facilities, will publicly dodge the issue unless there is a clear policy and regulatory framework.

São Paulo has also experimented with converting direct administration facilities to OSSs. The model implemented in São Paulo, although in an early stage of implementation, provides important lessons on the prospects and pitfalls of public hospital conversion in the Brazilian context. As practiced in São Paulo, conversion is limited by the availability of budgeted vacancies elsewhere in the system to absorb public employees who choose not to remain in the converted facilities. This problem may be partially offset by efficiency gains in the converted hospitals. Converted facilities also demonstrate significant quality improvements that contribute to patient satisfaction and community support. Several public agencies outside the health sector have successfully converted to OSSs. Evaluative research is needed to measure the impact of these experiences on costs, performance, and labor relations. How public employees in these agencies were converted to private contracts is another important area of inquiry.

Finally, international experience suggests that public hospital conversion is a long-term process involving careful planning, regulatory reform, and phased implementation. Experience demonstrates that conversion works best when it is part of a broader package of hospital reform. A number of successful models have emerged internationally that can be adapted to the Brazilian context. More specifically, experience demonstrates that the establishment of autonomous institutional structures and flexible employment regimes for health workers creates an enabling institutional environment for conversion. The next section describes a proposal to do just that by the Ministry of Health (Ministério da Saúde, MS).

State Foundations: The Way Forward for Public Hospitals?

In early 2007, as described in Barbosa (2007), the MS announced a proposal to convert public hospitals under direct and indirect administration to state foundations (*fundações estatais*, FS). The MS is drafting for submission to Congress framework legislation that would enable the establishment of FSs nationwide. The FS proposal borrows many elements from the OSS organizational form as practiced in São Paulo state. The organization would be a nonprofit private institution incorporated under private law, and it would have autonomous decision-making authority over all resources. Given its private status, the FS would apply flexible human resource management in which private labor law would govern all personnel management. Accountability arrangements would entail management contracts linked to a performance-based finance system, still to be devised. The model includes additional elements, such as governance boards with representatives from government (which would be in the majority), civil society, employees, and users, as well as professionalization of hospital management. Although the proposal may face legal and political challenges, based on the evidence presented in this and the previous chapter FSs represent a major structural reform that has strong potential to improve public hospital performance.

MS planners will have to deal with several challenges that could threaten the effectiveness of the model's implementation. First, there will be a need to develop guidelines and options for implementing the conversion of facilities under direct and indirect administration to FSs. Particular attention will have to be paid to personnel issues and costs. These guidelines should be based on an in-depth assessment of the international and national experiences presented in this chapter. Second, national and international experience shows that a major shortcoming of public contracting is poor contract monitoring, management, and enforcement, along with lack of transparency in government-contractor relations. States and municipalities will need considerable technical and management support to develop the required capacities. Furthermore, establishing and strengthening know-how in contract management takes time. This reality suggests a phased approach in which contracts are implemented initially for a small number of facilities and extended to additional facilities in subsequent phases once basic capacities are in place. Third, the information environment in many states and municipalities is deficient and could severely handicap robust contract monitoring, evaluation, and enforcement. Without timely information on performance (and costs), assessment—the first step toward corrective action—is impossible. Finally, the MS will have to take measures to avoid capture of FS governance boards by professional or political interest groups.

Annex 6A
Strengths and Weaknesses of the Public Sector Regime for Procurement, Labor, and Budgeting

The following summary is based on World Bank (2007).

Procurement

Framework legislation: Law 8666 (1993); Law 10520 (2002).

Strengths

Based on sound principles of competition, transparency, publicity, and equal treatment among competitors; allows for innovative features such as the reverse auction (*pregão*), which can be conducted electronically; auditing institutions function adequately.

Weaknesses

Excessively complex and detailed; emphasis is on formal components of tendering process rather than on components that would offer the purchaser greater advantage; most municipalities lack capacity to conduct procurement planning and implement rules in an efficient and timely manner; know-how for procurement of medical supplies and equipment is rare; inflexible interpretation of statutes contributes to proliferation of bidder complaints about inconsequential irregularities, a constant stream of disputes, and court injunctions; many (24) departures from competitive bidding are permitted, contributing to confusion and delays; hiring of individual consultants is difficult; there are no standardized bidding documents and no product standardization; the system is not useful for high-technology purchases; price negotiations do not take place; the system does not prevent collusion among bidders. Press reports suggest that Law 8666 has not reduced corruption in public procurement. Kick-backs on government contracts appear to be commonplace.

Human Resources

Framework legislation: Law 8112 (1990), complemented by local government legislation.

Strengths

Fosters personnel stability and protection against political interference; selection is based on a (limited) competition-based selection process; fosters recruitment of a core of public servants with specialized expertise in public goods (e.g., planning, regulation, disease surveillance).

Weaknesses

Managers are unable to directly select personnel (hiring is usually based on scores on multiple-choice tests that may not assess real skills and experience, and candidates are not interviewed to gauge organizational fit); all personnel within a technical category (physicians, nurses, etc.) receive the same starting wage; wage increases are made across-the-board, determined by government for all workers; lifetime employment is guaranteed after three-year probation; the firing process is long and convoluted; hiring is subject to irregular public competitions for civil service vacancies that can take up to six months to finalize; new positions are rarely created (and current positions are rarely eliminated) because a facility's staffing is rarely reviewed or updated, making it difficult for hospitals to adjust staff mix to technological innovations and changing demand; the system is not conducive to assessing outputs and results.

Budgeting and Finance

Framework legislation: Law 4320 (1964); Decree Law 200 (1967); annual budgetary law.

Strengths

Structured process for financial planning and budgeting; stimulates planning and budgeting culture; financial monitoring and control reduce possibility of misuse and fraud; structured units for planning and finance and for budgeting exist in most secretariats and large facilities.

Weaknesses

Excessively complex planning process; excessive number of ex ante controls and formal assessments; budget structure is often outdated and unrelated to policy priorities and programs; actual decision making regarding finance and budget often rests outside the health secretariats (i.e., within the finance secretariats); facility managers are granted little autonomy for reallocating available resources among line items; there is little participation by local or municipal councils in financial decision making; the emphasis on formal controls does not eliminate misuse and fraud; plans and budgets are not used as management tools; no evaluation of impact or effectiveness takes place ; "doing it right" often implies bypassing rules; finance and budget personnel are poorly qualified and poorly informed on technical issues and generally focus on following rules.

Annex 6B

Comparison of Summary Labor Regime Characteristics for Physicians by Organizational Arrangement in Public and Private Nonprofit Hospitals

Organizational arrangement	Labor regime	Employment tie	Hiring	Firing	Payment method	Entity determining compensation
Direct or indirect administration	Public: civil servants	Government (federal, state, or municipal)	Competitive process based on written examination.	Follows civil servant rules; long-drawn-out process	Salary (20–40 hours per week). Salary levels are rigid.	Government
	Private: outsourced cooperatives	Cooperative	Cooperative-established process according to private law. Usually a selective process based on review of résumé, references, and interview. Potential cooperative members pay a fee or share and are elected by assembly vote.	For salaried staff contracted under CLT, follows with-cause or without-cause due process.[a] For cooperative members, dismissal takes place through assembly vote.	Per hour or salary. Salary levels are set by cooperative. Cooperative members may receive income through distributions.	Cooperative
	Private: outsourced individuals	Government (federal, state, or municipal)	Temporary contracts, but generally renewed annually. Employment tie may last for many years.	For CLT, follows with-cause or without-cause due process.[a] For contracted workers, severance is immediate.	Salary or per hour. Salary levels are rigid.	Government

(continued)

269

Organizational arrangement	Labor regime	Employment tie	Hiring	Firing	Payment method	Entity determining compensation
Support foundations (affiliated with public hospitals)	Private	Support foundation[b]	Foundation establishes process according to private law. Usually a selective process based on review of résumé, references, and interview. Most are temporary contracts, renewed annually.	For CLT, follows with-cause or without-cause due process.[a] For contracted workers, severance is immediate.	Salary, based on number of work hours per week, usually 20–40 hours. Salary levels are highly variable.	Support foundation
OSS and autonomous administration	Private: CLT	Hospital or governance organization	Selective process based on review of résumé, references, and interview.	Follows CLT-determined with-cause or without-cause due process.[a]	Salary depends on number of work hours per week, usually between 20 and 40 hours. Salary levels are highly variable.	Hospital or governance organization

Source: Authors' elaboration.

Note: CLT, Consolidação das Leis do Trabalho. CLT differs from statutory employment in the following ways: (1) there is no guarantee of long-term employment; (2) the pension program is less robust, but contributions as a percentage of salary are higher for high- ncome workers; (3) severance pay is guaranteed on dismissal (in contrast to the public sector); (4) dismissal is a relatively rapid and straightforward process—employees can be fired with or without cause; (5) salaries are determined by the market rather than by government-defined salary categories and wage policies; (6) the selection process, usually determined by the organization, can involve a review of qualifications, interview, reference check, and so on but does not necessary involve selection based on a multiple-choice examination, as is the case for statutory employees; and (7) the employment relationship is between the hospital and employee. Statutory employees have employment relationships with a level of government).

a. With cause means that firing follows a standardized process set by CLT labor rules. Without cause means that firing takes place rapidly (it requires only one month's notice), but the employer must pay a severance allowance.

b. Because support foundations are affiliated with public hospitals, many physicians have employment ties with both the government owner (as civil servants or contracted workers) and the support foundation.

Notes

1. These variables were similar to those described in chapter 5 for organizational structures, but the survey questions and follow-up interviews sought to elicit evidence of how the structures and rule set were or were not put into practice. For the structure and measurement of the variables, see annexes 5C and 5D.

2. Scores on hospital behaviors were independent of scores for structures, which were generated from a separate set of survey questions. For example, a facility under direct administration could be rated "strategic" (managers bypassed hierarchical controls), or, conversely, an alternative facility could be deemed "administrative" (managers failed to take advantage of a flexible rule set and structure).

3. Health plans refer to an array of private insurers, including health maintenance organizations (HMOs), group medical organizations, cooperatives, and traditional insurers.

4. Incentive payment systems are usually an initiative of municipal and state governments but are oriented toward all employees.

5. For the performance analysis reported in chapter 5, this facility was transferred to the traditional group.

6. The results presented here draw mainly on a health expenditure tracking survey conducted in 2003 (World Bank 2007). Managers in 25 states and 18 urban municipal health secretariats and in 52 hospitals (37 public hospitals) were surveyed on their capacity and their problems in planning, budgeting, purchasing, and human resource management. Another source was diagnostic reports from eight consultancy firms contracted by the MS to diagnose and address management problems in a sample of 25 hospitals selected from throughout Brazil (MS/REFORSUS 2002).

7. Twenty-five percent of municipal facilities reported not having a stockroom.

8. Few hospitals report having autonomy in the purchase of equipment.

9. Developed in the 1960s, unit-dose drug distribution systems have become standard practice in hospitals in most OECD countries. Under this system, medication is dispensed to patients in ready-to-administer, prepackaged, single-dose packets prepared by the central pharmacy. Unit-dose systems have been found to reduce waste and medication errors (Murray and Shojania 2001).

10. The regulatory environment is also a critical factor in the establishment and sustainability of organizational forms that permit more effective labor management in health care organizations.

11. Professionals under temporary contracts have no institutional employment tie, are generally paid on an hourly or a part-time basis, and do not derive any benefits. Professionals who are cooperative members (*cotizados*) may be salaried or remunerated through allowances based on the number of hours worked, as well as the number of shares (*cotas*) held in the cooperative.

12. Facility directors have autonomy regarding the hiring and dismissal of emergency or temporary personnel. In some states and municipalities, managers can issue performance bonuses.

13. The results presented here are based on a survey of and interviews with managers in 5 states and 18 municipalities (World Bank 2007).

14. Planning instruments include the health agenda (*agenda da saúde*), annual plan (*plano anual*), multiyear plan (*plano plurianual*), regional plan (*plano regional*), and investment plan (*plano de investimento*).

15. For example, a municipality's annual health plan may be structured according to four major areas: service provision, management, strategic resources, and financing. These, in turn, are broken down into programmatic and geographic priorities. In contrast, the annual budget for the same year is structured either by line item, project, or activity, including facility maintenance, new construction, and equipment. Few, if any, of the areas and programs of the annual plan are mentioned.

16. High rotation of managerial staff is a symptom of politicized staffing under the direct administration model.

17. As noted, these organizational characteristics have been linked to superior performance in other health systems (Figueras, Robinson, and Jakubowski 2005).

18. No difference was found in the professional preparation of facility directors. Nearly all have training in hospital management or business administration. Both groups of facilities also reported possessing a similar complement of professional staff responsible for human resource, financial, contract, and procurement management.

19. For one OSS in the sample, these functions are centralized in a nonprofit private organization (*entidade privada não lucrativa,* EPNL).

20. Reluctance to contract out hotel services has also been observed in nonprofit but not for-profit facilities, confirming the distortion related to taxing contracted services but not in-house production.

21. Most member countries of the Organisation for Economic Co-operation and Development (OECD) are moving away from centralized management of employee staffing in public hospitals. International experience on human resource management is discussed in the conclusion to this chapter.

22. The risk here is that facility directors may hire friends and family. This is constrained in the case of the OSSs by governance organizations, state audits, and performance requirements.

23. The organizational arrangements presented in the table were described in chapter 5. Not all these organizational arrangements are shown in table 6.1, but Mendes and Costa (2005) included nearly all of them in their follow-on analysis of structures and behaviors of alternative and traditional facilities.

24. All federal hospitals and most hospitals under indirect administration manage their own budgets. The facility is considered an independent budgetary unit by government.

25. In contrast, private support foundations (FAs) generally have autonomy to secure additional revenues, including the sale of services, and to spend revenues on needed inputs, but they have little influence over spending patterns related to the facility's general (non-FA) budget. Any investment in equipment is done in coordination with hospital management.

26. This learning process related to contract process has been observed in Europe and elsewhere (Figueras, Robinson, and Jakubowski 2005; Preker and Harding 2003).

27. In both cases, conversion was implemented by the same OSS, the Paulist Association for Medical Development, under a management contract with a subnational government. The sources of this discussion include documentation provided by each facility and interviews with Dr. Nacime Mansur, OSS superintendent, on October 13, 2005; July 27, 2006; March 17, 2007; and June 21, 2007.

28. Overstaffing is typical of direct administration facilities in Brazil. It helps maintain total production at direct administration facilities, mitigating the effect of absenteeism and work shirking.

29. For example, a person hired as a nurse auxiliary must occupy that position (and pay level) until that staff member applies for and wins the concurso for another position. But vacancies rarely occur, and the state seldom opens a concurso. Meanwhile, the nurse auxiliary may have become a registered graduate nurse. Although the nurse was trained in management and did the job of a nursing coordinator for many years, according to the state, that person was still a nurse auxiliary and was paid an auxiliary's salary.

30. Because of the merging of services (e.g., laboratory and diagnostic services) in the hospital and emergency center, it was impossible to determine how conversion affected spending on emergency center services.

31. The facility received Level 2 ONA accreditation. As noted in chapter 8, most Brazilian hospitals are out of compliance with licensure regulations.

32. The 2005 exchange rate is used: US$1 = R$2.43. The budget includes indirect administration costs incurred by the municipal health secretariat for managing the facility

33. The data presented in table 6.2 should be interpreted with caution. They represent a simple comparison of relatively short (10-month) periods before and after conversion. A more robust analysis would account for longer before and after periods.

34. Analysis of time series data is needed to verify any trend in performance regarding efficiency and quality indicators. According to hospital registers, however, the neonatal mortality rate was 10.2 in 2004 and 11.2 in 2006, suggesting that quality enhancement measures implemented in late

2006 and 2007 contributed to the reduction in neonatal mortality to 5.5. Most of the neonatal deaths in 2006 occurred prior to conversion.

35. The only additional outlay was a one-time grant in 2005, representing 1 percent of the budget.

36. The 2006 exchange rate is used: US\$1 = R\$2.18.

37. As mentioned, the 2005 budget was actually higher: US\$84.6 million, including municipal indirect administrative costs.

38. The budget did include a proportion of the estimated administrative costs incurred by the municipal health secretariat to manage the facility. The OSS assumed many of these functions. The municipality no longer required a fully staffed hospital department in the health secretariat, but it did need a unit to manage and monitor the contract with the OSS. It issued an up-front payment of R\$700,000 to provide the OSS with working capital.

39. The OSS gained control over contracts with the firms to provide these services in the hospital; the municipality had managed the contracting poorly.

40. Over 85 percent of the overtime pay went to physicians and nurses. In theory, the overtime should have been sufficient to cover hospital services 24 hours a day, 7 days a week, but labor rigidities and poor personnel management resulted in a shortfall of professional staff in the evenings and on weekends.

41. A third case, not described here, consisted of an ambulatory center operated by São Paulo state. This 2,000 square meter facility with diagnostic units, pharmacy, and 54 consultation rooms was transferred to an OSS in late 2005. Upon conversion, 120 of the 540 employees requested transfers to other state facilities, partly because of incompatibility of working hours. Like the other facilities described, the center was in disrepair, requiring significant investments in plant and equipment. The facility was not able to retain the monetary value of the salaries of the transferred workers or to realize savings from elimination of overtime payments, as the municipal hospital had done. The state and the OSS agreed to an increase in the budget to pay for the cost of extending services and improving quality. The OSS used these additional funds to replace some of the transferred personnel (via CLT), upgrade and repair plant and equipment, train staff, introduce information systems, open new services, and extend service hours. Insufficient information was available for a full case study.

42. The PAS program was another, but failed, attempt at converting primary care units. PAS involved contracting cooperatives to deliver primary care services in São Paulo city. The lessons are described in box 4.2.

43. For Austria and Estonia, see Fidler et al. (2007); Palu and Kadakmaa (2001). For Australia, see Corden, (2003). For Portugal, see CAHSA (2006); Guichard (2004). For Spain, see Ibern (1998); Martín Martín (2003); CHC (n.d.). The discussion of Colombia draws on Humberto Arango, personal communication, 2006, and Toro et al. (2007).

44. In Austria most mayors were glad to turn over their hospitals to the holding company because the facilities' high costs and indebtedness were an increasing drain on municipal coffers. An undetermined number of municipalities had insufficient capacity to oversee or manage the facilities.

45. Any reduction or modification in infrastructure and service supply has to fit into the Austrian Hospital Master Plan governing hospital investments.

46. The microregulatory forms are more in line with broader financial and organizational reforms oriented toward obtaining more value for money, reflecting concerns about escalating costs and growing evidence of effective clinical practice.

47. More flexible procurement of drugs and supplies is also important but may not be critical. Several states have granted hospitals authority to procure a wide range of inputs, following public procurement law. More research is needed on purchasing performance after decentralization of public procurement functions to the facility level.

48. Other types of regulatory instruments that demand accountability from staff are evident in France, Germany, and the United Kingdom. For example, specification of clinical performance standards and performance targets is part of recent regulatory changes in the United Kingdom that are reflected in managerial instruments such as hospital business plans and management

contracts between regional purchasers and hospitals. In France and Germany instruments under implementation demand greater accountability from medical care organizations and their staffs, calling for scorecards, utilization reviews, public performance reports, and medical audits.

49. The researchers surveyed management functions and practices in three categories of facilities affiliated with philanthropic or charitable organizations (PCOs) and receiving public funding (as most PCOs do). The three categories are small individual facilities (most with fewer than 100 beds), large individual facilities, and medium-size hospitals belonging to a voluntary organization or a conglomerate. A fourth consists of facilities that do not receive SUS funds. No such information exists for hospitals operated by nonprofit foundations and private corporations.

50. A hospital with fewer than 50 beds was the outlier in this group.

51. Competitive pressures contributed to the introduction of modern governance and management practices in nonprofit hospitals in the United States, beginning in the late 1970s (Stevens 1989; Starr 1982).

52. Most hospitals would not pass licensure inspection under Brazilian legislation, if it were enforced by government.

53. These facilities operate at very low capacity and are of unknown or low quality.

54. A recent MS policy initiative (MS 2004f) seeks to convert small facilities to basic care centers, but whether this policy will be applied to private facilities is unclear. Part of the problem lies in the SUS's passive approach to contracting.

55. Nor do the OSSs offer the highly specialized care that is often not covered by private insurance but is demanded by the well-off. Such services are typically provided by much larger public teaching hospitals.

56. The state plans to introduce a DRG payment system that adjusts for severity of illness.

57. In 2003, because the state was late in providing the monthly allocation, several facilities could not meet the performance targets. The state and the OSSs renegotiated the contract—with lower targets.

58. Consultants and civil servants in the Service Contract Coordinating Unit are responsible for data analysis.

59. Similar data are generally not available at direct administration facilities, requiring expensive primary data collection.

7

Quality of Care: Still the Forgotten Component?

Quality is an issue at the forefront of national attention in Brazil, but it is discussed mainly in sensationalist press accounts of hospital problems, errors, and adverse events. As in many developing and developed countries, the absence of reliable data, systematic measurement, and institutional infrastructure for monitoring and evaluating quality frustrates most attempts to assess the quality of care in Brazilian hospitals. Because of lax regulatory enforcement, the voluntary nature of external controls, and the lack of accountability mechanisms, hospitals are not under pressure to introduce explicit, organizationwide quality improvement processes and procedures. True, there are many top-quality hospitals in Brazil, but the available evidence—from, usually, small-scale research—suggests that many hospitals are simply unsafe.

Nearly every government policy statement on health over the last 15 years has paid lip service to quality improvement, but few strategies and actions have materialized to systematically address quality issues in hospitals. The situation is similar in the private sector. Few private purchasers monitor the quality of care delivered by contracted providers.

Quality is the "forgotten component" of the Brazilian health system, concluded the World Bank in 1994 after analyzing the state of quality in Brazil's health services and the lack of systematic efforts, public or private, to monitor or improve quality. Despite advances since then, many of the report's findings are still valid. The good news is that some progress is taking place. For example, the recently instituted National Accreditation Organization (Organização Nacional de Acreditação, ONA) and other institutions have developed standards that serve as blueprints for delivering excellent care. Benchmarking systems based on systematic collection of performance indicator data are under development. Furthermore, a handful of hospitals has taken the lead in developing robust quality improvement programs that have great value as models throughout the country. Despite these small but promising experiences, there has been little progress toward systematically addressing quality issues, improving clinical processes, strengthening clinical management, or ensuring that evidence on best practice is incorporated into care delivery.

This chapter assesses the current state of quality in Brazilian hospitals. Chapter 8 then analyzes national and local quality performance improvement initiatives aimed at setting standards, measuring and assessing quality, and improving performance in hospitals.

Quality, Quality Improvement, and Costs

Quality is an abstract notion, easy to describe but difficult to operationalize. What is good health care is difficult to define and often depends on country-specific standards set by regulatory agencies. In any case, compliance with standards does not necessarily ensure good outcomes. Furthermore, quality is often a moving target for any health care organization: good outcomes one year may not guarantee good outcomes the next. Quality also has multiple, constantly changing dimensions. Accelerating advances in technology, rapidly evolving epidemiological profiles, the expanding pace and scope of medical research, and shifting regulatory environments make simple definitions difficult. Although the definition of quality care has changed over the years, quality assessment and improvement approaches are a good place to start. Two such approaches are examined here. The first is based on the classic quality assessment framework developed by Donabedian (1980). The second is the landmark *Crossing the Quality Chasm*, published in 2001 by the Institute of Medicine (IOM 2001).

Donabedian's framework is based on three components of quality: structure, process, and results. These components have become the cornerstone of quality assessment instruments and standards worldwide. The *evaluation of structure* consists of the assessment of the care providers' capabilities, including facilities, equipment, manpower, and financing. *Process evaluation* involves appraisal of the care process itself, ideally based on evidence. The *outcomes assessment* consists of identification of the end results of care processes, usually specified in terms of patient health, safety, or satisfaction. Later in the chapter, this framework is applied to assessment of quality in Brazilian hospitals.

The broader IOM approach encompasses both technical and patient-based criteria. It consists of six dimensions of quality care: patient safety, effectiveness, patient-centered care, timeliness, efficiency, and equity (box 7.1). The IOM has recommended that all health care organizations adopt these dimensions as major system objectives. Depending on the availability of data, several of these dimensions are used here to assess quality of care in Brazilian hospitals.

The IOM (citing Lohr 1990) defined quality as "the degree to which health services for individuals and populations increase the likelihood of desired health outcomes and are consistent with current professional knowledge" (IOM 2001: 232). Drawing in part on the IOM report, Dlugacz, Restifo, and Greenwood (2004) provide a more operational definition of quality care as "care that is measurably safe, of the highest standard, evidence-based, uniformly delivered, with the appropriate utilization of resources and services."

Hospital quality is increasingly viewed as a system and an organizational concern that includes institutional provisions for checks and balances, rather than as the duty of a particu-

---

Box 7.1
Major Dimensions of Quality Health Care

Quality health care has six principal dimensions:

> *Patient safety:* avoiding injuries to patients from the care that is intended to help them.
> *Effectiveness:* providing services based on scientific knowledge and refraining from providing services to those not likely to benefit from them.
> *Patient-centered care:* providing care that is respectful of and responsive to individual patient preferences, needs, and values and ensuring that patient values guide all clinical decisions.
> *Timeliness:* reducing waits and sometimes harmful delays for both the receivers and the givers of care.
> *Efficiency:* avoiding waste of equipment, supplies, ideas, and energy.
> *Equity:* providing care that does not vary in quality because of personal characteristics such as gender, ethnicity, geographic location, or socioeconomic status.

Source: IOM 2001: 5–6.

lar physician, manager, department, or facility (WHO 2003a; Scrivens 2002, 1997b; Shaw 2004a). Quality is a "system property" (IOM 2001: 4) that requires continuous assessment, management, and improvement of care processes accompanied by the appropriate standards, institutions, and systems to support these actions. Hospitals are complex systems character-ized by multiple interconnected functions, specializations, time-dependent processes, and intensive use of human resources. According to the IOM, ensuring quality requires redesign of care processes as well as intraorganizational interactions.

> Making environments safer means looking at processes of care to reduce defects in the pro-cess or departures from the ways things should have been done. Ensuring patient safety, therefore, involves the establishment of operational systems and processes that increase the reliability of patient care. (IOM 1999: 58)

> One of the greatest contributors to accidents in any industry including health care is human error. However, saying that an accident is due to human error is not the same as assigning blame because most human errors are induced by system failures . . . system errors pose the greatest threat to safety in complex systems because they lead to operator errors. (IOM 1999: 65)

Taking as a basis large-scale studies undertaken in 1997 in three U.S. states (Colorado, New York, and Utah), and extrapolating the findings to nearly 34 million hospital admis-sions nationwide, the IOM (2000) estimated that medical errors resulted in the deaths of 44,000 Americans annually. This figure is higher than annual deaths from motor vehicle accidents, breast cancer, or AIDS.[1]

These data are not meant to suggest that American medicine is of poor quality: similar studies to determine the adverse effects of medical errors have not been performed in other countries. The results of small-scale research reported in this chapter suggest the need to rigorously and systematically assess medical error–related events that have resulted in injury and death in Brazilian hospitals.

In addition to the adverse health consequences foisted on individuals, low quality also generates large, needless costs that jeopardize the affordability of the health system. Although research is limited, studies in Brazil, reported in this chapter, show that poor quality is associated with increased spending. In the United States, where much work has been done on the links between quality and costs, poor quality—as indicated by overuse, underuse, errors, adverse events, lost information, repetition of diagnostics and procedures, and readmissions—results in lost income for individuals and higher health spending. Using 1992 U.S. data, Thomas et al. (1999) put the total costs of adverse events (lost income, lost production, disability, and health care costs) at between US$37.6 billion and US$50 bil-lion. Additional health care costs alone represented more than half this amount. Thomas et al. reported that these outlays were higher than the costs of caring for people with HIV/AIDS in 1992. Other observers claim that poor quality may represent as much as 30 percent of U.S. medical spending (Lawrence 2003). The U.S.-based Leapfrog Group suggests that three measures—appropriate staffing of intensive care units (ICUs), performance of com-plex surgical procedures in high-volume facilities, and the use of computerized prescription systems—could significantly reduce errors, save lives, and yield savings of US$41.5 billion annually (Leapfrog Group 2006). Although the necessary data for making precise estimates are unavailable in Brazil, it is likely that substantial resources (and many lives) could be saved and resources reallocated by developing similar measures there.

Quality in Brazilian Hospitals

Two quality gaps exist in Brazil. The first is between Brazilian medical research and medical practice, and the second is between the quality of care provided at a few centers of excellence and in the bulk of other facilities. Although Brazil is taking the lead in many areas of medical research of global importance, the evidence in other areas suggests major quality deficiencies across these three components of care.

Quality Gaps

Brazilian hospitals play an increasingly important role in international biomedical and clinical research (table 7.1). For example, Brazil's contribution to world publications on cardiovascular research and cancer research increased by 59 and 61 percent, respectively, between 1989 and 1994 (Rodrigues, Fonseca, and Chaimovich 2000), and Brazilian-led innovations in stem-cell research, psychiatry, oncology, and embryology have cemented the country's reputation for world-class medical research.

Brazil has also launched innovative health initiatives such as the development of national guidelines and regulations for the practice of alternative medicine (including homeopathy and acupuncture) and the rolling out of a national policy on the use of generic drugs and drug advertising. At the same time, hospitals have developed internal policies for improved management and monitoring of procedures and outputs. For example, the Hospital das Clínicas in São Paulo has launched a training program for nurses to improve strategic planning and client-focused service provision. Perhaps the most significant initiative directed at quality improvement was the development of national and regional programs for hospital certification and accreditation (see chapter 8). Annex 7A presents an overview of quality-enhancing policy and managerial innovations by medical discipline.

Two centers of excellence deserve special mention. The Ludwig Institute in São Paulo is participating in the Human Cancer Genome Project and has identified 1 million sequences of the most common tumor genes in Brazil. It took less than a year to complete the task, after a similar project in the United States had taken more than three years to identify the first million sequences. The National Cancer Institute (Instituto Nacional de Câncer, INCA) in Rio de Janeiro is performing cutting-edge research on intelligent drugs that attack cancer cells. INCA and the Ludwig Institute are two among at least eight Brazilian institutions recognized worldwide for pioneering medical research on tumors, genetics, molecular biology, and biomedical engineering.

Although advanced research is being performed in Brazilian centers of excellence, the quality of care for most cancer patients in Brazil is lagging. According to data from the Brazilian Society for Clinical Oncology, a patient suffering from intestinal cancer in the United States will live for another 20 months after the onset of the most critical period of the illness. In Brazil the average survival period is only 12 months (*VEJA*, October 19, 2005, p. 74). In the United States and Europe 74 percent of breast cancer patients survive five years after treatment, compared with 51 percent in Brazil. Similar differences in survival rates were reported for other cancers.

The gap between the quality of care provided in a few elite hospitals and in most other hospitals is also significant. For example, survival rates for cancer treatment in the recognized centers of excellence such as those mentioned above are similar to those in high-income counties,

TABLE 7.1
Significant Developments in Brazilian Medical Research, 2000–5

Research specialization	Development and innovation	Location and year
Cloning	Therapeutic cloning (transfer of a nucleus from a cell to an ovule with no nucleus)	HC-FMUSP, 2004
Embryology	Discarded embryos used to treat degenerative and incurable illnesses, including dystrophy, Parkinson's disease, multiple sclerosis, and diabetes	HC-FMUSP, 2004
Infectious diseases	DNA vaccine used to prevent recurrence of tuberculosis	Municipal Department of Health, São Paulo, 2005
	Development of preparatory vaccine against bird flu (avian influenza)	Butantã Institute, São Paulo, 2005
Oncology	Development of technique for diagnosing bladder cancer using hyaluronic acid	UNIFESP, São Paulo, 2000
	Treatment of skin cancer using light-emitting diode as alternative to laser treatment	University of São Paulo (USP), São Carlos, 2003
	Discovery of protective effect of wine and grape juice in arteriosclerosis	Instituto de Coração, HC-FMUSP, São Paulo, 2004
Psychiatry	Treatment for obsessive compulsive disorder using cognitive techniques	HC–FMUSP, São Paulo (undated)
	Treatment for depression using a portable device to stimulate mood-regulating areas of brain	Research Institute, HC-FMUSP, São Paulo, 2005
	Pharmacological research into medicinal plants of Amazon and Atlantic Forest regions for use in psychiatric diagnosis and research	Institute of Applied Ethno-Psychology of the Amazon, IDEAA-Amazonas), 2005
Rheumatology	New treatment for rheumatoid arthritis, developed from a protein produced in the body	UNIFESP, São Paulo, 2004
Technological advances	Application of magnetic resonance device that facilitates routine examinations.	Beneficiência Portuguesa Hospital, São Paulo, 2005
	Refinement of use of three-dimensional X-rays for intensity-modulated radiation therapy (IMRT)	Albert Einstein Hospital, São Paulo, 2004
Transplants	Development of liver transplant technique using laser that helps detect alterations in human tissue composition	FMRP/USP, São Paulo, undated
Stem cell	Trunk cell transplant from a patient's bone marrow to spinal marrow.	University of São Paulo, 2003

Source: Author's elaboration based on information from federal and regional medical councils, 2005.
Note: FMRP, Facultade de Medicine de Ribeirão Preto; HC-FMUSP, Hospital das Clínicas da Faculdade de Medicina da Universidade de São Paulo; UNIFESP, Universidade Federal de São Paulo.

but this is not the case in most facilities. Some health facilities encounter major challenges just maintaining basic standards of infrastructure, staffing, and services, even as a few hospitals play host to world-class treatment and research and are staffed by outstanding medical professionals. The best hospitals are concentrated in the South and Southeast, in the cities of Rio de Janeiro, São Paulo, and Porto Alegre. They possess advanced medical technology and the most qualified medical and other health professionals (Noronha and Garcia Rosa 1999).

In a comparative analysis of cohort studies performed in Pelotas city in 1982 and 1993, Victora et al. (2000) found that although overall infant mortality rates for low-birthweight babies born to both well-off and poor mothers declined over the period, the difference between these two groups actually increased. The authors concluded that a quality-driven "equity gap" was at work here: the well-off had better access to higher-quality, newer technologies in neonatal care (generally adopted by non-SUS private hospitals) than did the poor, who frequented SUS facilities where these technologies were unavailable. The poorer-quality maternal and neonatal care in SUS hospitals used by black mothers is seen as a contributing factor to the significantly higher infant mortality observed in the black population in Brazil (Leal, da Gama, and da Cunha 2005; Barros, Victora, and Horta 2001; PNUD 2004).

A broader look at the hospital system from a national perspective highlights huge discrepancies in the provision of quality health care between and within hospitals. Widespread shortcomings in hospital structures, processes, and results are evident across state-run and private hospitals.

Measuring Quality

Gathering reliable data that show both achievements and problems in hospital quality in Brazil is challenging. To begin with, there is little consensus on how data should be collected and which measurements or indicators should be used. For example, each of the diverse quality assessment and accreditation systems applied in Brazil proposes slightly different methodologies for data collection, and each has its own supporters and detractors. None has had the unswerving support of the Ministry of Health (Ministério da Saúde, MS) over a significant period of time. No national institution systematically collects, measures, and reports information on quality of care.

In most hospitals information about quality, however defined, is simply not available. In others, data are gathered haphazardly, or the effort is centered on a single department or service and usually responds to the concerns of a small cadre of dedicated professionals. Collected data are rarely analyzed or used to inform policy decisions. In interviews conducted for this report, hospital managers expressed an interest in adopting data systems for measuring quality but lacked the know-how or had no real motivation to take such a program forward. Many are frustrated by the lack of a unified system to guide this kind of effort.

The remainder of this chapter uses the Donabedian framework of structure, process, and results to highlight some of the shortcomings apparent in the Brazilian health system. It draws on national facility surveys, state surveys, and small-scale research, focusing on areas for which data are available.[2]

Shortcomings in Structure

This section reviews problems in major structural components of quality: infrastructure, equipment, materials, and human resources. It includes a discussion of regulatory issues related to physician education, licensure and qualifications.

Physical Assets and Materials

The quality of infrastructure, equipment, and materials—a hospital's working tools—is an important determinant of care. The challenge for governmental authorities has been to ensure the standardization and systematization of these structures across the country through regulation. The discussion here draws mainly on the results of state and national assessment surveys of structural characteristics of samples of facilities, which sought to determine the extent of compliance with national and state facility licensure regulations.[3] The findings are consistent across all surveys: many facilities are not in compliance with licensure regulations—and are probably unsafe.

In the late 1990s the MS launched the National Hospital Services Assessment Program (Programa Nacional de Avaliação dos Serviços Hospitalares, PNASH), which sought to rate hospitals according to a set of structural standards prepared by the MS for physical structures, equipment, and human resources. Each hospital was to receive a rating (poor, bad, average, good, or excellent) according to an assessment instrument applied by MS inspectors. A score of 61 (out of 100) was considered a minimally acceptable level of compliance, meaning that the facility possessed adequate infrastructure, staffing, and equipment to treat patients. However, only psychiatric facilities were actually surveyed. In 2002, 252 psychiatric hospitals were inspected and rated, but a final report was never published. Evidently, a significant number did not meet the benchmark score of 61, and the MS was loathe to release this information.[4] Nevertheless, 29 psychiatric facilities with extremely low ratings were closed. The MS discontinued the PNASH in 2004.

In 2005 the MS launched a new assessment program, the National Health Service Assessment Program (Programa Nacional de Avaliação de Serviços de Saúde, PNASS). In that year PNASS collected data on 6,030 SUS-financed ambulatory and hospital facilities providing specialty services. The instrument was based on standards drawn from Brazilian licensure regulations.[5] As with the PNASH, facilities were ranked on a five-point Likert scale in which a weighted score of 61 (out of 100) was deemed minimally acceptable. The survey consisted of two parts: self-assessment by the facility, and an external assessment by inspectors drawn from local government health authorities. The results of the assessment by local authorities are presented in figure 7.1. Among the facilities, 39 percent were rated superior or good. More

FIGURE 7.1
PNASS Facility Assessment Scores, 2005–6 (in percent of hospitals)

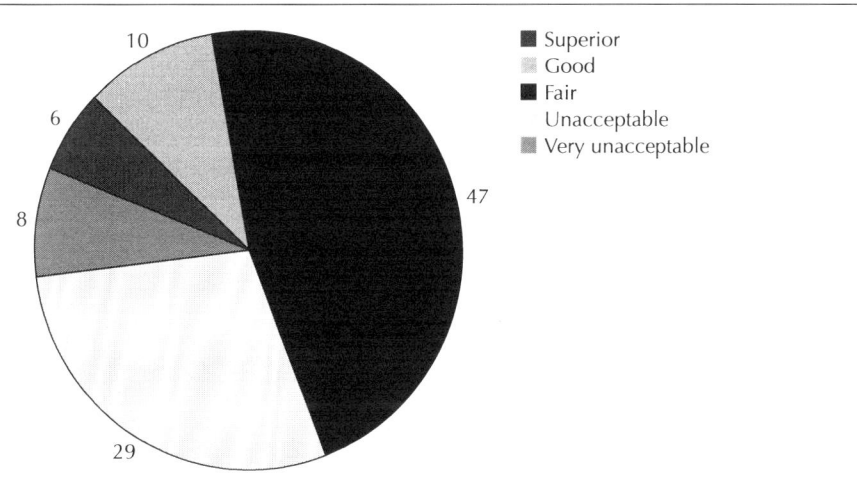

■ Superior
▨ Good
■ Fair
  Unacceptable
▨ Very unacceptable

Source: MS 2006d (preliminary data).

than a third (37 percent, not shown in the figure) were found out of compliance, scoring below the 61 benchmark. Nearly 40 percent of facilities did not undertake the survey, and it is safe to assume that most of them are out of compliance.[6]

It is highly likely that the external inspectors were excessively lenient in applying the standards to public facilities. All the inspectors were drawn from state and municipal health administrative units and therefore were internal to the SUS system. In fact, the inspectors' ratings were higher than those derived from the self-assessments.

It is common knowledge in Brazil that state and municipal sanitary authorities responsible for regulatory enforcement irregularly inspect or enforce licensure regulations. Inspections generally follow press reports of malpractice or adverse events.[7] As suggested by the survey described above, many facilities operate without a valid license. Furthermore, where inspections occur, authorities concentrate on private, for-profit hospitals; they infrequently inspect publicly operated or SUS-financed nonprofit facilities. Prestigious for-profit facilities serving the well-off are regularly inspected for compliance with licensure legislation and sanitary codes, while public hospitals serving low-income populations are rarely, if ever, inspected. Conflicts of interest may be a factor, since public officials participating in inspection teams are also responsible for overseeing public facilities.

The voluminous and convoluted nature of licensure and sanitary codes in Brazil undermines their impact and effectiveness. For example, the PNASS survey instrument is based on 123 sanitary regulations, resolutions, directives, laws, and norms spanning an 80-year period. Many are out of date and irrelevant to a modern hospital. Understanding the precise requirements can be a daunting chore. Streamlining and simplifying the regulations would facilitate implementation.[8]

Surveys provide aggregate information on the degree of compliance with regulations mandating minimal structural standards. But what does this mean with respect to the condition of the facilities and their service units? State-based surveys offer some answers.

A commonly used measurement of structural quality involves the state of buildings and infrastructure within a hospital complex. In 2002 and 2003 the São Paulo State Regional Medical Council (Conselho Regional de Medicina do Estado de São Paulo, CREMESP) surveyed more than 1,000 hospitals, emergency care centers, and maternity units in the state.[9] CREMESP (2004a) defined a hospital's physical environment as "adequate" when it complied with minimum state and national standards for licensing (e.g., cleanliness, adequate between-bed space for free circulation, beds connected to an oxygen supply network, nursing station located in all first-aid rooms). In the survey, conducted on-site by independent inspectors, an instrument based on these regulations was used. Summary results are presented in table 7.2.

In more than half the hospitals the physical area for patients was considered substandard. Public hospitals scored better than private facilities. Nonprofit hospitals scored particularly low; only 30 percent ranked as adequate. Most of the nonprofits were small, with fewer than 50 beds. A higher proportion of private for-profit facilities than of public and nonprofit hospitals was deemed adequate.

Barbosa et al. (2002) undertook a separate national survey of 69 private philanthropic hospitals ranging in size from fewer than 50 to more than 300 beds. Of these, 13 percent had no established system of works and repairs for the maintenance of hospital buildings and equipment,[10] and 22 percent had no professional maintenance staff. Larger hospitals and

TABLE 7.2
Physical Conditions in São Paulo Hospitals, by Ownership, 2003
(*N* = 743)

| | Ownership | | | | | | |
| | Public | | | Private | | | |
Physical area	All	State	Municipal	All	Nonprofit	For-profit	Total
Adequate (%)	50.0	45.7	46.5	44.0	30.3	62.8	45.4
Inadequate (%)	47.6	51.4	50.5	53.9	68.8	33.3	52.5
No information (%)	2.4	2.9	33.0	2.1	0.9	3.9	2.2
Number (total)	164	35	101	579	337	231	743

Source: CREMESP 2004a.

conglomerates (more than 600 beds) fared better; only 9.3 percent of 86 sampled facilities reported not having a professional responsible for maintenance.

Barbosa et al. also found that most nonprofit hospitals were operating laboratories and radiology units without a valid operating license. The review showed that 80 percent of the sampled hospitals had the required license for their laboratories but that only 58 percent had a license for radiology units. In a separate survey of 81 hospitals belonging to private nonprofit conglomerates, about a fourth did not have licenses for their laboratories or radiology units. Larger facilities were worse than smaller ones in that respect; of the 15 large hospitals (more than 500 beds) that were surveyed, 10 had valid licenses for their laboratories and 11 for their radiology units.[11]

Returning to the CREMESP survey, 667 surgical theaters were inspected to ascertain whether they had the minimum equipment for performing safe surgical and anesthetic procedures. The results indicate that nearly one-third of private and one-fifth of public hospitals had less than half the minimum equipment (table 7.3).[12] At the other extreme, 34 percent of the private hospitals and 40 percent of the public facilities had surgery theaters with at least 90 percent of the minimum necessary equipment.

TABLE 7.3
Surgical Theaters with Minimum Required Equipment in São Paulo State, by Ownership, 2003
(*N* = 667)

| | Facility type | | | | | |
| | Private | | Public | | Total | |
Proportion of minimum required equipment (percent)[a]	No.	%	No.	%	No.	%
<50	170	31.5	24	18.9	194	29.1
50–90	183	33.8	47	37.0	230	34.5
>90	183	33.8	50	39.4	233	34.9
Not available	4	0.7	6	4.7	10	1.5
Total	540.0	100.0	127.0	100.0	667.0	100.0

Source: CREMESP 2004a.
a. Minimum required equipment for surgery rooms includes operating lamp, laryngoscope handle and blades, anesthesia needles, endotracheal tubes, respirator, pulse oximeter, electrocardiogram (ECG) monitor, capnometer monitor, medical vacuum system, oxygen, and nitrous oxide.

TABLE 7.4
Equipment in Intensive Care Units in São Paulo State, by Ownership, 2003
(N = 359)

Minimum required equipment present	Facility type		Total
	Public	Private	
No (%)	48.6	58.6	56.5
Yes (%)	51.4	41.4	43.5
Number of facilities	74	285	359

Source: CREMESP 2004a.

Intensive care units were also found to be underequipped. To conform to Brazilian regulations, an ICU must have a minimum amount of equipment relating to various procedures. As displayed in table 7.4, the CREMESP study found that of the 359 ICUs for which data were available (information was not available for 17), only 44 percent had the necessary equipment at the time of inspection. Private facilities performed slightly better than public ones, with 59 percent possessing the required equipment, compared with 49 percent of the public ICUs. The same study found that 14 percent of ICUs did not meet the minimum requirements in support services, including gas meter, clinical laboratory, and hemotherapeutics.

The quality of record keeping in hospitals is poor (table 7.5). About two-thirds of all hospitals and 72 percent of private hospitals had incomplete records, according to the CREMESP survey. Public hospitals did slightly better, with 56 percent.

The deficient structural condition of hospitals does not appear to be limited to São Paulo state and may be much worse in other states. Further evidence of unenforced licensure legislation comes from an assessment of state-financed hospitals in a Central-West state conducted by independent surveyors certified by the ONA. Facilities were assessed according to ONA's three levels of standards. The first level was roughly equivalent to compliance with licensure legislation on structural characteristics of the hospital. To obtain ONA Level 1

TABLE 7.5
Adequacy of Record Keeping in Hospitals in São Paulo State, by Ownership, 2003
(N = 743)

State of record keeping	Public			Private			Total
	All	State	Municipal	All	Benevolent and philanthropic	For-profit	
Patient records appropriately filled out (%)	31.7	42.9	23.7	16.6	10.7	23.4	19.9
Records incomplete (%)	55.5	42.9	62.4	71.8	80.7	60.2	68.3
No information (%)	12.8	14.2	13.9	11.6	8.6	16.4	11.8
Number	164	35	101	579	337	231	743

Source: CREMESP 2004a.

approval, a facility must demonstrate to the independent surveyor team that its structures are "reliable and organized."

No hospital surveyed met ONA Level 1 standards; all 15 hospitals reviewed fell well short of the minimal standards in almost every area (table 7.6). Only for standards related to "leadership and administration" did more than half of the hospitals meet the necessary requirements. None reached the required standards for "infrastructure and logistical support" or "professional services and assistance." The entire hospital network in this particular

TABLE 7.6
Qualification of SUS Hospitals in a Brazilian State for ONA Level 1 Accreditation, 2002

ONA component	Number of hospitals	Number of qualified hospitals	Qualified hospitals (%)
Leadership and administration			
Management	15	15	100
Administration	15	10	67
Quality assurance	15	0	0
Professional and support services			
Clinical corps	15	0	0
Nursing	15	0	0
Services relating to patient and client care			
Internment	15	0	0
Referrals	13	1	8
Ambulatory care	9	0	0
Emergency	15	0	0
Surgical center	15	0	0
Anesthesiology	15	0	0
Obstetrics	13	0	0
Intensive care	6	0	0
Hemotherapeutics	13	7	54
Rehabilitation	5	1	20
Diagnostic support services			
Clinical laboratory	14	0	0
Diagnosis for image	15	1	7
Support and supply services			
Medical archives	15	1	7
Control of infections	11	2	18
Pharmacy	15	2	18
Laundry	15	0	0
Hygiene	15	1	7
Diet and nutrition	15	0	0
Infrastructural services and logistical support			
Works and repairs	15	0	0
Electrical systems	15	0	0
General maintenance	15	0	0
General security	15	0	0

Source: Gastal et al. 2005b.

state satisfied neither the minimum requirements for patient safety nor the standards pre-scribed by law to permit them to open their doors for business. Whether similar conditions exist in other states is unknown.

Several studies have examined the structural conditions of maternity hospitals in Brazil. Costa et al. (2004) assessed structural aspects of 28 hospitals providing maternity services in Minas Gerais in 1996. The researchers applied a point-based assessment model that rated the "safety" of the facilities in terms of general infrastructure, perinatal infrastructure and personnel, and technical resources for perinatal care. Thirteen (46 percent) were found to have adequate conditions for maternal and perinatal care for low-risk cases, while only six (21 percent) were deemed adequate for medium- and high-risk cases. Disturbingly, at least 50 percent of the facilities did not have hygienic delivery rooms, neonatal resuscitation units, ICU incubators, lactaries, maternal recovery rooms, or back-up electrical generators. The authors concluded that the hospitals found to have deficient structural conditions were "cer-tainly exposing [patients] to unnecessary and avoidable risks" (Costa et al. 2004: 709). The situation has probably improved since 1996, and as a result of the research findings, five of the hospitals were decertified in 1998 and no longer receive SUS patients. In Teresina city, in a study sponsored by the United Nations Children's Fund (UNICEF), Borba et al. (2001) examined the state of obstetrical and prenatal care in SUS maternity hospitals and found the overall situation to be one of "grave deficiencies." Finally, an in-depth analysis of four maternity hospitals in Rio de Janeiro city reported that none had the capacity to perform an emergency cesarean section in 30 minutes or less because of lack of surgical supplies, anes-thesia, or surgical gowns (Garcia Rosa and Hortale 2000).

Human Resources

In addition to deficiencies in infrastructure and record keeping, the CRESMESP survey found evidence of shortcomings in human resources. These include staff shortages, lack of techni-cal support, and underqualified or unqualified personnel. Looking at senior positions, the survey found that 16 percent of the hospitals did not have a clinical director currently on staff (in public hospitals, 33 percent did not). Of the facilities that did have a clinical director, in only 47 percent was the director elected by the hospital medical corps, as required by Brazil-ian regulations (Resolution CFM 1352/92).

The data from nonprofit hospitals surveyed by Barbosa et al. (2002) showed that a large proportion had senior staff in place and only 4 percent lacked a clinical director. The same study of 69 facilities, however, revealed vacancies in many other posts. Of note was the dearth of directors or technical support personnel in various areas, including diagnostic and treatment services, quality, and surveillance.

The CREMESP survey included inspection of 564 maternity units. In 13 percent of these, deliveries were performed by an unqualified staff member such as an auxiliary nurse or attendant. This problem appears to be related to hospital size: in more than half of the cases in which staff members lacked the required qualifications, the facility had fewer than 50 beds. The same study found, in a sample of 492 facilities, that the medical records in mater-nity and nursery units were not adequately completed in 78 percent of cases, including 83 percent of private facilities and 58 percent of public facilities.[13]

Elsewhere in Brazil, the situation may be worse than in São Paulo, but absence of informa-tion and small sample sizes limit generalizations. For example, Costa et al. (2004) reported that

11 of 28 sampled maternity units in Minas Gerais did not provide 24-hour pediatric services in the delivery room, and half did not provide 24-hour nursing services in delivery rooms.

Physician Education, Licensure, and Performance Assessment

Quality of care in hospitals is a product of well-run organizations and the quality of professional practice. This discussion of the quality of physicians focuses on regulatory measures to certify physicians and maintain their continuing competence. As in many other countries, medical practice is self-regulated in Brazil, delegated by law to federal and regional medical councils.

Physician certification in Brazil consists of graduation from a medical school and registration with state medical boards. There is no formal process—no board exams or systems—to assess knowledge or potential performance. Despite repeated calls by CREMESP and other organizations for a national medical exam to determine physician licensure, such a measure has yet to gain acceptance. Yet available evidence suggests that some medical schools do not adequately prepare their students for practice. A 2004 study by the Brazilian Medical Association reports on the deterioration of standards in medical education (Bueno, Loures, and Pieruccini 2004). A number of factors have contributed to this decline: increased availability of private courses, despite an oversupply of doctors; regional differences in the availability of medical schools, with a high concentration of universities and doctors in the South and Southeast; and lack of consensus between the Ministries of Health and Education on student numbers and quality standards in medical schools. These issues are reviewed in box 7.2.

CREMESP has supported a volunteer assessment exam of medical students for many years. The exam is generally given to students in their final (sixth) year of study or to recent graduates. In late 2005, 1,003 sixth-year students from 23 medical schools in São Paulo state took the exam. According to CRESMESP (2006), these represented about half the state's sixth-year medical students.[14] The exam consisted of 120 questions in basic science, bioethics, public health, and seven medical specialties. Of the group, 68 percent had a passing score of 60 or higher, and the average score was 73.3. Large variations, however, were observed across medical schools. For example, 40 percent or more of the students from more than half the schools failed, as did between 60 and 80 percent of the students from five schools.

Students taking the exam in 2006 and 2007 fared worse; only 62 and 44 percent of test takers passed in those years.[15] In 2007 more than 50 percent of students from 13 of 23 medical schools represented failed.[16] The CREMESP report laments the deteriorating conditions of medical education in São Paulo.

> The increasing educational deficit exposes the population to health risks [related] to the low quality of care. [given] the high concentration of physicians in many cities . . . São Paulo does not need more physicians, rather [it needs] better physicians. (CREMESP 2007: 7)

The only other state medical council to apply a similar exam is that of Espiritu Santo. In 2007, 78 students representing 53 percent of six-year students attending medical schools there took the exam. All passed. How well students are prepared by medical schools in other states is unknown.

Indirect evidence of poorly trained physicians can be drawn from registers of formal grievances filed by patients. CREMESP maintains a record of such complaints for São Paulo state. The number of physicians who are subjects of a formal grievance increased from 1,029 in 1995, when the register was started, to 3,569 in 2006. According to CREMESP, the rate of

Box 7.2
What Is Happening to the Quality of Medical Education in Brazil?

A debate rages within the Brazilian medical profession about the measurement of the quality of medical education. The National Examination for Medical Courses (Exame Nacional de Cursos, NEC) is the most widely applied testing instrument.[a] Scores are measured on a scale of A to E, where A is rated as 1 standard deviation above the general average score, B is from 0.5 to 1 above the average, C is from 0.5 below to 0.5 above the average, D is between 0.5 and 1 below, and E is more than 1 standard deviation below the average.

Results from the NEC between 1999 and 2002 suggest a polarization, with the incidence of both the top scores and the lowest scores increasing: grade A results went from 12 percent in 1999 to 17 percent in 2002, and grade E results rose from 9 to 14 percent. Furthermore, regional differences appear to be growing: in 1999, of a total of 13 medical schools in the Northeast, 5 scored A or B, but by 2002 none scored better than C. During the same period of time, the number of medical schools scoring A or B in the Southeast region remained more or less stable (15 in 1999 and 16 in 2002, out of a total of 44 in 1999 and 48 in 2002).

A different system for measuring quality in medical education, the Evaluation of Supply Conditions (Avaliação das Condições de Oferta, ACO), grades medical schools according to standards for the teaching staff, teaching methods, and facilities. The results for 1999 and 2000 support the NEC finding that standards in private universities are much lower than those in public institutions. The quality of teaching was rated "inadequate" in 12 of the 34 private universities (35 percent), with none scoring "very good." Only 7 of the 138 public universities (5 percent) were rated "inadequate," and 30 (22 percent) scored "very good."

Between 2000 and 2003, 20 new medical schools were established in Brazil. Bueno, Loures, and Pieruccini (2004) argue that this unrestricted growth in the number of schools, at a time when the number of doctors per capita is well above internationally recommended levels, is contributing to the deterioration in medical teaching and thus in hospital standards. Declining standards in teaching, combined with stark regional differences between universities, inadequate infrastructure, and poorly prepared faculties, are eroding the quality of health services and making it harder for people from poor, rural areas to access quality health care.

Source: Bueno, Loures, and Pieruccini 2004.

a. As stipulated in Law 9.131 (1995), all students are required to take the test that is used to assess the quality of medical schools. Application of the test to medical school graduates is irregular, however, and passing the NEC is not required for certification.

grievances (the number of cases divided by the number of active physicians) also rose over this period, from 1.7 to 3.9 percent. Information on grievances in other states is unavailable.

After many years of debate, Brazil has taken the first steps toward encouraging physician competence. Recognizing that it is no longer tenable for a young physician to be certified for life, in 2005 the Federal Council of Medicine approved a mandatory recertification process for specialists. The measure, however, applies only to specialists certified after January 1, 2006; participation is voluntary for specialists certified before that date. Recertification, which is required at five-year intervals, is awarded by a to-be-formed national commission and involves a point-based system. Candidates earn points by self-reporting their courses completed; seminars, symposiums, and conferences attended; postdoctoral degrees earned; scientific papers published; and residency programs coordinated during a five-year period. Failure to participate leads to loss of license.

Such a recertification system, based on point awards for continuing medical education, has been criticized for its unknown and perhaps weak connection to physicians' actual performance. Recertification programs elsewhere are moving away from point-based systems and toward the inclusion of additional measures such as competency exams,[17] reviews of patient complaints and disciplinary actions, appraisal of practice patterns, and patient and peer assessments (Norcini 1999; Newble, Paget, and Mclaren 1999; Swinkels 1999). Granted, these measures are costly, unpopular, and difficult to construct, but they are considered more robust for improving physician performance than simple point-based systems. Brazil's nascent physician recertification system is an important first step toward fostering physician accountability for providing quality care, but it is too soon to tell whether the process will weed out bad physicians and improve patient protection.

Unlike the recent strides toward recertifying physicians, disciplinary mechanisms to protect patients from physician malpractice have advanced little and appear ineffective. Federal and regional medical councils are responsible for assessing, judging, and disciplining physicians for malpractice and ethical violations. All physicians must belong to a regional council, which exists in every state. Members of the councils' ethics or disciplinary tribunals are physicians elected by their colleagues. Disciplinary actions originate with a complaint to the regional council. An action can result in exoneration, confidential warning or censure, public censure, or a 30-day license suspension. The regional councils do not usually make public the number of cases processed or the results of disciplinary tribunals. Although the number of cases processed appears to be increasing in some jurisdictions, the councils have traditionally been lenient with physicians and do not fulfill their mandate to protect the health and safety of the public. Anecdotal evidence suggests that councils rarely suspend medical licenses and are more likely to issue a confidential warning or censure. Because there is no public or government participation in the boards, lines of accountability appear diffuse.

Regional councils do not evoke licenses but can recommend revocation. Only the Federal Council of Medicine can revoke a license, on recommendation by a regional council. A physician receiving a temporary suspension by a regional council has the right to appeal the decision to the Federal Council of Medicine. The federal body, however, rarely upholds a serious disciplinary action; as table 7.7 indicates, between 2001 and 2005 only around 9 percent of cases in Brazil received serious disciplinary action (temporary suspension or revocation of a medical license). In contrast, state medical boards in the United States suspended or revoked licenses in, on average, 58 percent of cases between 2001 and 2005; the states of California and New York suspended or revoked medical licenses in 55 and 60 percent of cases, respectively. In 2005, as reported in *O Globo* (August 21, 2006), the Regional Medical Council of Rio de Janeiro State (Conselho Regional de Medicina do Estado de Rio de Janeiro, CREMERJ) processed 93 cases, issued 3 temporary suspensions (3.2 percent), and recommended 5 revocations (5.4 percent). The sanctioned physicians have the right to appeal to the Federal Council of Medicine, with a high probability of leniency (see table 7.7).

In sum, Brazil has yet to develop a regulatory system that protects the public against ill-trained or incompetent physicians. There are no systems for certifying medical school graduates, and self-regulation, as a means of detecting and curtailing medical malpractice, does not work. Physician regulation remains just as much a "prisoner to the interests and self-protectiveness of the medical profession" today as it was more than a decade ago (World Bank 1994: 139).

TABLE 7.7
Disciplinary Actions against Physicians in Brazil and the United States, 2001–5

Country or state	2001	2002	2003	2004	2005
Brazil					
Cases (number)	141	184	239	231	344
License suspension, 30 days (%)	4	3	3	4	8
License revocation (%)	4	8	4	4	2
United States					
Cases (total number)	4,758	4,946	5,342	6,261	6,213
License restriction (%)	25	25	25	21	22
License revocation (%)	35	36	34	34	32
California state					
Cases (state number)	495	569	572	651	624
License restriction (%)	26	25	29	24	23
License revocation (%)	34	33	36	33	35
New York state					
Cases (state number)	503	461	508	534	534
License restriction (%)	19	21	28	38	29
License revocation (%)	51	49	46	42	39

Source: Brazil: Conselho Federal de Medicina 2006; United States: Federation of State Medical Boards 2006.

Shortcomings in Processes and Results

Measuring processes involves assessing the quality of mechanisms and procedures for delivering health care in hospitals. Few Brazilian studies directly address this issue, and information on results is even scarcer.[18] Researchers trying to assess quality processes and outcomes in Brazilian health care invariably encounter shortcomings in the data that are available. Data are seldom collected systematically, access to records is limited, and the available databases are unreliable or incompatible with each other, making comparisons almost impossible. Even among hospitals that subscribe to the same programs for accreditation or for certification (by an external agency), methods for evaluating processes and data collection often vary, and different indicators may be used to assess the same process.

Because data on quality of care were so poor, a literature review of 1,100 publications and reports on quality of care in Brazil between 1997 and 2002 was commissioned for this volume. The review revealed that few studies based quality assessments on data analysis by applying rigorous methods. Most research was small in scale and focused on a specific service or department in a large facility or teaching hospital. Moreover, the review identified a large number of authors but only a few with consistent research production on the topic (only five authors had published more than four articles).[19]

The findings from these small-scale studies are summarized in box 7.3 and are presented in greater detail in annex 7B. Although the findings focus on processes and results, problems related to structure are also reported. Applying the framework developed by the IOM (2001), the review found a wide range of quality problems: errors and delays in diagnoses; failure to follow recommended practices; failure to conduct treatments, procedures, and diagnostics

Box 7.3
Problems with Quality and Possible Causes: Insights from a Literature Review

The literature review commissioned for this report and conducted by Kisil (2003) and Sampaio (2004) identified the following problems in Brazilian hospitals and some likely causes. See appendix 7B for details on the literature consulted.

Errors or delays in diagnosis
- Patient's difficulties in finding or accessing specialist services to obtain accurate diagnoses
- Diagnostic failures at patient's initial examination and doctors' difficulties in prioritizing the most serious cases
- Overuse of preop examinations

Failure to follow recommended procedures
- Use of outdated therapies and techniques

Failure to carry out operations and examinations using appropriate procedures
- Leniency of medical boards in punishing cases of malpractice; revocation of medical licenses very rare
- Absence of publicly available documents that reference and index cases of medical error
- Lack of comprehensive and systematic evaluations of clinical quality among medical professionals
- Shortcomings in midwifery and neonatal care, perhaps attributable to the presence of unqualified health workers

Failures in the selection and administration of treatments
- Lack of standardization in use of medicines
- Doctors' failure to follow protocols for prescribing medicines, with a tendency to choose the most expensive available

Faults in dosage or method of using drugs and in administration of prescribed drugs
- Inappropriate environment for prescribing and dispensing drugs
- Lack of attention to detail; distraction; safety faults during drug preparation
- Medicines prescribed for children not provided in appropriate form or dosage for consumption by minors

Unnecessary delays in treatment or in sharing examination results
- Perhaps attributable to shortcomings in structure, services, and equipment

Use of incorrect or inappropriate treatment
- Time- or money-saving treatments applied for convenience of staff, or at request of patient for reasons of social status (e.g., high rate of cesarean sections)

Failure to use recommended prophylactic treatments
- Failure of health managers and planners to use cheaper and more accessible treatments, even when there is a consensus that certain treatments should be standard

(continued)

Box 7.3 *(continued)*

Lack of monitoring, revision, and control system
- Lack of systemic evaluations of data on service providers
- Absence of mandatory hospital committees
- Shortcomings in professional qualifications; lack of literature in Portuguese

Problems with equipment
- Lack of training on use of new and existing equipment
- Absence of essential equipment in certain health facilities

Lack of a staff training system
- Short-term contracts, low wages, and internal conflicts giving rise to absenteeism
- Problems of communication and interaction between teams
- Lack of continuity of administrative personnel

---

using appropriate protocols; problems in the selection and administration of treatments; errors in dosage or use of drugs and in the administration of prescribed drugs; avoidable delays in treatment; failure to use recommended prophylactic treatments; and lack of a system for monitoring, revision, and control.

The studies point to a variety of shortcomings in processes throughout the hospital system. For example, a study by Pereira, Franken, and Sprovieri (2000) of iatrogenia in cardiology highlights a significant number of incidents of therapeutic failures, unwanted side effects of medication, complications with therapeutic and diagnostic procedures, and medical malpractice.[20] A 2001 study of maternal deaths in a university hospital concluded that 91 percent of such deaths were avoidable and that in more than half the cases medical negligence was the cause (Almeida 2001). Apart from the ethical and public health issues raised by such reports, Carvalho et al. (1991) point out that avoiding unnecessary deaths is important because they distort medical statistics and limit the use of these data in improving public health policy. One large-scale study of coronary surgery in 131 hospitals in Brazil showed a mortality rate of 7.2 percent, much higher than in the United States (2.8 percent), Canada (2.5 percent), or France (3.2 percent) (Noronha et al. 2003; WHO 2003a).

Although information related to process quality is not always readily available, the research highlighted some of the causes of poor quality of care in Brazilian hospitals. Among the most important are absence of systems for monitoring and quality control; no or poor understanding of protocols or clinical guidelines; failure to follow such protocols where they do exist; absence of functioning networks to provide continuous care; low technical and managerial capacities among service providers; absence of well-organized management structures; and deteriorating and obsolete buildings and infrastructure.

The absence of standardized practice norms or of treatment protocols or norms appears to be another process shortcoming that contributes to low quality. In 1997 and 1998, CREMESP conducted random surveys of maternity and neonatal units in hospitals in São Paulo state. As table 7.8 shows, less than 20 percent of facilities had norms for maternal admissions or protocols for predelivery rooms, and only about a third had delivery room protocols. The survey found that most university hospitals had standardized processes but that most private facilities did not.

TABLE 7.8

Presence of Standardized Practice Norms or Treatment Protocols, Maternity Services in São Paulo Hospitals, by Ownership, 1997–98

(percent)

Service	Public (N = 16)	Private (N = 73)	University (N = 10)	Total
Admissions	20	12	70	19
Predelivery room	21	10	70	18
Delivery room	33	20	100	31

Source: CREMESP 2000.

In Brazil a growing body of research on perinatal mortality relates structures and processes to results.[21] The following findings merit attention:

- In a cohort study of 40,953 births and 825 perinatal deaths in Belo Horizonte city, Lansky, França, and Kawachi (2007) reported that perinatal mortality rates were higher in SUS public and private hospitals than in non-SUS facilities.[22] This relation held for both low-birthweight and normal-birthweight babies. The researchers sought to understand this difference while controlling for confounding variables. First, they found significant differences in the cause of death. For example, preventable intrapartum asphyxia was two to four times higher in SUS facilities, whereas immaturity was the main cause in private non-SUS facilities. Perinatal mortality from acquired hospital infections was also higher in SUS facilities. When maternal education and birthweight—two factors associated with perinatal mortality—were controlled for, SUS facilities were found to be independently associated with higher perinatal mortality. Lower-quality facilities also proved to be independently associated with higher perinatal mortality.[23] In addition to untimely access, the authors attributed the higher perinatal rates in SUS facilities to "disorganized" perinatal care involving ineffective obstetric management and facility shortcomings in "responding adequately to situations such as birth complications" (Lansky, França, and Kawachi 2007: 872). Lack of quality monitoring and absence of routine audits were additional deficiencies observed by the authors.
- Drawing on the database created for the above-mentioned research, in a second but more focused study of 118 perinatal deaths and 492 births in SUS hospitals in Belo Horizonte, Lansky et al. (2006) sought to understand how hospital-based obstetric care processes affect outcomes.[24] Half of the deaths were attributed to preventable interpartum asphyxia, and 85 percent of these cases had inadequate fetal monitoring. Sixty percent of the deaths occurred in low-complexity facilities without adequate neonatal care; only 6 percent were attended in a facility with a neonatal ICU. Hourly fetal monitoring and maternal monitoring was not conducted in 82 and 84 percent of the cases, respectively. A partograph was not used in 37 percent of cases of death, compared with 21 percent of the controls.[25] In a regression model that controlled for a number of confounding variables (e.g., birthweight, mother's age, prenatal care, gender of infant, and illnesses during pregnancy), nonuse of a partograph was found to be independently associated with perinatal mortality.[26]
- Finally, pioneering research in Brazil examined the interaction between structure and process in hospitals and the impact of this interaction on neonatal mortality. Rattner

(2001) studied neonatal care, low birthweight, and preventable neonatal mortality across 51 hospitals in São Paulo state. According to the results, if improvements in structure (e.g., plant, material resources, number and specialization of human resources) took place without implementation of sound processes such as application of treatment guidelines, the risk of negative outcomes such as avoidable neonatal mortality would increase. The implication of the findings is that there is a synergy between structure and process: a more pronounced reduction in avoidable mortality will be achieved if investments are made simultaneously in both structures and processes. If investments focus on infrastructure and equipment alone, without concomitant (and probably continuous) attention to care processes, the impact on health variables may be negative (see box 7.4).

Case Study: Hospital Infection Rates and Measurement

Marçal dos Santos et al. (2005) reported the findings of a 2003 national survey of 27 state hospitals, 1,009 municipal hospitals, and 4,148 private hospitals that attempted to assess the incidence and control of hospital infection (HI) rates.[27] The authors were unable to quantify HI rates for the entire sample because internal methods for measuring the rates were often flawed. For example, many hospitals did not calculate correctly the number of hospital discharges, failing to add up total patients discharged, transfers, and deaths. In other instances these data were incomplete. In addition, many hospitals did not gather sufficient details relating to the seriousness of the infections or the exposure period, making intrahospital and interhospital comparisons impossible. The authors considered the data reliable for only 13 percent of cases.

Only one-third of hospitals report having measures for controlling an outbreak of an infection, and about half report having a program to control HI (figure 7.2).[28] About three-fourths

FIGURE 7.2
Hospital Infection Control, by Hospital Complexity
(N = 4,148 hospitals)

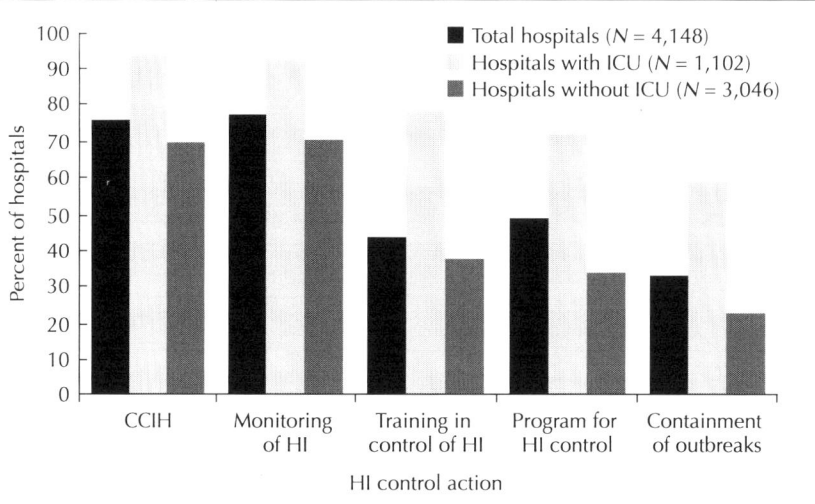

Source: Marçal dos Santos et al. 2005.
Note: CCIH, *comissão de controle de infecção hospitalar* (committee for the control of hospital infections).

Box 7.4
Bad Processes as a First-Order Problem: Interaction between Structure and Practice in Neonatal Wards

Rattner (2001) asked: What is the interaction between structures and processes? If processes in hospitals are not of a high standard but investments in structure are made, can improved health quality outcomes still be achieved? Or might the reverse happen? If, for example, investment is made in new equipment, what will be the effect if staff members do not know how to use the equipment properly or to interpret the results? What happens when processes are sound but are not supported by the requisite structures?

Rattner assessed structures and processes, their interaction, and the impact on preventable neonatal mortality. The results show that process investments, at whatever level of structure, will have a positive but not significant impact. Rattner did, however, find a significant correlation between structure investments for varying levels of processes, as shown in the figure. Even for a small sample size of 51 hospitals, the risk of a negative outcome (neonatal mortality) can actually increase if process quality is poor and at the same time investments in structure are made.

The figure shows that where process levels are low (P10 on the *x*-axis), large investments in structure triple the risk of avoidable neonatal mortality, with a confidence interval of between 1.43 and 6. Data points with positive or higher risk are displayed above the line labeled 1, while data points with lower risk (i.e., greater protection) are found below that line. Where processes are good (P75, meaning a 75 percent possibility of a quality process, or P90, meaning a 90 percent possibility), large investments in structure have a positive impact, reducing avoidable neonatal deaths. At P90, indicating an extremely good process, large investments in structure will have a protective effect of 0.28, meaning that the avoidable neonatal mortality rate will be reduced by 72 percent.

Effects of Investments in Structures on Neonatal Mortality Risk at Different Process Levels

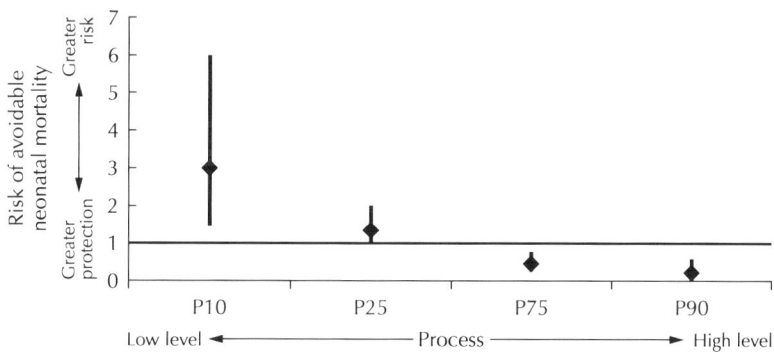

Note: The P values represent the degree (in percent) of compliance with criteria specified by the São Paulo state health secretariat. The greater the P value, the better the care in terms of process.

have appointed infection control committees and claim to monitor HI regularly. Less than half report training staff to control HI. Data not shown in figure 7.2 indicate that public hospitals operated by the federal government were the best performers, private hospitals were the next best, and state and municipal hospitals were the worst. For example, only 56 percent of municipally operated hospitals reported having an infection committee, and 30 percent reported having a program to control HI.

In 1995 the government adopted the internationally recognized NNISS/CDC system for diagnosing and tracking hospital infections.[29] As of 2003, however, only 17 percent of hospitals were using it. A separate system launched by the MS in 1998 has been adopted by 51 percent of hospitals. Disturbingly, 37 percent of hospitals reported having no defined criteria for identifying and monitoring infections.[30]

Marçal dos Santos et al. (2005) were able to determine infection rates for 182 (out of 636) hospitals with ICUs because these facilities took greater care in applying reporting criteria and methods. They facilities reported more than 9,000 cases of hospital infections and 1,320 HI-related deaths (table 7.9). Based on a total of nearly 100,000 discharges, the global rate of hospital infection was calculated at around 9 percent and related deaths were estimated at 14 percent. The real figures are probably higher because only 29 percent of the original sample of 636 hospitals provided reliable data. Moreover, hospitals that rigorously monitor HI are more likely to have programs for reducing HI incidence. For comparison, Prade et al. (1995) estimated a 15.6 percent HI rate in Brazil.[31]

The quality of results depends on process quality. High HI-related mortality may, in part, be attributed to the fact that the establishment of HI control committees has not got off the ground in many hospitals.[32] Marçal dos Santos et al. (2005) found that 76 percent of hospitals had appointed members of the hospital infection committee required under Brazilian hospital regulations; 24 percent had not (figure 7.2). Larger hospitals and those with greater capacity (that is, with ICUs) showed a greater tendency to adopt such systems.

Nomination of members does not mean that the HI committee actually monitors infections. In 1999 hospital infection committees were found to be inactive or nonexistent in more than half of 6,387 hospitals. A fully operational HI control program would ensure compliance with basic health care standards and control the application of hospital antimicrobial and germicidal agents, which, if used indiscriminately, can increase bacterial resistance, thus adding to global health costs (Prade et al. 1995).

The example of hospital infection committees highlights another problem with some of the current processes and results measurements. Although all hospitals are required by law to have an HI committee, the emphasis is on the formal requirement of simply having one, not on whether it is functioning—actually working to detect and control HIs.[33] The high infection rates in all hospitals, including the three-quarters that have an infection committee, stand as testament to this dichotomy between the requirement and the practice.

TABLE 7.9
HI Incidence in Adult ICUs, Brazil (excluding São Paulo), 2001–3

Hospitals with adult ICU (number)	636
Hospitals providing data (number)	182
Hospitals providing data (%)	29
Cases of HI (number)	9,197
Hospital discharges (number)	97,946
HI-related deaths (number)	1,320
HI rate (%)	9
HI-related deaths (%)	14

Source: Marçal dos Santos et al. 2005.

The 2004 CREMESP study referred to earlier confirms the results of Marçal dos Santos et al. (2005). CREMESP checked more than a thousand hospitals and emergency units in São Paulo for the presence of the HI committee mandated by law. The findings, presented in table 7.10, revealed that in 67 percent of the facilities no such committee existed. Only 32 percent of the hospitals in the study had all the committees required by law, and in 38 percent of these, one or more committees were found to be nonfunctional. A breakdown of the data for public hospitals shows that state hospitals are more compliant with the law than municipal hospitals, nearly 90 percent of which had no committees.

The importance of developing these activities is reinforced by internationally recognized work estimating that 40 to 60 percent of infections are preventable through well-conducted HI-control programs (IHI 2007). Simple policies on cleanliness can significantly cut the infection rate. For example, Broomfield Hospital in the United Kingdom reduced infections in its orthopedic unit by two-thirds in one year by adopting improved practices for hand cleaning, hygiene, and laundering of doctors' scrubs, barring caregivers from wearing jewelry, and enforcing other practices for limiting the transmission of bacteria from infected patients to inanimate objects and then to other patients (McCaughey n.d.).

Finally, monitoring and reducing hospital infections is important not only because of the mortality from infections but also because of the increased costs involved in treating infected patients. A study of 136 patients in an ICU in Recife, Pernambuco state, found that the average hospital stay was 2.8 days for patients who did not develop infections but 8.4 days for those with hospital infections. The average daily treatment cost was R$1,486.24 for uninfected patients but nearly twice as high (R$2,820.82) for patients who picked up infections in the hospital (Costa et al. 2003).[34]

Patient Satisfaction

An important measure of results is patient satisfaction. Interviews with facility managers suggest considerable interest in monitoring clients' opinions of services, yet few hospitals systematically ask for their opinions. The main reason for the dearth of assessments of patient satisfaction is the lack of standardized methodology: those hospitals that do survey patients use diverse methods and instruments, and interhospital comparisons are almost impossible.

TABLE 7.10

Existence and Functioning of Mandatory Hospital Committees, São Paulo State, 2003

| Status of mandatory hospital committee | Hospital type | | | | | | Total |
| | Public | | | Private | | | |
	All	State	Municipal	All	Nonprofit	For-profit	
In existence and active (%)	14.6	48.6	5.7	23.0	20.4	24.5	19.8
In existence but inactive (%)	7.3	20.0	4.4	15.3	14.2	16.5	12.2
Nonexistent (%)	77.3	31.4	89.0	60.7	64.5	57.9	67.1
No information (%)	0.8	0	0.9	1.0	0.9	1.1	0.9
Number (total)	384	35	318	627	338	278	1,011

Source: CREMESP 2004a.

Few of the hospitals that seek to measure patient satisfaction use the results to influence hospital policy or to make changes arising from recommendations. For example, interviews with directors of six hospitals found that five use a customer satisfaction appraisal, but only one said that the results are consulted; the other four reported that they were rarely consulted (Kisil 2004).

Patient satisfaction is an area in which the MS has taken an interest. In 1998 and 2002 the MS and the National Council of Secretaries of Health (Conselho Nacional de Secretários de Saúde, CONASS) jointly sponsored national surveys of patient satisfaction with SUS services, assessing perceptions of health services among users and nonusers of the SUS. Unfortunately, all the data were aggregated by region, and so state, municipal, and hospital information is not available for comparisons.

The 2002 survey reported adequate client satisfaction with hospital care but identified several problems (CONASS 2003a). According to the findings, 30 percent of households reported a hospital stay in the two years prior to the survey, and nearly 70 percent of these stays were in SUS-financed hospitals. About 72 percent of respondents rated their stay as "good" or "very good" and 14 percent as "very bad," "bad," or "neither good nor bad." Nearly 12 percent of SUS-hospital patients thought inpatient care was "getting worse"; 29 percent saw "no change." The main problems related to SUS services mentioned by the respondents included waiting lines for ambulatory consultations (41 percent), diagnostic services (14 percent), and inpatient care (7.5 percent); disrespectful or discourteous treatment (5 percent); and poor physician preparation (5 percent).[35]

Summary Assessment

The available evidence on hospital quality in Brazil indicates serious shortcomings in the three main areas of analysis: structure, process, and results. A significant number of hospitals are unsafe, as evidenced by their failure to meet licensure standards or comply with regulations for controlling hospital infections. Small-scale research suggests that clinical processes are deficient, resulting in a assorted errors, adverse events, and suboptimal practices.

Apparently, the press does a better job of monitoring quality than system stakeholders such as the SUS, insurers, or providers. The media, however, do not offer the best means of monitoring quality of care. Despite widespread recognition that data on quality are essential for assessing and improving hospital care, the surveys and literature reviewed in this chapter suggest that measuring and comparing quality is not a priority topic of analysis.

It is tempting to attribute these quality issues to lack of resources. Yet research from both developed and developing countries shows that variations in quality across organizations are not linked to spending levels (Peabody et al. 2006; IOM 2001). Although some facilities may need an injection of resources to raise quality, higher spending does not necessarily improve care or outcomes. There is general consensus among students of quality that lack of standardization of clinical processes and practices, and failure to use clinical evidence to inform those practices, are main drivers of variations in costs and quality. In the comparative analysis of hospitals under different organizational arrangements in chapter 6, one group of hospitals outperformed another in quality performance even though both had similar levels of spending.

Hospital quality is also affected by the quality of professional practice. Mandatory recertification is getting under way, but it applies only to physicians licensed after January 1, 2006, and will therefore have an impact only on future generations of physicians. Although the Brazilian model of recertification through mandatory continuing education has been adopted by a number of countries (Allsop and Jones 2005), the link between education and performance is unconfirmed.

Brazil lacks a system for certifying the competence of medical school graduates, and its regulatory mechanism for detecting and dealing with poor medical practice is ineffective. As noted in a World Bank report more than a decade ago, physician regulation remains a "prisoner to the interests and self-protectiveness of the medical profession" (World Bank 1994: 139). Obligatory certifying examinations and effective disciplinary processes, as well as measures to improve medical education, are essential for improving the overall quality of medical care in Brazil. Certifying exams would give medical schools an incentive to improve the quality of their teaching and curriculum. Standardization and supervision of medical school curriculums, with links to licensing requirements, is an additional measure. It is generally acknowledged that physicians should at least keep up with new knowledge of treatments and technologies. Including representatives of broader civil society and government in the councils would be a step in the right direction toward improving the accountability of the councils to the public.

Hospital quality in Brazil is often based on subjective assertions and marketing strategies claiming "prestige," "trust," or possession of the "latest technology." Without data on processes and outcomes, such claims are difficult to support. Perhaps the most worrisome findings are that the quality of care provided in most hospitals is unknown and that little is being done in systematic fashion to measure and assess quality performance.

This situation is beginning to change. Since the second half of the 1990s various approaches for assessing quality in hospitals have been developed. The roll-out of these approaches is still slow and somewhat piecemeal, but their adoption by more hospitals would be a sign that the importance of hospital quality is being recognized. In addition, a number of facilities have launched successful quality improvement programs. The next chapter examines some of these recent initiatives.

Annex 7A
Policy and Managerial Innovations Across Medical Disciplines, 2000–2005

Medical discipline	Changes and advances	Location and year
Alternative medicine	Development of national guidelines and regulations for use of alternative medicines (physiotherapy, homeopathy, and acupuncture) in SUS hospitals	National Council of Health, 2005
Phonoaudiology	Development of a dysphasia valve	Albert Einstein Hospital, São Paulo, 2000
	Rehabilitation of cancer patients who have difficulty in speaking, chewing, swallowing, or hearing	Brazilian Cancer Association, 2003
	Conductive education for sufferers from cerebral paralysis	HC-FMUSP, São Paulo, 2004
Nursing	Strategic administrative planning and customer focus for nursing	HC-FMUSP, São Paulo, 2004
	Systematization of procedures	HC-FMUSP, São Paulo, 2003
Pharmacy	Implementation of national policy on use of generic drugs and monitoring of drug advertising	ANVISA, 2000
	Revision of legislation to test the effectiveness and side effects of new medicines	ANVISA, 2001
Physiotherapy and occupational therapy	Rehabilitation: improved mobility of patients in intensive care to end dependence on supported breathing	Albert Einstein Hospital, São Paulo, 2005
	Early diagnosis of impaired sight among premature children to prevent blindness	UNICAMP, São Paulo, 2004
	Hemodynamic effect of surgical hypertension in patients after surgical cardiopaths (respiratory)	Instituto de Coração, HC-FMUSP, São Paulo, 2004
Psychology	Participation of psychologists in Management of Quality program, helping with changes in understanding of mental processes.	Instituto de Coração, HC-FMUSP, São Paulo, 2003
	Home-based psychotherapy	PUC-SP, São Paulo, 2002
	Joint groups for promotion of community health	HC-FMUSP, Ribeirão Preto, 2002

Source: Data from federal and regional professional councils, 2005.
Note: ANVISA, Agência Nacional de Vigilância Sanitária (National Agency for Sanitary Surveillance); HC-FMUSP, Hospital das Clínicas da Faculdade de Medicina da Universidade de São Paulo; PUC-SP, Pontifícia Universidade Católica de São Paulo.

Annex 7B

Process Shortcomings in Brazilian Hospitals and Possible Causes

Shortcomings and possible causes	Supporting evidence from microstudies
Diagnosis	
Errors or delays in diagnosis	
• Patient's difficulties in finding or accessing specialist services to obtain accurate diagnoses	Studies by Sánchez Cenurión (1993), Ferreira (1999), and Almeida (2001) criticize lack of clarity and of hierarchy within health provider layers and networks, giving rise to delays in patient referrals.
• Diagnostic failures at the time of a patient's initial examination, and doctors' difficulty in prioritizing the most serious cases	Shortcomings in medical training, organization of staff, and working environment were found by Garcia Rosa and Hortale (2000).
• Overuse of preoperation examinations	Arieta et al. (2004) suggest that reducing the number of preoperation examinations by up to 60 percent would not alter the results of subsequent surgical procedures.
Failure to follow recommended procedures	
• Use of outdated therapies and techniques	Prade (2002) shows that open drainage of urine is still common despite the proven risk of its increasing hospital infections up to 24-fold.
Treatment	
Failures in the selection and administration of treatments	
• Lack of standardization in use of medicines	Only 35 percent of philanthropic hospitals were found to use the same system of standardization of medicines; dispensing of medicines in individual doses was found to be consistent across only 54 percent of the same hospitals (Barbosa et al. 2002).
• Doctors' failure to follow protocols for prescribing medicines, with a tendency to choose the most expensive available	Akashi (1998) found that doctors in one tertiary hospital would more commonly prescribe the most expensive antihypertensive drugs, while international and national guidelines recommended a different drug.
• Medicines prescribed to children not provided in appropriate form or dosage for consumption by minors	A university hospital study on the use of intravenous medicines for children found that out of 8,245 doses administered in one month, none of the 41 drugs were in an appropriate dosage for pediatric use. This gave rise in some cases to increased doses, risks of contamination, and massive wastage: the estimated cost for 24 hours of intravenous treatment was US$46.23, of which US$6.71 was the cost of drugs administered to the patient and US$39.52 was for drugs discarded because they were not required for a pediatric dosage (Peterlini, Chaud, and Pedreira et al. 2003).

(continued)

Shortcomings and possible causes	Supporting evidence from microstudies
Treatment (continued)	
Faults in dosage or method of using drugs and in administration of prescribed drugs	
• Inappropriate environment for prescribing and dispensing drugs. • Lack of attention to detail; distraction; safety faults during drug preparation	Studies found that 35 percent of prescriptions were illegible and 95 percent of prescriptions lacked one or more items (Bohomol 2003; Silva 2003).
Unnecessary delays in treatment or in sharing examination results	
• Perhaps attributable to shortcomings in structure, services, and equipment	Garcia Rosa and Hortale (2002) attribute the long delay between deciding on and performing a cesarean section to problems related to structure, service, and equipment.
Use of incorrect or inappropriate treatment	
• Time- or money-saving treatments used for convenience of staff or at patient's request, for reasons of social status	Various studies show alarmingly high rates of caesarean births in Brazil (Gomes et al. 1999; Gouveia 1996).
Prophylaxis failures	
Failure to use recommended prophylactic treatments	
• Failure of health managers and planners to use cheaper and more accessible treatments, even when there is consensus that certain treatments should be standard	According to widespread consensus in the medical world, antenatal corticosteroid therapy should be used in cases of premature births. A study of seven maternity wards in Rio de Janeiro showed that such therapy was used in only 4 percent of premature births, when a 100 percent usage rate was expected (Krauss da Silva et al. 1999).
Systemic shortcomings	
Lack of monitoring, review, and control system	
• Lack of systematic evaluations of data on service providers in the national system of information • Absence of mandatory committees • Shortcomings in professional qualifications; lack of literature in Portuguese	In 67 percent of 1,011 facilities visited, the obligatory hospital infection prevention committee was not in place; in 35 percent of hospitals that had appointed such committees, no record of their activities was available (CREMESP 2004a). Lack of such committees in many hospitals contributes to high rates of hospital infections: 15.6 percent in Brazil, compared with between 3 and 5 percent in the United States (Santos 1996) and a global average of 8 to 10 percent (Prade et al. 1995). Translations of key medical texts tend not to use Brazilian examples (Prade 2002).
Problems with equipment	
• Lack of training on use of new and existing equipment • Absence of essential equipment in certain health facilities	Fully equipped and functioning ambulances were present in only 25 percent of private facilities and 25 percent of public facilities in São Paulo state; barely 50 percent of emergency rooms were considered appropriately equipped (CREMESP 2004a).

Shortcomings and possible causes	Supporting evidence from microstudies
Lack of a staff training system	
• Short-term contracts, low wages, and internal conflicts giving rise to absenteeism • Problems of communication and interaction between teams • Lack of continuity of administrative personnel	Barboza et al. (2003), Cecílio (1994), and others attribute suspension of and delays in carrying out surgical procedures to high absenteeism. Low nursing salaries mean that many nurses take second jobs and thus find themselves overburdened in their workload (Nakao et al. 1986; D'Innocenzo 2001).

Source: Sampaio 2004; Kisil 2003.

Notes

1. The IOM maintains that the magnitude of the problem (medical errors) is much greater than is currently acknowledged because hospital patients represent a small portion of patient contacts with the health care system.
2. Most of the findings draw on literature reviews and analyses commissioned for this paper (Sampaio 2004; Kisil 2003, 2004; Gastal et al. 2005a, 2005b). Small-scale research, reviewed by Kisil (2003), is also an important source.
3. Licensure sets the minimally acceptable operating standards for health care organizations. The standards usually focus on infrastructure, staffing, and equipment.
4. The unsatisfactory results were discussed at a meeting of the National Health Council in 2004.
5. The instrument was derived from and is very similar to the Level 1 instrument used by ONA to assess compliance with licensure regulations.
6. A self-selection bias may have affected the results. Participation in the PNASS survey was voluntary, and facilities that chose to opt out may be more likely to exhibit poor quality.
7. The PNASH survey described above was applied to psychiatric facilities in part because of a series of press reports denouncing conditions in such facilities.
8. Recent diagnostic instruments developed by the ONA and the MS specify licensure standards and their regulatory source (ONA 2005; MS 2004b). These instruments greatly facilitate the assessment of regulatory compliance by both hospitals and authorities.
9. The sample represented 95 percent of facilities in the categories registered with CREMESP.
10. Such a system was in place in 53.6 percent of the hospitals; 24.5 percent had an incomplete system.
11. Pupo (2004) found that larger facilities generally score better on assessment instruments which review their structural capacities. In contrast, smaller hospitals have numerous shortfalls in infrastructure; staffing; life-support, surgical, and sterilization equipment; postanesthesia recovery; and advanced diagnostic and therapeutic services. Smaller facilities also lack medical ethics committees.
12. All private facilities were under contract with the SUS and received a significant proportion of financing from public sources.
13. A CRESMESP survey conducted in 1997 and 1998 of a sample of 99 delivery rooms and neonatal units in São Paulo hospitals found many structural deficiencies. Many hospitals failed to comply with minimal standards for equipment and staff required by Brazilian licensure legislation (CRESMESP 2000).
14. Since the test is voluntary, the test takers are not representative of the student body of any medical school.
15. In 2006 688 students took the test; in 2007, 998 did.
16. Students from 23 of the 31 medical schools in the state participated in the exam.
17. A candidate who does not accumulate sufficient points has the option of taking a competency exam.

18. There is considerable evidence that well-formulated care processes result in better-quality care (Desai, O'Connor, and Bishop 1997; Griffin and Kinmouth 1998).
19. A few caveats are in order on the results of the literature review. Because of the dearth of studies, the variety and incomparability of methods, the use of different nomenclature, and the small size of the sample or care setting, interpretation and synthesis were difficult. The available information does not allow for concrete answers to the following questions: How generalizable are the findings to the universe of Brazilian hospitals? How frequently do the errors occur in the system as a whole? Are there systemic factors that systematically contribute to poor quality? What is the overall cost of poor quality?
20. Iatrogenia refers to medical complications induced inadvertently by a physician or surgeon or by medical treatment or diagnostic procedures.
21. The perinatal period commences at 22 completed weeks (154 days) of gestation, the time when birthweight is normally 500 grams, and ends at 7 completed days after birth.
22. In Belo Horizonte 97 percent of births take place in hospitals; this is similar to the average for Brazil.
23. Quality was measured by a structural point-based system developed by Costa et al. (2004) in which hospitals are placed in one of three categories—high, intermediate, or low.
24. The sample was drawn randomly from an universe of 40,953 births and 825 perinatal deaths and therefore is representative of Belo Horizonte. The quality of obstetric care was determined on the basis of an analysis of medical records. The authors noted that the study was limited by the poor quality and incompleteness of medical records. This is an important finding in itself.
25. A partograph, which is recommended by the WHO, depicts labor progression and helps identify when intervention is warranted.
26. Other variables found to be independently associated with perinatal mortality included lack of prenatal care, low birthweight, illnesses during pregnancy, and newborn illnesses.
27. This survey was supported by the National Agency for Sanitary Surveillance (Agência Nacional de Vigilância Sanitária, ANVISA). The survey response rates are as follows: states, 100 percent; municipalities, 18 percent; private hospitals, 70 percent.
28. All hospitals are mandated to possess an HI control program by Federal Law 9431 (1997).
29. NNISS/CDC stands for the U.S. National Nosocomial Infections Surveillance System and the Centers for Disease Control.
30. Similarly, a significant number of hospitals were found not to use materials to combat infections. When asked about the use of antimicrobials, germicides, and other materials, 53.5 percent of hospitals replied that they did use such measures, 40.8 percent said they did not, and 5.7 percent did not give an answer (Marçal dos Santos et al. 2005). Failure in so many hospitals to use appropriate measures to combat infections can give rise to increases in the number and types of such infections and to multiresistant forms, thus prolonging periods of hospitalization and increases in morbidity, mortality, and support costs.
31. International comparisons are difficult because of differences in definitions and methodology. In addition, the Marçal data refer only to ICUs. In the United States surgical infection rates range between 2 and 5 percent (Qualis Health 2006). Pennsylvania, one of the few U.S. states that systematically track hospital infections, reported 7.5 hospital-acquired infections per 1,000 admissions in 173 general acute hospitals in 2004 (PHC4 2005).
32. Hospital infection committees are mandated by MS regulations (Portaria 196, June 24, 1983).
33. In addition to the HI committee, every hospital in Brazil is required to have committees overseeing medical ethics, the control of hospital infections, the revision of medical records, and accident prevention (*comissão de ética médica, comissão de controle de infecção hospitalar, comissão de revisão de prontuário médico, comissão interna de prevenção de acidentes*).
34. These cost estimates are consistent with international data. The NNISS/CDC system estimates that surgical site infections prolong hospital stays by 7.5 days and increase costs between US$2,734 and US$26,019 per infection.
35. Eighty-nine percent of respondents reported using the SUS.

8

Quality Assessment and Improvement

The capacity of any country to measure, assess, and raise the quality of care is critical to systemwide improvement of health care delivery and patient outcomes. Facilities acting alone are often ill prepared or lack incentives to take on such complex tasks. Systematic policy and institutional support for quality and patient safety is at an early stage of development in Brazil. For the most part, quality enhancement initiatives based on proven methods have occurred infrequently, and mostly at an operational rather than national policy level.

Over the last 15 years, however, a number of voluntary and government-supported initiatives have sought to establish accreditation, benchmarking, and quality improvement programs as a means of assessing and raising the quality of hospital care. The most important of these efforts include a government-sponsored accreditation system, a certification program and benchmarking system established by a state medical society, a quality-based purchasing scheme developed by a private purchaser, and several government-led national and state programs. Though important advances, most of these initiatives are isolated, stand-alone efforts. Broad implementation by hospitals (and health care purchasers) has been limited. Some of these efforts were short-lived. None has been evaluated.

At the provider level, some hospitals have become serious about quality assessment and improvement. Most of these efforts are linked to participation in accreditation and certification programs. In some, quality enhancement is related to an effort to improve the hospital's financial standing. Although an undetermined number of facilities have developed quality enhancement initiatives in a specific service or department, less than an estimated 2 percent of Brazilian hospitals have implemented *organization-wide and continuous* quality improvement programs. Only a handful of these collect, analyze, and report data on their results.

To anticipate a major argument of this chapter: Brazil has yet to develop national quality performance policies, an assessment and reporting infrastructure, and accountability mechanisms to drive and support quality enhancement systemwide. Unless these building blocks for quality performance are developed, quality will likely remain the forgotten component of the Brazilian health system for the foreseeable future.

Hospital Accreditation and Certification in Brazil: Adoption, Challenges, and Opportunities

Brazil leads Latin America in the development of accreditation systems. A review of progress on hospital accreditation across 19 countries in Latin America found that Brazil was one of only 5 countries in the region that had not only established a national commission on accreditation and produced a manual of standards but had also begun implementing the program nationally. Indeed, Brazil was the only country in South America to have gone that far (Novaes 1999). This section reviews the development of hospital accreditation systems in Brazil. Box 8.1 defines the terminology used here.

Box 8.1
Accreditation, Licensure, and Certification

Accreditation is a formal process by which a recognized body, usually a nongovernmental organization (NGO), assesses a health care organization and verifies that it meets applicable predetermined and published standards. Accreditation standards, usually regarded as optimal and achievable, are designed to encourage continuous improvement efforts within accredited organizations. An accreditation decision about a specific health care organization is made following a periodic on-site assessment by a team of peer reviewers external to the organization or system. Accreditation is typically conducted every two to three years.

Accreditation is often a voluntary process in which organizations choose to participate, rather than one required by law and regulation, and in this sense it differs from licensure. A number of countries, however, are making accreditation mandatory.

Licensure is a process by which a governmental authority grants permission to an individual practitioner or health care organization to operate. Licensure regulations usually aim to ensure that an organization meets minimal standards to protect public health and patient safety.

Certification is a process by which an authorized body—a purchaser, or a governmental or nongovernmental organization—evaluates an organization and recognizes that it meets predetermined standards or criteria. When applied to an organization, or a part of an organization such as a laboratory, certification usually implies that the organization has additional services, technology, or capacity beyond those found in similar organizations.

Source: Rooney and van Ostenberg 1999.

Hospital accreditation in Brazil stems from voluntary initiatives launched by hospitals in the 1980s with the aim of establishing accreditation criteria that would be distinct from the licensing requirements set out by the Ministry of Health (Ministério da Saúde, MS). In 1986 the Brazilian College of Surgeons, after deliberating on the training and certification of new surgeons and the quality of hospitals, created the Special and Permanent Committee for Qualification of Hospitals (Noronha and Garcia Rosa 1999).

Around the same time, the Pan-American Health Organization (PAHO) and the World Health Organization (WHO) began work on initiatives for the establishment of health standards specifically adapted to local contexts. Impetus for such moves came from the first Latin America Conference on Hospital Accreditation, in 1989, which concluded that no country in Latin America was using hospital accreditation as a way of improving hospital quality. Major steps were subsequently taken at an accreditation seminar organized by PAHO in Brasília in 1992 (Novaes and Neuhauser 2000).

During the 1990s four Brazilian states launched independent accreditation initiatives. The São Paulo Association of Medicine and the Regional Board of Medicine introduced the Control of Hospital Quality program (Controle de Qualidade Hospitalar, CQH). In Rio Grande do Sul the private sector established a hospital accreditation program, and in Paraná the state Health Department also started a program. The Rio de Janeiro initiative involved a joint effort by the National Academy of Medicine, the Brazilian College of Surgeons, and the Institute for Social Medicine of the State University of Rio de Janeiro.

From 1995 onward, the MS sought to build on these state initiatives by fusing the separate schemes into a national accreditation system. Combining experiences from the four pioneering states, as well as from other countries, the Brazilian Program for Quality and Productivity (Programa Brasileiro da Qualidade e Produtividada, PBQP) was launched in 1997 to define specific standards for an assessment process for accrediting hospitals. *Manual Brasileiro de Acreditação Hospitalar* (Novaes 1999), published in 1998 under the PBQP, was the first set of nationwide standards for accreditation throughout Brazil.

The National Accreditation Organization

In November 1998 the MS approved a proposal for a national hospital accreditation commission, the National Accreditation Organization (Organização Nacional de Acreditação, ONA). The ONA was responsible for developing rules, norms, and procedures to accompany the standards and took the lead in creating technical norms, developing a code of ethics, training surveyors, and certifying surveyor institutions and firms. Box 8.2 describes the ONA governance structure.

The ONA takes a phased approach to accreditation. Hospitals must pass Level 1 (dealing mostly with structural aspects) before passing to Level 2 and then must pass Level 2 (focusing on processes) before passing to the third and highest level of accreditation, which targets outcomes (Zeribi and Marquez 2004). Level 2 is known as "full accreditation," while Level 1 is known simply as "accreditation." Both are valid for two years. Level 3, valid for three years, means that a hospital is "accredited with excellence." Accredited facilities must maintain standards throughout the validity period, and regular evaluations are carried out to ensure that standards are kept up. During the application process, if an institution falls short of achieving a level by a small margin, it has 90 days to rectify the problems indicated by the evaluation before a second assessment. Each level requires a separate assessment process

---

Box 8.2
Governance Arrangements in the ONA

The ONA, a private, nongovernmental organization authorized by the MS (Portaria 538, 2001), enjoys widespread institutional support. As with the development of accreditation systems in other countries, many stakeholders were involved in its founding, The ONA was the product of a collaborative process involving medical societies, trade associations, and public and private institutions.

Oversight is conducted by an independent board (*conselho de administração*) consisting of representatives of medical societies; trade associations such as private and nonprofit hospitals, medical cooperatives, and private insurers; government institutions—the MS and the National Agency for Sanitary Surveillance (Agência Nacional de Vigilância Sanitária, ANVISA); the National Council of Secretaries of Health (Conselho Nacional de Secretáríos de Saúde, CONASS); and the Council of Municipal Health Secretaries (Conselho Nacional de Secretários Municipais de Saúde, CONASEMS). More recently, the National Agency for Health Insurance (Agência Nacional de Saúde Suplementar, ANS) has joined the board of ONA, with a view to expanding the accreditation system to facilities under contract with private health insurers.

The ONA offers the most widely recognized and implemented accreditation system in Brazil. The system was built on regional accreditation initiatives, with the technical support of the Pan American Health Organization and the MS.

Source: Gastal et al. 2005b.

with distinct sets of standards (ONA 2004). The ONA does not conduct accreditation surveys itself; these are contracted out to private organizations trained and certified by the ONA.[1]

In addition to its organization, another feature that distinguishes the ONA from other accreditation systems applied in Brazil is its emphasis on compliance with licensure regulations. Recognizing that most Brazilian hospitals are out of compliance, Level 1 focuses on attaining full compliance with the minimal standards called for in the regulations. Thus, Level 1 accreditation can better be described as licensure. A recently published self-assessment instrument ties each Level 1 standard to the supporting regulations (ONA 2005).

From Level 2 upward, ONA standards focus on processes and results. They are consonant with international standards and are designed to enable comparisons between sites and over time. As with accreditation systems elsewhere, the standards provide a picture of the overall quality of the entire organization. During an evaluation, a single hospital department or service is assessed not in isolation but as part of the overall institution. A hospital can thus receive accreditation only after each unit has passed the assessment. The ultimate goal is to improve the quality of care for all patients. An example of the requirements of one such component, obstetrics, is provided in annex 8A.

Other Accreditation Systems

In addition to the ONA system, two other accreditation systems are active in Brazil: the Rio de Janeiro–based initiative known as the Brazilian Accreditation Consortium (Consórcio Brasileiro de Acreditação, CBA), and the Sao Paulo–based CQH. Both drew on the standards developed by the internationally recognized Joint Commission on Accreditation of Healthcare Organizations (JCAHO), as had the ONA system. Unlike the ONA, neither is officially affiliated with government. A brief description of the two systems follows.

- *CBA.* The CBA was formed in 1998, with assistance from the JCAHO, on the basis of earlier accreditation programs developed by four hospitals.[2] The National Academy of Medicine, the Brazilian College of Surgeons, and the State University of Rio de Janeiro, joined by the Cesgranrio Foundation, together drew up a set of standards based on JCAHO standards for hospitals. The resulting manual, completed in 1999, has been used to evaluate hospitals, principally in the state of Rio de Janeiro.

- *CQH.* The CQH Seal of Quality Program was launched in 1991 in São Paulo state to monitor and control hospital infections across member institutions in the state through regular visits by external evaluation teams. The CQH is a joint initiative of the Medical Association of São Paulo (APM) and the Regional Medical Council of São Paulo State (Conselho Regional de Medicina do Estado de São Paulo, CREMESP). The CQH is the oldest existing quality assessment system in Brazil that exhibits a classic framework of structure, process, and results. As with accreditation under all systems in Brazil, a hospital applies voluntarily to the CQH program and is visited by a team of independent evaluators that assesses the extent to which the institution meets the quality processes and standards specified in the CQH manual. Full compliance with these leads to the award of a Seal of Quality (Selo de Conformidade).

Each of the three accreditation systems described above draws on international standards, particularly those of the JCAHO model. All specify similar standards, particularly for processes and results. As is typical of accreditation programs worldwide, adoption is voluntary. The assessment processes themselves are rigorous, are directed to the entire organization, and are performed by multidisciplinary but independent teams of trained professionals. Of the three systems, the ONA standards are arguably the most closely tailored to Brazilian reality, inviting progression, in three stages, from compliance with the minimal standards to the highest standard of excellence. All three systems are robust; table 8.1 summarizes their main distinguishing features. Unlike the ONA, in which accreditation is government endorsed, or the CBA, in which accreditation is carried out with the participation of international surveyors and is internationally recognized, the CQH Seal of Approval program is locally authorized and is applied mostly in São Paulo state. Thus, the CQH can best be described as an independent certification system.

Although Brazil offers a range of accreditation and certification systems, uptake has been disappointingly meager. As table 8.2 shows, only 55 of the more than 6,500 hospitals in the country were accredited in 2003. Most of the 38 that applied under the ONA qualified at Level 1; 3 received CBA accreditation and 14, CQH accreditation.

Most accredited hospitals are medium-size (fewer than 100 beds) specialized institutions located in the South or Southeast. Of the 55 accredited hospitals, 38 are located in São Paulo state, and only 2 have fewer than 50 beds. Accredited hospitals are likely to be private institutions: 44 of the 55 are private, 9 are public, and 2 are military hospitals. In sum,

TABLE 8.1
Comparison of the Three Main Hospital Accreditation Systems

Accreditation system	ONA	CQH	CBA
Composition	National-level bodies representing public and private sectors, purchasers, and medical societies	São Paulo Medical Association and Regional Medical Council of São Paulo State	National Academy of Medicine, Brazilian College of Surgeons, University of Rio de Janeiro State, and the Cesgranrio Foundation
Basis of standards	PAHO/WHO/JCAHO	JCAHO	JCAHO
Assessment team	Evaluators from independent certified assessment institutions	Independent CQH inspectors	External inspectors from CBA and Joint Commission International (JCI)
Focus	Structure (health safety), process, and results	Process and results	Process, functions, and results
Validity of certification	Level 1, two years Level 2, two years Level 3, three years	Seal of Quality, two years	Accreditation of institution, two years
Follow up	Scheduled and unscheduled visits and follow-up through one-off sentinel visits[a]	Follow-up visits and reporting of postcertification indicators	Follow-up and sentinel visits[a]

Source: Schiesari 2003.

a. A sentinel visit is a response to an unexpected event involving death or serious physical or psychological injury or the risk thereof. Serious injury specifically includes loss of limb or function. A sentinel event signals the need for immediate investigation and response (JCAHO).

TABLE 8.2
Number of Accredited Hospitals, by Type and Location, 2003

Indicator	Total	ONA	CBA	CQH
Total	55	38	3	14
By type				
Public	10	7	0	3
Private	44	30	3	11
Military	1	1	0	0
By region				
North	0	0	0	0
Northeast	3	3	0	0
Central-West	3	2	0	1
South	8	7	1	0
Southeast	41	26	2	13
By state				
São Paulo	38	23	1	13
Minas Gerais	3	3	0	0
Rio Grande de Sul	6	5	1	1
Other	8	7	1	0

Source: Gastal et al. 2005b.

accreditation is not affecting critical parts of the hospital sector—small hospitals, with fewer than 50 beds, which account for nearly two-thirds (65 percent) of the country's hospitals, and public hospitals, which represent more than a third.

Hospitals appear to have few incentives to complete the requirements for accreditation. Accreditation is not yet on the policy agenda of the Unified Health System (Sistema Único de Saúde, SUS), despite MS support for the founding of the ONA, nor is accreditation a key consideration among private purchasers.[3] There appears to be considerable interest in participating in the CQH Seal of Quality program; institutions contracted by CQH to perform inspections have made 142 separate certification visits. Since the initiation of the CQH in the early 1990s, more than 100 hospitals have participated in its programs, many for more than 10 years. Yet over this period, only 23 have been awarded the seal. Of these, 14 still had the seal in 2004, and 9 did not. The CQH has not explored the reasons for this apparent difficulty in achieving certification, or why some health facilities that had received the seal lost their certification.

One concern voiced by both public authorities and managers of public and private facilities is about the costs involved in meeting accreditation and licensure requirements, especially investments in plant and equipment. A review of investments made to attain accreditation suggests, however, that costs may not be a major barrier. Gastal et al. (2005b) surveyed 18 hospitals that had achieved ONA Level 1 (licensure) between 2002 and 2004 regarding the costs of investments.[4] Hospitals reported making an array of investments in personnel, consultancies, staff training, information systems, infrastructural investments, equipment, furniture, and assessment costs.[5] The average and maximum amounts spent, by category, are shown in table 8.3. Of the 18 hospitals, 88 percent had invested in infrastructure, highlighting the weakness of this particular area. About 44 percent had invested in technical assistance, for an average R$32,800, including the cost of assessment.

TABLE 8.3
Costs and Investments Involved in Achieving ONA Level 1, 2002–4
(R$ thousands, 2004; N = 18)

Cost type	Average	Maximum
Infrastructure	98.4	300.0
Medical equipment	91.2	400.0
Information systems	62.7	638.0
Personnel	49.5	620.0
Furniture	23.9	150.0
Other equipment	20.1	100.0
Certification	18.6	50.0
Consultancies (technical assistance)	14.2	86.0
Other	13.7	67.3
Training	12.2	100.0
Average	293.8	1,750.2

Source: Gastal et al. 2005b.
Note: US$1 = R$2.98 (2002–4 average).

The average investment of nearly R$300,000 (US$100,000) reported in the survey represents less than 1 percent of the annual budget of the medium-size public hospitals analyzed in chapter 6. Even the average maximum payment of R$1.8 million represents only about 5 percent of spending in these facilities.[6] In comparison, between 1998 and 2004 the government's REFORSUS investment project, cofinanced by the World Bank and the Inter-American Development Bank, invested US$410 million in about 1,000 hospitals, mainly for equipment and works.[7] Those investments were not linked to securing accreditation or even to participating in accreditation programs.

Other research corroborates that cost may not be an important barrier to expansion of accreditation. An international literature review on implementation of accreditation systems found that only 1 of the 10 documents reviewed mentioned financial cost as a reason for failure or unwillingness to carry out the program (Neto 2004). Major obstacles reported included lack of interest by management, refusal by staff to participate, and difficulties in changing organizational culture or practices, often resulting in internal conflicts.

Additional factors may contribute to the difficulties in expanding accreditation. First, the existence of multiple accreditation systems may create confusion among hospital managers about which is the "best" choice. Anecdotal evidence suggests some unnecessary rivalry among the three systems. Any accreditation program requires a critical mass of participants, which helps motivate other organizations to take part. A unified national program, ideally supported by the MS with broader hospital participation, would put pressure on nonparticipants.

A second challenge for Brazilian accreditation systems is keeping up with the changes arising from an ever-shifting political landscape. A new MS team may view the last initiative as the work of the outgoing administration and therefore seek changes or a new system altogether. For example, in 2004 the MS broke its agreement with the ONA for reasons that were not entirely clear. Some observers suggest that the ONA fell out of favor because it was the creation of a previous government and therefore unwelcome. Others speculate that the government backpedaled on the expansion of accreditation to avoid political fallout from assessments that might reveal the dismal conditions in most public and SUS-financed private hospitals. In recent years the MS has done little to promote accreditation of any kind.

The third and perhaps most important question about accreditation programs is one of incentives. As in many other countries, accreditation in Brazil is voluntary.[8] Participation depends on leadership by facility management or governance bodies. Lack of incentives to seek accreditation remains the major obstacle to further expansion. There are three kinds of incentives that could be emphasized to make accreditation attractive: economic incentives, in the sense that public and private purchasers (the SUS, insurers, prepayment plans) can require that hospitals with which they have contractual relationships be accredited in order to ensure good quality standards; the use of accreditation as a marketing tool to attract more business; and efficiency incentives, since good quality can result in cost savings.[9] Many private, and often prestigious, facilities accredited by the CBA use accreditation for marketing purposes. These facilities, however, appear genuinely interested in providing high-quality care; they were the first in Brazil to develop and implement quality improvement programs throughout their organizations.[10]

Experiences from other countries suggest that making accreditation a requirement for financing, or providing hospitals with financial incentives to attain accreditation status, can be a robust driver for adoption. In the United States public payers such as Medicare and Medicaid require that hospitals be accredited if they are to receive any funding. Accreditation is also required for public and social insurance funding in Belgium and in Catalonia, Spain.

A recent and innovative program to link accreditation to payment, now under way in Brazil, presents a model for others to follow. UNIMED/BH is a private medical cooperative in Belo Horizonte (BH) that operates a prepayment plan and contracts 40 hospitals to provide services to its members. In 2005 UNIMED/BH launched a program offering proportional reimbursement for hospitals that attain each level of ONA accreditation.[11] For example, reimbursement rates are increased 7 percent if the facility signs an agreement to participate in the ONA process (e.g., conducts a self-assessment, undergoes an external assessment, and adopts a time-bound action plan to attain Level 1 accreditation). Reimbursement increases by another 7 percent for Level 1 accreditation and by an additional 9 and 15 percent, respectively, for Levels 2 and 3. According to UNIMED, the aim is for all 40 hospitals contracted by UNIMED in or near Belo Horizonte to reach Level 3 accreditation over a three-year period (2005–8). Importantly, UNIMED also finances the cost of assessment and cofinances training required to upgrade the skills of professional staff. Facilities that do not reach at least Level 1 accreditation after two years will be dropped from the UNIMED network. If successful, these measures by a single purchaser will nearly double the number of accredited hospitals in Brazil.

Accreditation and Performance

What are the benefits of accreditation, and how are these benefits attained? Accreditation alone does not guarantee good quality: it is one tool in an overall system for measuring, assessing, and improving quality. It evaluates an institution's organizational structures, processes, and performance in relation to established standards.

Worldwide, accreditation systems are increasingly linked to the development of systems and programs to improve care at the hospital level in a continuous process (Scrivens 1997b). For example, in the 1990s the JCAHO modified its standards to take a more systemic approach based on continuous quality improvement. Donahue and van Ostenberg (2000: 244) comment concerning the revisions, "the focus of accreditation standards is on the internal capacity of an organization to create and sustain systems and processes needed to evaluate and monitor the competence of its health professional staff."

Accreditation forces hospitals to examine their competencies, assessing and comparing the care they provide against the standards (Scrivens 1997a, 1997b; WHO 2003a; Shaw 2004a, 2004b; Dlugacz, Restifo, and Greenwood 2004; Daucourt and Michel 2003). This is achieved through an initial diagnostic, usually a self-assessment, and then through the application of management methodologies to guide the improvement process. Thus, participation in an accreditation program usually requires a hospital to develop a quality improvement program and implement it internally. In a sense, compliance with the standards becomes the driver for a quality improvement process throughout the organization.

An array of quality management tools can be used to facilitate change, and a number of leading hospitals in Brazil have achieved and maintained quality improvement programs using one or more of these tools. The Gastal et al. (2005b) survey of accredited hospitals asked managers to evaluate the management tools they used to improve quality. Their responses are synthesized in table 8.4. The most popular processes or tools applied in the sampled hospitals include PDCA, 5W2H, total quality management (TQM), and 5S. Most of the tools identified in the survey have been borrowed from the manufacturing, engineering, and service industries and adapted by hospitals worldwide to organize and guide their quality improvement efforts (Neto and Bittar 2004).

The findings show that many of the hospitals surveyed measure client satisfaction, act on their findings (35 hospitals of 37), and implement a program to standardize care processes and patient flows throughout the organization (33 of 37). The ONA standards serve as guidelines for internal standardization. How client satisfaction is measured and improved and how standardization is achieved can vary across facilities. In most cases assessment of client satisfaction and process standardization were not stand-alone activities but were part of a broad, organizationwide quality management process.

Schiesari (2003), reviewing quality improvement programs in five Brazilian hospitals during the accreditation process, found similar results to those reported in table 8.4. Significantly, she reported that the sample facilities formed working groups to address an array of concerns, including training, auditing, implementation of standards, reduction of adverse events, measurement of client satisfaction, and development of performance indicators.

The successful implementation of such programs relies on the buy-in of senior management, the structuring of staff incentives, and continual training. The study by Kisil (2004), who interviewed directors of five leading hospitals, supported many of the findings from the surveys reported above. Kisil identified various areas of best practice, including the formation of a team trained in quality improvement programs to guide the process; regular collection of data relating to sentinel indicators and storage of this information in a database that allows for analysis and production of reports; identification of stakeholders who are encouraged to participate in the process and in dissemination of information about quality; education of all staff about the need for quality; establishment of practical, real targets

TABLE 8.4
Hospital Management Tools Used to Gain Accreditation, with Effectiveness Ratings, 2002–4

Management tool[a]	Number of hospitals using the tool (N = 37)	Effectiveness rating (average), on a scale of 1 to 5	Description
Measurement of client satisfaction	35	4.7	An assessment, usually a survey, employed to measure client satisfaction, reduce the incidence of complaints, and improve planning.
Process standardization	33	4.6	Applied within the organization to guarantee that all methods and procedures are carried out in the same way; permits critical analysis of these methods with the aim of improving them.
PDCA	27	4.3	Management method used to promote ongoing improvements through four phases, from which PDCA takes its name: planning, doing, checking, and acting. A continuous and cyclical methodology, it aims to consolidate standardization of practices.
5W2H	24	4.3	Used to map and standardize processes, to put together action plans, and to establish procedures based on indicators. The abbreviation refers to the five Ws (who, what, when, where, and why) and the two Hs (how and how much).
Total quality management (TQM)	20	4.3	Introduced to Brazil from Japan by industrial organizations. Not a tool in itself, but a series of practical management methods; used to draw on knowledge and practices that are essential to the organization. Principal focus is on the management of processes.
5S	20	4.0	Mobilization of staff, incorporating new working practices and attitudes aimed at reducing waste. The five Ss are derived from the Japanese terms for discard, arrange, clean, standardize, and discipline.
Balanced scorecard (BSC)	20	3.7	Allows an organization to analyze strategies and plans on the basis of a system of indicators that affect performance, in line with the current and future vision of the organization. Strategies and objectives are broken down into five subsections: finance, client and market, process, learning and growth, and society.
ISO 9000	16	3.4	A standards-based assessment process that aims to ensure compliance with quality norms in all phases of the production cycle of a good or service. The standards, set by the International Organization for Standardization (ISO), emphasize an organization's quality processes and capabilities, especially the maintenance of a quality management system. ISO 9000 is mainly used in the Brazilian health sector for certifying laboratories and diagnostic units. Certification is by an independent body.

(continued)

TABLE 8.4 *(continued)*

Management tool[a]	Number of hospitals using the tool (N = 37)	Effectiveness rating (average), on a scale of 1 to 5	Description
National Prize for Quality (Premio Nacional de Qualidad, PNQ)	15	2.8	A standards-based assessment process that focuses on management processes rather than results. Derived from the Malcolm Baldridge National Quality Award in the United States, the PNQ is based on specific criteria or standards of innovation and excellence in quality management. Originally designed for service industries, PNQ has been applied to the health sector. One hospital has won this prestigious award.

Source: Gastal et al. 2005b.

Note: Managers responsible for quality improvements were asked to identify and rate their management tools for improving quality using a Likert scale of 1 to 5, where 1 means not at all effective and 5 means very effective. Responses were received from 37 ONA-accredited hospitals.

a. Tools applied by at least 40 percent of ONA-accredited hospitals that provided information.

for improvements over time that serve to demonstrate progress; and management of quality processes involving three interrelated activities—planning of quality, control of quality, and improvements in quality.

Experience from accreditation programs in developed and developing countries shows that well-designed accreditation systems contribute to improved quality of health services. Although few accreditation programs have been evaluated with the use of rigorous methodologies, accredited facilities more often comply with standards than do unaccredited facilities (Shaw 2004a). Accreditation and the quality enhancement programs employed to achieve it can lead to improved health care quality. Compliance with standards is related to improved care processes associated with outcomes such as reductions in hospital infection rates, medical errors, and adverse events (Heerey and Necochea 2005; Scrivens 2002; Shaw 2004a, 2004b). This is particularly true when the accreditation scheme is integrated into an overall quality measurement and improvement program (WHO 2003a). In addition, the processes of training personnel, adapting systems, and developing indicators can in themselves improve hospital quality, irrespective of whether accreditation is sought or achieved.

In Brazil evidence is emerging that accredited or externally certified hospitals surpass unaccredited facilities in quality and efficiency. In 2005 the CQH conducted a comparative analysis of hospitals that participated in the Seal of Quality Program between 1999 and 2003.[12] The findings are presented in table 8.5. For nearly all efficiency and quality indicators selected for the study, certified facilities significantly outperformed their uncertified counterparts. The differences in efficiency are noteworthy: certified hospitals had significantly lower lengths of stay (LOSs) and higher occupancy rates than uncertified facilities. Absenteeism, personnel turnover, and hospital infection rates, however, were not much different.

In sum, the available evidence suggests that successful adoption of facility accreditation or standards-based certification programs such as the CQH is associated with significantly greater efficiency and quality.

TABLE 8.5
Efficiency and Quality in Hospitals with and without the CQH Seal of Quality, Selected Indicators, 1999–2003

Indicators showing significantly better performance by facilities with CQH seal	With seal	Without seal	p
Efficiency			
Average length of stay[a]	3.5	4.1	0.000
Bed turnover interval[b]	1.6	2.4	0.000
Bed occupancy rate[c]	68.7	63.0	0.000
Bed turnover rate[d]	6.2	5.5	0.000
Surgical cancellation rate[e]	2.5	5.4	0.000
Quality			
Institutional mortality[f]	1.46	2.74	0.000
Surgery mortality rate[g]	0.26	0.93	0.000
Readmission rate[h]	1.4	2.1	0.011
ICU readmission rate (during patient stay)[i]	5.8	10.9	0.008
Hospital infection (HI) rate, neonatal ICU[j]	21.3	26.5	0.006
HI rate, maternity[k]	2.0	1.1	0.000

Indicators showing no significant performance between groups of facilities			
Efficiency			
Absenteeism rate[l]	4.6	4.0	0.382
Personnel turnover rate[m]	2.4	5.8	0.442
Quality			
HI rate[n]	2.5	2.6	0.298
HI rate, surgery[o]	1.4	2.3	0.145

Source: Nishikuni and Minuci 2006.
Note: Based on annual statistical reporting to the CQH by an average of 146 hospitals during the five-year period; of these, 13 (on average) possessed the Seal of Quality and 133 did not. ICU, intensive care unit.
a. Average number of days that inpatients (exclusive of newborns) remained in the hospital.
b. Average number of days that an available bed remained empty between the discharge of one inpatient and the admission of the next.
c. Percentage of total inpatient beds occupied over a given period.
d. Mean number of patients "passing through" each bed during a period (indicates the use made of available beds).
e. Number of surgical cancellations as a percentage of total surgeries over a given period.
f. Deaths after 48 hours of internment as a percentage of total inpatient discharges.
g. Deaths as a percentage of total surgical interventions.
h. Readmissions as a percentage of inpatient discharges.
i. Readmissions as a percentage of ICU discharges.
j. Episodes as a percentage of ICU discharges.
k. Episodes as a percentage of obstetric discharges.
l. Absent staff-hours as a percentage of total contracted staff-hours.
m. Number of separated workers as a percentage of total contracted workers.
n. Episodes as a percentage of inpatient discharges.
o. Episodes as a percentage of surgical discharges.

Case Study: Quality Turnaround at Santa Casa Hospital

Only a few Brazilian hospitals run effective quality improvement programs, with measurable before-and-after results. The Santa Casa Hospital in Rio Grande de Sul state is one of them. The case study, based on on-site interviews and documents, examines internal processes related to institution-wide organizational change that was carried out so successfully as to win the National Quality Prize.

Santa Casa de Porto Alegre (SCPA) is a nonprofit, philanthropic institution with six hospitals (1,349 beds) handling 5,000 inpatient stays and 75,000 outpatient visits annually. SUS-financed patients make up 86 percent of the SCPA clientele. Most of the other patients are privately insured. In addition to providing medical services, SCPA is a research and education center that offers undergraduate and graduate programs in medicine and nursing. The organizational structure consists of a governance board, board director, and executive director.

SCPA almost closed in the 1970s and 1980s, saddled with dilapidated infrastructure, high costs, low investment, weak management, lax maintenance, and persistent stock-outs—the same problems confronting many nonprofit (and public) hospitals today. In 1983 a professional management team was hired to reorganize the complex. The reorganization was phased in on a 20-year schedule. During 1983–87 changes in the board of directors and senior management and upgrades of basic infrastructure brought financial recovery, improved the hospital's credibility among suppliers, and won recognition for SCPA as a teaching hospital. The plan for 1988–92 entailed modernization and redefinition of the organizational structure, implementation of a strategic planning process, increased emphasis on productivity, new investment policies, transparency of information policy, and improved use of information technologies. By 1993 the hospital culture was ready to pursue a quality improvement agenda that would raise hospital performance from "adequate" to "excellent."

The 1993–2003 schedule began with the roll-out of a Quality Management Program (Programa de Gestão da Qualidade, PGQ), with financial support from private philanthropic foundations and the state of Rio Grande do Sul. The main actions under the four-stage PGQ were as follows:

- *Stage 1: Mobilize the management team for quality control.* Establish a quality board, a quality unit, and problem-solving groups (PSGs) to fulfill strategic and executive functions within the program. The PSGs initially focused on infrastructural problems and used the method of identification, analysis, and solution of problems. Now the PSGs monitor processes to improve quality, products, and services.
- *Stage 2: Develop human resources through education and training.* The education component included internal and external seminars, conferences on quality control with other companies, and visits to companies that used the 5S tool (see table 8.4) and were benchmarks for quality.
- *Stage 3: Plan for the quality management program.* This exercise, conducted by the quality board, addressed management, operational support, medical infrastructure, and clinical production. At this stage, the hospital joined the state Quality Management Program.
- *Stage 4: Implement quality management.* This work entailed consolidation of the 5S program and execution of the routine and results-oriented management program. Nineteen quality assessment areas are now regularly monitored, and a quality prize is awarded bimonthly to the highest achievers.

In 2002 SCPA became the first hospital to win the prestigious National Prize for Quality (PNQ), which recognizes achievements in quality management. Some difficulties remain, but Santa Casa is now considered a center of excellence, especially for maternal and neonatal medicine and for pioneering work in organ transplants. What is interesting about the SCPA experience is that before implementing the Quality Management Program, the facility had undergone 10 years of organizational and managerial reforms (and infrastructure upgrading) to create an enabling institutional environment for continuous improvement of quality and performance.

Implementation of the quality management program at Santa Casa Hospital was not without its challenges. Difficulties arose because Santa Casa was breaking new ground in modernizing organizational arrangements and management structure and introducing systematic quality improvement. There were few examples to follow, and information on standards, processes, and benchmarks was sparse. Santa Casa's nearly complete dependence on limited, and sometimes unreliable, government funding was another factor that contributed to slowing the process.

Nonetheless, today Santa Casa is a success story. The hospital has a solid information system for measuring and analyzing results. Data are systematically collected for an array of indicators and are used to monitor, assess, and improve financial performance, quality, production, and efficiency. Client satisfaction, monitored through regular patient surveys, has soared, from 18 percent in 2001 before the PGQ to 94 percent in 2004 (table 8.6). Other noteworthy before-and-after results shown in the table are reductions in surgery cancellations and in mortality. Worker dissatisfaction, as reflected in turnover, has increased slightly, but absenteeism is down slightly.

Nonquantitative indicators also highlighted improvements in other areas. One of the recommendations before the implementation of the quality management program was to provide a more patient-friendly service. Current practices point to improvements in this area, including increases in the number of blood donors. According to SCPA managers, waiting time for emergency consultations has decreased from 13 hours to 8 minutes.

TABLE 8.6
PGQ Results at Santa Casa Hospital

(percent)

Indicator	Before PGQ, 2001	With PGQ, 2004
Patient satisfaction	18.0[a]	94.0[b]
Coworker satisfaction	87.7	81.3
Surgery cancellation	18.2[c]	10.6
Absenteeism	2.0	1.9
Staff turnover	1.3	1.7
Mortality	4.2	3.6

Source: Internal hospital documents.
a. 1998. b. 2003. c. 1999.

Other Quality Assessment and Improvement Initiatives

Elsewhere in Brazil, and around the world, other types of performance monitoring and benchmarking systems are being implemented, and governments are sponsoring various national quality improvement programs.

Performance Monitoring and Benchmarking

Routine collection of data on clinical indicators with the object of monitoring and comparing processes and results over time is another principal element of an effective quality assessment and improvement system. Data collection is often complementary to standards-based accreditation, providing information on quality outcomes on a regular basis, while accreditation provides information from site surveys at two- or three-year intervals.[13]

Systematic collection and analysis of data on quality have yet to take hold in most Brazilian hospitals. Policies and systems oriented toward measurement and evaluation of quality, review and comparison of quality performance, and public disclosure are lacking. Furthermore, there is no national institutional infrastructure for developing and implementing such policies, if they did exist. But in this, Brazil is not unique.

A review of quality enhancement programs in hospitals in Australia, the United Kingdom, and the United States concluded that there was "a paucity of reliable and valid clinical data and limitations in the quality and usability of available administrative data sets" (McLoughlin et al. 2001: 461). The study pointed to a lack of consensus on how data should be gathered, which also holds in the Brazilian context.

Benchmarking involves comparing hospitals against performance measures (box 8.3). Sometimes hospitals find performance measures from another, similar hospital more compelling than standards because meeting them appears feasible and the hospitals are motivated to "beat" their peers. Two recent monitoring and benchmarking initiatives provide hospitals with a comparative tool for measuring quality. The first was launched in the 1990s by the CQH. The second is a very recent effort under the auspices of the ONA.

CQH Benchmarking System

The CQH operates a benchmarking system for hospitals registered in the Seal of Quality program. In 2002 this system consisted of 29 indicators, including efficiency, production, absenteeism, mortality, and infection rates (CQH 2003).[14] A subset of the indicators, published quarterly, can be used as benchmarks for participating and nonparticipating hospitals. The extent to which these indicators are used for comparison and quality improvement purposes is unknown. In a review of the CQH database, only about two-thirds of participating hospitals, including all those awarded the Seal of Quality, regularly provided the full dataset. Additional limitations include the lack of stratification of hospitals by size, location, ownership, and complexity, making it harder to make meaningful comparisons.[15]

ONA Training Program on Quality-Performance Indicators

Following up on a series of workshops with accreditation surveyor organizations and hospital representatives held in 2005, the ONA produced an Internet-based course and manual to

---

Box 8.3
Benchmarking

Benchmarking is based on the idea that learning from the experience of others is the most effective way to improve service quality. It is intended to enable comparisons between different organizations on specific references, processes, practices, or performance measures. Comparison of an institution with the best in the industry can motivate it to match or exceed the leader's record. References might include client satisfaction, outcomes, and staff motivation. Higgins (1997: 61) defines benchmarking as

> a continuous systematic process for evaluating products, services and work practices of organizations that are recognized as representing best practice for the purpose of organizational improvement. The benchmarking focus may be internal, external or functional, comparing performance to a particular function or process with the best performance regardless of the industry.

Implementation of a benchmarking program involves both operationalizing a system and managing it. Operationalization consists of three steps: defining the benchmarks, deciding who or what will serve as the reference body or organization against which comparisons will be made, and finding and gathering relevant data. Management includes doing what needs to be done (e.g., training) to ensure that the benchmarking process is carried out effectively.

Mello and Camargo (1998) distinguish four types of benchmarking: *internal,* involving comparisons between similar procedures within an organization; *competitive,* involving comparison with the best direct competitor; *functional,* involving comparison of the same procedures or functions in different sectors between organizations that carry out similar processes; and *generic,* involving comparison of working processes with other organizations that have innovative working methods. They cite the example of a U.S. hospital in which benchmarking with another institution resulted in a 30 percent reduction of operating costs. The same hospital carried out an internal benchmarking process that discovered big differences in lengths of stay for patients admitted for the same procedures (hernia repair), but with different surgeons. Doctor 2's patients stayed in the hospital an average of four days longer than Doctor 1's and cost an average of $4,794 more to treat.

---

guide health professionals and hospital managers in developing, implementing, and tracking performance indicators for their institutions (ONA 2006). This modest effort responds to the failure to define and apply performance indicators in the Brazilian health sector. Whether the initiative will result in a systematic and nationwide benchmarking program remains to be seen; that depends on the emergence of strong motivation for the expansion of accreditation and of systematic data collection in general.

MS Quality Improvement Efforts

Over the years, the MS has launched several innovative programs to improve the quality of SUS-financed services. Many of these programs have been short-lived. They have usually been linked to the political cycle, and none has been evaluated. Of equal concern is the lack of a national quality improvement policy and strategy. Despite mounting evidence of quality shortfalls, the national health authorities are making no coherent and sustained effort to address quality concerns. The following are brief descriptions of recent MS programs, some terminated and others ongoing, that attempt to assess and improve quality.

Collaborative Centers Program

In mid-2000 the MS launched an innovative hospital mentor program, Programa de Centros Colaboradores, that paired high-quality hospitals with facilities seeking to improve quality. The mentors were known as collaborative centers (CCs); the recipients, as client hospitals (HCs). The CCs were responsible for providing the HCs with training and technical assistance in 10 managerial and clinical areas.[16] Through on-site inspections, the MS selected 30 CCs—large hospitals (with more than 250 beds), located mostly in the South and Southeast regions. The HCs were chosen on criteria such as size (more than 100 beds), importance in the regional network, and quality improvement needs. Sixty HCs were selected, located mostly in the North and Northeast regions. The program was discontinued in 2003, and no attempt was made to evaluate it. Staff members from participating hospitals suggest that several problems led to the program's demise: insufficient funding, lack of knowledge of and experience with quality assessment and standards, and inability of HC professional staff to spend sufficient time at CCs to understand institutional contexts and provide continuous support.

Program to Humanize Hospital Care

The Programa Nacional de Humanização de Assistência Hospitalar (PNHAH), launched in 2001, sought to introduce more patient-friendly care in SUS-financed hospitals by monitoring and improving client satisfaction with services. The program also supported training to improve professional-patient interaction in hospital settings. Initially, 94 hospitals participated in the PNHAH, and client satisfaction surveys were carried out in each. The ultimate goal was for each hospital to earn an MS "humane hospital" award. The program, as originally conceived, appears to have been discontinued. Research for this volume uncovered no information about its results or its impact in the 94 participating hospitals.

In 2003 the MS launched a national policy, HumanizaSUS, that includes elements of the PNHAH but is much broader in scope (MS 2004c). HumanizaSUS is directed to all SUS-financed services. The policy aims to reduce waiting lines, allow all patients to know the professional responsible for their care, guarantee that all patients are provided with information about their conditions, and promote health worker participation in management and training decisions. Information on program results is unavailable.

National Hospital Services Assessment Program

In 1998 the MS launched the Programa Nacional de Avaliação dos Serviços Hospitalares (PNASH) to assess, rate, and compare hospitals according to a set of mostly structural standards. The standards and corresponding instruments were prepared by the MS, and MS inspectors conducted the survey. As reported in chapter 7, the PNASH was implemented only in psychiatric facilities (but resulted in the closure of 29 facilities). The program was discontinued in 2003 and was redesigned in 2004, as described next.

National Health Service Assessment Program

The Programa Nacional de Avaliação de Serviços de Saúde (PNASS) was the result of a redesign of the PNASH. It is a quality assessment and monitoring system with several interconnected parts (MS 2004b). The first consists of an assessment of mainly structural characteristics, based on standards specified in government facility licensure regulations and norms and similar to the ONA Level 1 standards. As in the PNASH (described in more detail in chapter 7), facilities are scored on a 100-point weighted scale and are grouped into five categories: superior, good, fair, unacceptable, and highly unacceptable. The assessment is a two-step process: a self-assessment and, following that, an inspection conducted by local SUS authorities. The second and third dimensions of the PNASS consist of client and worker satisfaction surveys of random samples of respondents. The final dimension involves the analysis and comparison of a subset of efficiency and quality indicators culled from available databases—those of the Authorization for Hospitalization (Autorização de Internação Hospitalar, AIH) and the MS Health Facility Registry (Cadastro Nacional de Estabelecimentos de Saúde, CNES).[17] According to the MS, the PNASS will be applied twice a year to all SUS-financed facilities providing specialty services, and the results are to be made available to state and municipal authorities. The results of the first survey, conducted in 2005, were reported in chapter 7.

The PNASS represents an important step in establishing systematic assessment of facilities, if it is carried out twice a year, as intended. Unlike the "external control" and "compliance" orientation of the PNASH, the PNASS is oriented toward creating an assessment culture at the municipal and state levels, which in the SUS are responsible for licensure, oversight, and monitoring of service provision. Whether this culture will be attained is difficult to determine so early in implementation. Several potential shortcomings in its implementation are evident. First, local government authorities are responsible for inspection. Because the PNASS focuses on SUS-financed units, the inspectors are not independent parties, engendering a conflict of interest that is likely to bias assessment. Second, there are no incentives—financial, regulatory, or other—for facility managers to raise standards, increase client satisfaction, or improve indicators. Again, it is up to local authorities to decide if, how, and when to act on the survey results. Unlike the PNASH, in which the MS used the results to close facilities where conditions were unacceptable, the PNASS does not make any attempt to sanction facilities that are out of compliance with the law (e.g., with licensure legislation). Third, there are no plans for public dissemination of the facility-based data, which reduces pressure to improve performance through public accountability.

Letter Writing and the National Hotline Programs

Since 2002 the MS has operated two consumer feedback mechanisms to gauge patient satisfaction with SUS facilities. CartaSUS elicits and processes letters from patients treated at SUS facilities, and Disque Saúde, is a toll-free consumer hotline for registering grievances. The MS Office of the Ombudsman is responsible for both programs. In 2002 and 2003 CartaSUS received more than 470,000 letters and forwarded them to state and municipal health secretariats. According to the MS review of 8,685 grievances mentioned in letters received in 2002, 3,202 cases (37 percent) were not responded to in a timely matter, and an additional 1,793 (21 percent) were considered "inconclusive" in terms of corrective actions taken. Through Disque Saúde, the MS received 1.3 million phone calls in 2003. Grievances are channeled to state and municipal authorities and are not made public; follow-up is unknown.

Both programs have potential to be effective systems for cataloging and analyzing consumer feedback. However, information is not systematically compiled for analysis. Worse, little or no attempt is made to follow up on responses or on corrective actions taken by local authorities. Anecdotal evidence suggests that the Office of the Ombudsman does little more than channel complaints and grievances to local authorities.

Care Coordination Across Provider Levels

Individual health facilities may adopt quality measures, but the effectiveness of the overall system does not depend solely on accreditation, benchmarking, or legislation applicable to individual hospitals. Of equal importance is the ability of hospitals to work with other providers that offer complementary care. These include primary care centers, ambulatory specialty centers, diagnostic services, emergency response units, and home care services (Shortell et al. 2000a, 2000b). Clinical coordination through the formation of networks or formal relationships among clinical settings helps improve efficiency and quality (Aiken, Sochalski, and Lake 1997; Gittell et al. 2000; Knaus et al. 1986; Shortell et al. 2001, 2000b; Lawrence 2003). Why does the Brazilian system, in its current form, not facilitate care coordination across different levels and medical care organizations?

The Case for Interorganizational Coordination

The future trajectory of the Brazilian health system is away from acute hospital care and toward coordination or integration of service provision across a range of providers and practice settings. This transformation will be a long-term endeavor. Dramatic increases in the proportion of the chronically ill population, and in the sophisticated and expensive care required for these patients, have important implications for medical care. The health system in Brazil, as elsewhere, is organized to provide care for acute illnesses that are resolved quickly, but a different response is required for noncommunicable diseases (NCDs).[18] Care for patients with NCDs must be provided continuously, throughout the patient's life, rather than in intermittent visits.[19] Delivery systems need to be (re)organized to enable care to be delivered by a multidisciplinary team and, usually, across an array of medical care organizations, with careful allocation of tasks among team members and ongoing management of patient contact. There is also growing consensus that care is best coordinated through some type of organized and integrated network.

In networks, providers of different types—hospitals, specialty ambulatory units, pharmacies, diagnostic units, emergency centers, mobile units, and primary care units—come together in a formal and sometimes legal arrangement to manage health care delivery. This often occurs in accordance (or under contract) with purchasers. There is no consensus on the "best" or "right" way to configure or structure a health care network; it is highly dependent on institutional and market environments as well as systemic characteristics. In member countries of the Organisation for Economic Co-operation and Development (OECD), no single model of system integration has emerged, and it is unlikely that a single model will prevail in Brazil. Box 8.4 summarizes key features of organized networks.

Referral Systems: An Enabling Environment for Network Formation?

Since the late 1990s, the MS has sought to establish a system to organize and manage patient flows, referrals, and counterreferrals among SUS-financed facilities providing basic, diagnostic, specialty, emergency, and inpatient care.[20] The main mechanism for setting up the system involved the creation of intermunicipal screening and appointment centers (*centros de regulação*, CRs). Staffed by physicians, phone operators, and information technology personnel, these centers are located in predefined macro- and microregions and usually serve a

Box 8.4
What Is an Organized Regional Network?

An organized delivery system such as a network should ideally "focus on meeting the population's health needs; match service capacity to meet those needs; coordinate and integrate care across a continuum [of providers]; have information systems to link patients, providers, and payers; be able to provide information on cost, quality outcomes, and patient satisfaction to multiple stakeholders; use financial incentives and organizational structure to align governance, management, physicians, and other caregivers; be able to improve continuously the care that it provides; and work with others to ensure that the community's health objectives are met" (Shortell et al. 2000b: 19).

From a more operational standpoint, at the very least any arrangement should allow for the following cross-provider functions: facile exchange and sharing of patient-related information; use of clinical guidelines for case management; application of standardized referral and counterreferral rules; defined roles and competencies of providers, with a concern for achieving scale efficiencies; and collection, analysis, tracking, and sharing of performance, health, and cost data.

The application of clinical pathways is considered best practice for coordinating care among providers. The Institute of Medicine (IOM 2001: 135) describes clinical pathways as "blueprints for care [that] set forth a set of services needed for patients with a given health problem and the sequence in which they should take place." Equally important is the need to manage information technology that enables physicians and other medical professionals to share clinical information about patients and track their progress.

In 2005 the Joint Commission on Accreditation of Healthcare Organizations published a manual on accrediting integrated delivery systems (JCAHO 2005). Though oriented toward integrated systems in the United States, the manual presents standards for eight functions considered essential for quality care within such systems: rights, responsibilities, and ethics; continuum of care; education and communication; health promotion and disease prevention; performance improvement; leadership; human resource management; and information management.

---

number of municipalities. Most are managed by the states or by large urban municipalities. CRs receive, review, authorize, and monitor requests for specialty outpatient appointments, diagnostic exams, referrals, and emergency care among all facilities located in a defined catchment area. The CRs are supposed to be equipped with phone banks and information technology. The latter provides prompt information on the availability of beds, appointment slots, ambulances, and so on in a defined geographic area.

In theory, the CRs should be based on the formation of a "hierarchical and regionalized" provider network (MS 2006b: 13–14) and on the use of clinical pathways (see box 8.4) that "order the flow of patients among care levels based on definitions of each level's [facilities'] resolutive capacity"(17). For example, using information on the availability of beds, appointment slots, and length of waiting lists among facilities in a defined catchment area, and in accordance with the protocols and definition of the types and volume of care provided at each facility, the CRs approve and authorize requests for ambulatory specialty consultations, emergency care, and elective and emergency hospital admissions, including some high-complexity procedures. If the request is justified, the CRs make the appointment or direct the cases to the appropriate facility in an organized network. The CRs are also responsible for following up on each case by tracking patient progress, while reducing unnecessary inpatient stays and subsequent specialty visits.

Implementation has been slow and uneven. In practice, most CRs serve as appointment or emergency call centers. Schilling, dos Reis, and de Moraies (2006) reported that in a survey of all cities with more than 100,000 inhabitants, only 97 (38 percent) had established CRs by 2005. Most of these CRs were considered incipient because they functioned mainly as call centers to obtain emergency transport or to secure specialty, surgical, and diagnostic appointment slots and inpatient beds. For example, of 67 capital cities and cities with more than 250,000 inhabitants, 42 percent reported having CRs for elective admissions, but 57, 70, and 60 percent reported having call centers for emergency admissions, specialty outpatient consultations, and diagnostic exams, respectively. Use of clinical pathways is uncommon. Only 24 (35 percent) reported *preparing* clinical pathways, suggesting that CRs simply matched supply with demand rather than assessing, screening, and managing requests for higher-level services. On a more positive note, most municipalities that possess CRs or call centers have invested in information technology to facilitate a timely matching process for emergency and elective admissions, specialty appointments, and diagnostic exams.

CRs have the potential to contribute to greater vertical and horizontal coordination of health care. Clearly, even the use of call centers to match demand and supply for high-volume services is an important achievement. To fulfill their potential, CRs need rule-based referral systems and multidisciplinary teams functioning within formal intermunicipal network arrangements. In other words, the actual management of patient flows through CRs is encumbered by the absence of organized networks (see below),[21] by the lack of clinical pathways for coordinating and standardizing patient care across providers, and by the weakness of intergovernmental agreements whereby each level of government agrees to provide a defined level and volume of care at facilities under its purview to all residents of a predefined catchment area.[22]

An example of a successful referral system is the National Regulatory Center for High Complexity Care (Central Nacional de Regulação da Alta Complexidade, CNRAC) operated by the MS. CNRAC organizes, authorizes, and finances requests from throughout Brazil for approximately 600 high-technology treatments not uniformly available in the country or offered by a limited number of facilities. Teams of recognized specialists at prestigious institutions appraise, screen, and authorize referral requests (*laudos médicos*) in their fields of expertise (e.g., cancer, orthopedic-traumatology, cardiology, neurology, neurosurgery), based on established clinical pathways. In 2005 CNRAC approved and financed 5,638 cases in authorized facilities—up from 232 in 2002, the system's first year (MS 2006c). In addition to improving equitable access to high-complexity care, CNRAC has established a rational mechanism for assessing and screening referral requests for scarce and expensive care.

Obstacles to Network Formation in the SUS

Under the SUS system, responsibility for delivering health services is distributed among states and municipalities according to the complexity of the service provided. Primary and secondary care is generally the responsibility of municipal governments, while tertiary and referral care belongs to state governments and, to a lesser extent, the MS.

MS regulations enacted in 2002 (NOAS/SUS 01/02) mandated the formation of regional health care networks, that provided increasingly complex care at the microregional, macroregional, and regional levels. The thinking behind the system was to establish a network based on a care pyramid model—from primary care at the bottom to highly complex care at the top. For a number of reasons, however, meaningful networks and care coordination have not emerged.

First, the structure of the SUS, under which responsibilities are divided among municipalities, states, and the MS, ensures that each level of the system is independent. The federal government does not apply indirect instruments such as funding requirements as means of organizing the delivery system to perform more effectively. Given the absence of such instruments, one level (e.g., the federal MS or the states) has little influence on the response by another level (the municipalities) to a health need that may affect all levels. (This problem is common among decentralized systems.) The incentive structure encourages each level to look inward, toward itself and its constituents, and not outward, to the other components. This situation is compounded by the tendency of the municipality, as a political body, to be concerned about the needs of the voters within its remit rather than about broader concerns that may be shared with other municipalities. It is in the interest of local politicians to channel resources toward the quality of services within their own municipality and not toward linkages with others.

Second, the financing system encourages fragmentation among health facilities. Each municipality manages its own spending and delivery, regardless of the source of funding.[23] The model gives municipalities an incentive to provide more health services within their remit are than needed for their small populations (75 percent have fewer than 20,000 inhabitants)—and no incentive to form networks to facilitate care coordination and reduce service duplication. Municipalities thus seek to expand health care at the local level, even if the result is underutilization, as evidenced by the low bed occupancy rates in most municipal hospitals. In sum, municipalities have little incentive to work with other municipalities within networks. This situation severely limits the effectiveness of a response to the rising incidence of NCDs and to the need for an integrated and continuous care system.

Network formation is further restrained by the absence of a discrete organization to oversee its development: a central hub for the management of network development has not been defined under the legislation (Shortell 2000b). Under the national Health Care Operational Norms (Normas Operacionais de Assistência à Saúde, NOAS), the one body mandated to lead network formation—the Regional Health Directorate—has no formal powers. As a result, networks are informal arrangements and commonly operate in the gray area between the municipal and state levels. Although network development exists on paper, the practical steps for establishing networks have not been thought through.

The pyramid model of acute health care organization, in which primary care is subordinated to higher-level care, plays down the importance of basic care services (Mendes 2002). As a result, the quality of services at the primary care level—the most important level for meeting patient demand—has received relatively little priority.[24] As the burden of NCDs and the need for interaction between levels and components of the health system grow, the pyramid structure becomes less effective because care for these conditions requires horizontal rather than vertical coordination with the primary health care facility acting as the central node for referral to other health facilities. Although lack of a national policy may work against network creation, a few states and municipalities, among them Curitiba city and Minas Gerais state, are experimenting with network arrangements.

A Municipal Network in Curitiba

In the early 1990s the Municipal Health Secretariat of Curitiba city (Paraná state) restructured the administration of health services, paving the way for experimentation with network arrangements. Starting in 2001, the secretariat began to integrate different levels of care. This effort included such innovations as the introduction of electronic medical records, the establishment of a central laboratory, and the use of electronic patient ID cards. The network consists of 107 health units, 29 hospitals, 5 emergency units, and 40 specialty facilities. It includes public and contracted private facilities in the city of Curitiba, but not in other municipalities in the metropolitan region.

The integration process was supported by staff training in clinical management and the development of a series of clinical pathways or guidelines. Each health facility was expected to use the guidelines as the basis for strategic planning.[25] In addition, the secretariat signed a management contract with each health unit, establishing targets, performance incentives, and a monitoring system (World Bank 2006a).

To give an example, according to city officials the centralization of laboratory services, coupled with an effective collection and delivery service for samples, improved efficiency and quality in laboratory testing. Mendes (2005) cites the example of hypertension patients, who before the establishment of guidelines were treated with medication whether or not they needed it. After the development of guidelines for treating hypertension, practitioners adjusted their treatment of patients according to the seriousness of each case.

Regional Networks in Minas Gerais State

The Program to Improve Quality of Hospital Care (Programa de Fortalecimento e Melhoria da Qualidade dos Hospitais, PROHOSP) in Minas Gerais state is similar to the programs in Curitiba, but it focuses on hospitals, and its scope is statewide (SES-MG 2003, 2005). Typical of many states in the South and Southeast regions of Brazil, Minas Gerais faced problems of hospital oversupply and size. Of the state's 614 hospitals in 2002, only 20 percent had more than 100 beds. The average occupancy rate was less than 50 percent, and smaller hospitals operated at less than 30 percent occupancy. Hospital care was fragmented across a large number of facilities. In many smaller facilities, structural conditions were unsafe. In others, the volume of complex procedures handled was too low for expertise to develop, and outcomes were poor. The state also estimated that it was inefficiently spending large sums of money on admissions for low-complexity conditions instead of treating them at the more affordable primary level. Table 8.7 shows spending on admissions for conditions treatable in ambulatory care (CTAC) in 2002.[26] The state estimated that 28 percent of all hospital admissions were for such conditions, at a cost of R$120 million (US$41 million), or 21 percent of hospital spending. These conditions represented 33 to 47 percent of admissions in hospitals with fewer than 100 beds.

In 2005, under the state Health Regionalization Plan, PROHOSP began to rationalize the supply of hospital care on the basis of a regional network model.[27] The program established 13 macroregions and 75 microregions, covering all of the state's 853 municipalities. Management units to guide network development were installed in the macroregions.

PROHOSP directed state investment financing to only a subset of 130 "pole" or referral hospitals in the macro- and microregions.[28] The idea was to reduce the supply of smaller

TABLE 8.7

Minas Gerais State: Spending on Admissions for Conditions Treatable in Ambulatory Care, by Hospital Size, 2002

Size (number of beds)	Number of hospitals	Admissions for CTAC	Spending on CTAC (R$ millions)
0–30	144	43.2	10.7
31–50	168	37.5	20.7
51–100	182	32.0	37.8
101–200	81	26.2	28.8
201+	30	13.6	22.4
Total	614	28.1	120.4

Source: SES-MG 2005.
Note: US$1 = R$ 2.93 (2002 average).

facilities while increasing the resolutive capacity of larger hospitals. Minas Gerais is investing in larger hospitals (more than 100 beds) or in hospitals with the technical capacity to serve as regional referral centers. The state plans to convert an undetermined number of smaller hospitals to ambulatory or emergency care centers. Eventually, all financing for admissions in nonpole facilities will be discontinued, and many facilities are likely to shut down.

The state also established referral systems within the centros de regulação (CRs) in each macroregion and in nearly all microregions, linking and coordinating care among the pole hospitals and between these hospitals and ambulatory facilities.[29] Using information technology, each CR assesses and authorizes requests for emergency transport and care, elective admissions, specialty consultations, diagnostic exams, and high complexity care within and across the macro- and microregions. The CRs also track patient progress after admission to hospitals. According to the state, the CRs have contributed to a reduction in unnecessary admissions, patient stays, emergency care, and interhospital transfers. In 2006 the CRs managed about 70 percent of all hospital inpatient care, contributing to a 50 percent reduction in hospital average length of stay (SES-MG 2007).

Finally, Minas Gerais created an innovative financial system to strengthen primary care delivery, especially in the poorest areas. The municipal health secretariats, the recipients of the new state financing, signed management contracts with the state and with the pole hospitals, accepting such targets as reducing hospital mortality rates and developing stock control systems. The secretariats monitor performance quality in each hospital. The program is supported by an education strategy in which managers and staff receive training in hospital management and craft individual hospital plans at the end of each course.

Summary Assessment and Recommendations: A Framework for Systematic Quality Improvement

National, local, and facility-based systems and programs for improving quality have been examined in this chapter. Though limited in scope, the establishment of assessment, accreditation, and benchmarking systems in the last 15 years marks important steps in Brazil's progress toward raising quality. Facility-based quality improvement programs, combined with local attempts at network formation, demonstrate that concern about quality is taking hold. Whether these isolated efforts will result in a national movement for quality improvement remains to be seen.

Recent international experience—responding to emerging research and increasing government concerns about a "quality gap" (IOM 2000)—suggests that quality improvement requires a combination of actions in three categories: system support, accountability mechanisms, and organizational development (figure 8.1). Although overlap exists across these categories and among the elements within them, consensus is building that actions in each area are required to stimulate, implement, and maintain high-quality service delivery.

Category 1: System Support

Continuous quality improvement requires a systematic approach with a robust national support infrastructure. Major elements include formulation of national policies or strategies to enhance quality; establishment of institutions (public or private) to measure and monitor quality, provide guidance to health care organizations, and strengthen their capacity; and provision of support for systematic research on patient satisfaction and evaluation of clinical practices.

National policy initiatives appear to be an important starting point for national debate and action on quality of care. Recent initiatives have put quality on the national agendas in the United Kingdom (Department of Health 1998), the United States (President's Advisory Commission on Consumer Protection and Quality in the Health Care Industry 1998), and Australia (Commonwealth Department of Health and Aged Care 1999; AHAMAC 1996). Recommendations made in these reports precipitated an array of activities that can be viewed as the foundation for establishing national-level structures and institutions specializing in quality performance evaluation, monitoring, and capacity building. The goal of these activities is

FIGURE 8.1

Building Blocks for a National System of Quality Assessment, Management, and Improvement

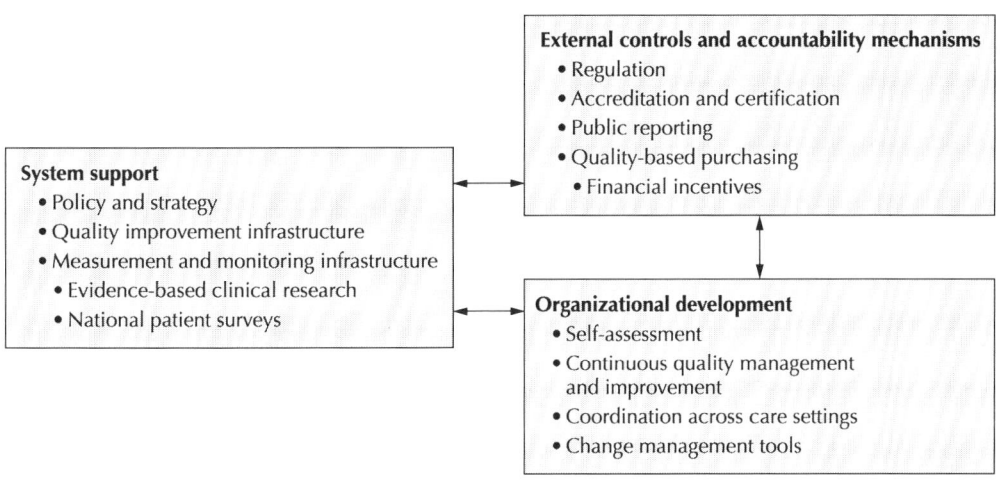

Source: Authors.

to encourage and reinforce quality improvement at the organizational or service delivery level. The institutions in the three countries, and their mandates, are presented in annex 8B. Annex 8C describes important features of the U.S., U.K., and Australian experiences in establishing national institutional arrangements for measuring, monitoring, and improving quality.

Through broad stakeholder involvement, each country established bodies with a blend of national mandates reflecting country-specific priorities, public interest, and institutional arrangements. These mandates typically called for the following actions:

- Measure, monitor, and compare performance.
- Establish performance measures; establish, assess, and strengthen performance data and databases.
- Develop and disseminate clinical guidelines.
- Assess clinical evidence and assist health care organizations in converting evidence into practice.
- Promote a national agenda for research and development related to quality.

As shown in this chapter, systems and institutional arrangements for monitoring quality through measurement of results and outputs are nascent in Brazil, and little progress has been made toward establishing a national infrastructure to support quality performance.[30] Over the next several years Brazil faces four challenges:

- Develop a national quality improvement strategy.
- Achieve consensus on standards for the definition, collection, and analysis of clinical data from Brazil and other countries.
- Create a national agenda for research on quality.
- Establish national (and independent) bodies to measure and monitor quality performance, provide technical support to medical care organizations, increase capacity for safety and quality improvement, and conduct systematic quality research.

Each of these recommendations should be developed with strong stakeholder involvement by medical colleges, consumer groups, professional organizations, and research institutions. The ONA-based performance indicator initiative and the CQH benchmarking system are important steps in the right direction, but without strong national support and expansion, implementation will probably be limited to the same few facilities that have already been accredited and have implemented quality improvement efforts.

Category 2: External Controls and Accountability Mechanisms

This category consists of a set of external checks and balances, including incentives built into the health care system to meet established quality standards and performance targets. These include regulation, accreditation, certification, public reporting, and quality-based purchasing. Many of these elements exist in Brazil but are weakly enforced or thinly implemented.

Quality Regulation

Quality regulation sets the basic ground rules that specify minimally acceptable performance standards for health care professionals and organizations. *Licensure* is mandatory and is based on inspection by government. Although Brazil has a well-formulated hospital licensure framework, it is rarely enforced and fails to weed out poor and sometimes dangerous facilities. Many facilities do not comply with the laws on minimal structural standards and would be forced to close if compliance were enforced.

Accreditation

Unlike licensure, accreditation seeks to establish optimally achievable standards through independent review. It focuses on the entire organization. These standards provide a framework for delivering quality care that facility managers can use to improve performance (Dlugacz, Restifo, and Greenwood 2004). The distinction between facility licensure and accreditation has become increasingly blurred (Scrivens 2002). In the United States many states use accreditation as part of quality standards regulation. France and Italy mandate accreditation for all hospitals, and Canada does so for teaching facilities. Spain (Catalonia), Belgium, and the United States have used accreditation as a certification tool—a requirement for receiving public or social insurance funding. Others reimburse accredited facilities at higher rates, as in the case of UNIMED/BH, described above.

Accreditation systems are well developed in Brazil, but they are voluntary, and their use is unacceptably low. There is no link to government licensing regulations or to overall quality-based certification requirements that determine contractual and financial arrangements between payers (the SUS and private insurers) and hospitals. Although government was instrumental in creating the ONA accreditation system, it appears loath to expand it. This reluctance may reflect fear that universal accreditation may bring to light poor conditions in public facilities.

An active government is often viewed as a competent government. In keeping with Brazil's focus on people and their well-being, eligibility for SUS financing should be linked to licensure and, eventually, accreditation. Without such a link, and the concomitant financial incentive, most Brazilian hospitals will remain substandard and potentially unsafe into the foreseeable future.

New regulatory interventions are needed to improve outcomes from complex procedures performed in hospitals. As elsewhere, Brazilian hospitals that perform few complex procedures have worse outcomes than high-volume facilities (see table 3.10). New York state provides an example of a proactive regulatory program: survival rates from coronary artery bypass graft surgery rose after the state restricted the number of hospitals performing such procedures to high-volume facilities (Chassin 2002, 1997).

Public Reporting

Although standards remain critical to the assessment of factors contributing to good and bad quality, accreditation itself is probably an insufficient driver of continuous quality improvement. Public reporting, based on continuous indicator monitoring and comparison, has become an increasingly common mechanism to complement standards-based assessment systems (Rooney and van Ostenberg 1999; McLoughlin et al. 2001; Scrivens 1997a, 1997b). Accreditation provides a snapshot of standards-based quality during a specific period—the days during which the assessment survey is conducted. It reveals little about the period (usually three years) intervening between surveys. In other words, accreditation is no substitute for systematic outcome evaluation, drawing on central databases that store information on key performance indicators.

Public reporting can be seen as a type of external benchmarking in which organizational performance is compared across facilities or with recognized best-practice facilities. Annex 8D reviews international experience related to hospital performance report cards.

There is little demand in Brazil for public disclosure of comparative performance, probably as a consequence of the weaknesses in available data and the absence of institutional platforms. A public reporting system comparing performance across hospitals and linked to systematic performance monitoring is needed to complement standards-based initiatives such as accreditation.

Quality-Based Purchasing

Quality-based purchasing involves using the purchaser-provider contract (or agreement) as a quality enhancement and enforcement tool. In addition to specifying quality requirements in the contract, quality-based purchasing can also entail the use of financial and other incentives to guarantee that the provider meets quality standards and has established practices to monitor and improve quality. Purchasers also have a cost incentive: it is well-known that quality problems related to misuse and overuse result in higher costs (IOM 2001). Variations in quality are closely related to cost variations. Standardizing the delivery of care, based on available evidence, improves quality while reducing cost variations. The UNIMED/BH initiative to pay higher reimbursement rates for accredited facilities is an example of quality-based purchasing. Annex 8E reviews quality-based purchasing in OECD countries.

Category 3: Organizational Development

Health care organizations such as hospitals are the interface between the health care system and patients. Within the hospital, clinical teams in an array of departments provide frontline care. Improving quality means changing the behaviors of these frontline teams, as well as cultivating within the organization an enabling environment to facilitate their work. Drawing on industrial management techniques, systems analyses, and engineering concepts, strategies and tools have been developed to evaluate and improve quality-of-care processes at the organizational level. These strategies and the corresponding change instruments are collectively referred to as continuous quality improvement (CQI). CQI is an organizational and managerial approach for upgrading quality through identification, prevention, and correction of errors via continuous assessment, monitoring, and strengthening of care delivery processes at the facility level. It is also a systems approach that involves work processes in all departments and therefore entails changes throughout the hospital. In short, CQI targets changes in the process or the environment in which quality problems arise.

Basic tenets of the CQI approach in health consist of leadership, systematic assessment of performance, effective teamwork, proactive change, use of information technologies, focus on improving *all* care processes; incorporation of evidence into practice; and coordination of care across provider settings (Lighter and Fair 2004; Dlugacz, Restifo, and Greenwood 2004; IOM 2001; Lawrence 2003).[31] CQI is often implemented in conjunction with management techniques and methods such as PDCA, TQM, 5S, and ISO (see table 8.4) that are used to guide the change process. Considerable knowledge of CQI features and management tools already exists in Brazil but is limited to a relatively few, mostly private hospitals that have introduced institutionwide CQI-based improvement programs. An undetermined number of facilities have redesigned specific care processes (e.g., maternal care, emergency care), usually managed by an individual physician, but similar changes have not permeated all delivery settings in the hospital. Few systematic attempts have been made to evaluate these initiatives, identify lessons and best practices, and share experiences.

Several aspects of an overall CQI program require strengthening to facilitate expansion of quality improvement programs in Brazilian hospitals. Notable among these are data-driven assessment, information technology, and coordination across providers.

Data-Driven Assessment

The key to quality improvement is the continuous assessment of performance data. It is nearly impossible to alter care processes without information and analysis. Data reveal problems as well as areas for improvement. Robust data are powerful, objective tools for pinpointing problem areas. They are the starting point for working with staff to recognize and correct problems and to put in place processes to prevent their recurrence.[32] In a number of Brazilian hospitals, even elementary data such as descriptive statistics on bed use and length of stay are lacking or unreliable. Data on quality, including outcomes, processes, adverse events, and accidents broken down by department, treatment, or procedure, are rarely or irregularly collected by facilities. Information is collected to comply with regulations, not for change and improvement.

Nearly all Brazilian hospitals have some sort of computerized information that can be used to initiate rudimentary data collection and analysis.[33] If not, simple surveys of medical and technical staff and patients can be effective starting points.[34] It is critical to start such surveys, based on specific questions, observed problems, or organizational and systemic priorities. This tailored approach will help avoid the collection of piles of information that become unmanageable or, worse, sit unanalyzed.

Information Technology

With the explosion in medical research over the last 15 years, incorporating evidence into practice is nearly impossible without the assistance of information technology. Some observers suggest that "modern medicine cannot be practiced effectively and safely without information-technology support" (Lawrence 2003: 91). As is true elsewhere, most Brazilian hospitals have yet to exploit available and increasingly inexpensive information technology to improve quality. Some facilities have installed advanced systems typically found in recognized centers of excellence in OECD countries, but progress has been slow for most of the others.

There is growing evidence that information technologies contribute to improvements in quality and efficiency.[35] Most observers would agree on the information technologies that offer the greatest advantages in terms of quality improvement: (1) clinical decision support systems that assist physicians and nurses in patient diagnosis and monitoring, screening for medication interactions, and compliance with guidelines; (2) automated knowledge bases that distill medical literature and present treatment recommendations, identify best practices, and assess outcomes of different treatment methods; (3) electronic medical records;[36] and (4) Internet-based technologies for communicating with patients (e.g., telemedical consultations and computerized medication reminder systems to improve compliance), as well as for facilitating communication among clinicians and extending training opportunities.

It cannot be overemphasized that information technology is a tool; by itself, it will probably not assist quality improvement in Brazilian hospitals unless it is used within an effective accountability framework, applied as part of a package of CQI features,[37] and linked to a national information infrastructure. Any promotion of, or public investment in, information technology requires careful analysis (e.g., of standards and applications), as well as a roll-out strategy to ensure uptake. In many hospitals the institutional environment is not yet conducive to major investments in information technology.

Coordination Across Providers

As in all middle- and upper-income countries, in Brazil chronic diseases are by far the leading cause of illness, disability, and death. More than half of the country's disease burden relates to just five conditions: cancer, diabetes, and neuropsychiatric, cardiovascular, and chronic respiratory disorders. The cost of treatment over a five-year period (2005–9) was estimated at US$34 billion, about 5 percent of GDP in 2003 (World Bank 2005a). Both the number of people affected and the resources required for treatment will accelerate over the next 20 years.

Chronic conditions are best treated through integrated and continuous treatment arrangements across provider settings in which health care professionals work as a team. Acute stand-alone facilities that do not coordinate care with other providers or with the patient and family are ill prepared to address chronic conditions effectively and efficiently.[38]

In Brazil, despite the outwardly integrated nature of government (municipal)-operated systems, many facilities operate as islands that have limited referral linkages with primary care, ambulatory, and diagnostic services. Many specialists in these facilities act as "independent craftsman" rather than as members of a care team and an organization that integrates and supports care delivery.

Forming functional, integrated, and territorially based networks that take a team approach to delivering care needs to be placed high on the policy agenda in Brazil. This will require restructuring the SUS into a more region-based (rather than municipal-based) model. The redesign of the delivery system will include the redefinition of institutional roles, identification of team-based tasks, and organizational arrangements to support and oversee the care team while ensuring that the patient gets the needed care. Municipalities and states now have few incentives to stretch across borders to establish working network relationships. If this status quo is maintained, it is unlikely that Brazil will be able to address or afford its chronic disease challenge.

Annex 8A
An Example of ONA Standards and Performance Elements: Obstetrics

The following standards are from ONA (2004).

Level 1 standard. The service is staffed by a qualified multiprofessional team and includes separate and equipped areas to provide prepartum, birth, postpartum, and newborn care.

Performance elements

- Qualified, multiprofessional team, trained in neonatal resuscitation
- Equipment and installations meeting requirements for obstetric care and newborn procedures
- System in place for maintenance and checking of equipment
- Conditions for ensuring cleanliness of hands
- Standard procedures in place for isolation of patient as required
- List of obstetricians organized in shifts for each day of the week, with contact details
- List of nonobstetric specialists, with contact details for emergencies
- System of documentation in place

Level 2 standard. Manuals specifying up-to-date norms, routines, and procedures are available; training and continuous education programs are realized; basic statistical information to support clinical management and decision making is collected.

Performance elements

- Manual of norms, routines, and procedures documented, up-to-date, available, and being applied
- Participation in a regional system of perinatal care, to allow for transfer of high-risk patients, as required
- Program of ongoing training and education, with evidence of improvements
- Process for patient orientation
- Process for ongoing patient care and follow-up of cases

Level 3 standard. Data on patient satisfaction are collected and analyzed; the service actively participates in an institutional program on quality and productivity; the service is integrated into the organization's information system; and data on performance indicators are available to enable evaluation and comparison with reference benchmarks.

Performance elements

- System of information based on specific obstetric indicators that permit analysis and comparison
- Cycles of improvement showing systematic impact
- System of analysis of client satisfaction—internal and external
- System of planning and continued technical improvement of staff, care services, and specific procedures

335

Annex 8B

Government Initiatives to Build National Capacity for Continuous Quality Improvement, 1997–2001

Strategies	United States	United Kingdom	Australia
Public reports describing quality problems and calls for improvement	*Quality First: Better Care for All Americans* (President's Advisory Commission on Consumer Protection and Quality in Health Care 1998) *Crossing the Quality Chasm: A New Health Care System for the 21st Century* (IOM 2001) *To Err is Human: Building a Safer Health System* (IOM 2000)	"The New National Health Service: Modern and Dependable" (Department of Health 1997) "A First-Class Service: Quality in the National Health Service" (Department of Health 1998) "An Organization with Memory: Report of an Expert Group on Learning from Adverse Events in the NHS" (Department of Health 2000)	Reports of expert national committees *The Final Report of the Taskforce on Quality in Australian Health Care* (AHAMAC 1996) National Expert Advisory Group on Safety and Quality in Australian Health Care. *Implementing Safety and Quality Enhancement in Health Care* (Commonwealth Department of Health and Aged Care 1999) "Safety First: Report to the Australian Health Ministers' Conference" (ACSQHC 2000)
Establishment of national bodies or programs to improve capacity for measuring and monitoring performance	National Forum for Quality Measurement and Reporting	National Clinical Assessment Authority National Patient Safety Agency National Performance Framework	National Health Performance Committee
Public reporting of performance, national and local	National Quality Report developed for 2003 by Agency for Healthcare Research and Quality (AHRQ) Voluntary and mandated reporting at local levels	Public reporting on some elements of performance down to local levels Development of National Service Frameworks	Annual Performance Reports as part of Australian Health Care Agreements Annual Reports of National Health Performance Committee and its predecessor
Establishment of national bodies to improve capacity for safety and quality improvement	Refocusing of AHRQ	National Institute for Health and Clinical Excellence Commission for Health Improvement National Service Frameworks in priority disease areas National Health Service Modernization Agency	Australian Commission on Safety and Quality in Health Care National Institute of Clinical Studies National Health Priority Action Council
Systemic use of incentives	Federal (Centers for Medicare and Medicaid Services) and state requirements for measurement, reporting, and improvement as conditions of participation in Medicare and Medicaid	Performance agreements at Treasury level Clinical governance within agency contracts Mandated compliance with National Service Frameworks	Quality Improvement and Enhancement Funds as part of Australian Health Care Agreements A variety of federal and state requirements at local and national levels (e.g., incentive payments to general practice for improved patient outcomes for diabetes and asthma)

Source: McLoughlin et al. 2001.

Annex 8C

Setting the Policy and Institutional Framework for Systematic Quality Measurement and Improvement: Examples from the United States, the United Kingdom, and Australia

Systematic performance measurement and monitoring is a common theme in the United States, the United Kingdom, and Australia. Information collection, analysis, and dissemination are viewed as critical tools for driving quality performance systemwide. The U.S. Institute of Medicine called for the establishment of a "comprehensive health information infrastructure," defined as "a set of technologies, standards, applications systems, values and laws that support all facets of individual health, health care and public health."[39] Another common aspect was the establishment of national-level institutions to develop and implement quality enhancement strategies, even though health financing and organization vary considerably across the three countries. Some of these bodies were public, others private, and still others public-private partnerships. Each body was formed after broad consultations with stakeholders.

The U.S. Agency for Healthcare Research and Quality (AHRQ) has developed sets of quality indicators for national tracking, public reporting, and quality-based purchasing arrangements, as well as for health care organizations establishing quality improvement systems. Extensive lists of indicators are available for four areas: preventive care, inpatient care, patient safety, and pediatrics. The table on the next page presents, as an example, inpatient indicators classified by mortality, volume, and utilization.

The United Kingdom is implementing a framework for improving quality that consists of two main strategies, the national service framework (NSF) and the national performance framework (NPF). Both are part of a performance-based public service agreement between the Treasury and the Department of Health. NSFs are standards and corresponding implementation strategies for improving quality in specific areas of care such as coronary heart disease, cancer, pediatric intensive care, and diabetes. They are produced by panels of experts under the auspices of the National Institute for Health and Clinical Excellence (NICE), an independent institution created to facilitate the development and implementation of these standards for defined services or care groups (e.g., cancer patients). The targets or milestones are the basis for measuring progress within an agreed timeframe.

The NPFs include performance indicators that will be used to measure and compare performance in regions, hospitals, and primary care groups across six areas: health improvement, access, effective and appropriate care, efficiency, patient satisfaction, and health outcomes. Specific indicators include death rates, emergency readmissions for elderly people,

Volume indicators
Esophageal resection volume
Pancreatic resection volume
Abdominal aortic aneurysm (AAA) repair volume
Coronary artery bypass graft (CABG) volume
Percutaneous transluminal coronary angioplasty (PTCA) volume
Carotid endarterectomy (CEA) volume
Mortality indicators for inpatient conditions
Acute myocardial infarction (AMI) mortality rate
AMI mortality rate, without transfer cases
Congestive heart failure (CHF) mortality rate
Acute stroke mortality rate
Gastrointestinal hemorrhage mortality rate
Hip fracture mortality rate
Pneumonia mortality rate
Mortality indicators for inpatient procedures
Esophageal resection mortality rate
Pancreatic resection mortality rate
AAA repair mortality rate
CABG mortality rate
PTCA mortality rate
CEA mortality rate
Craniotomy mortality rate
Hip replacement mortality rate
Utilization indicators
Cesarean delivery rate
Primary cesarean delivery rate
Vaginal birth after cesarean (VBAC) rate
VBAC rate, uncomplicated
Laparoscopic cholecystectomy rate
Incidental appendectomy in elderly rate
Bilateral cardiac catheterization rate

Source: AHRQ 2006.

treatment costs, and length of stay. These indicators can be included in performance agreements between NHS executive and regional authorities and between the latter and hospital trusts. A statutory body, the Commission of Health Improvement (CHI), was established to develop indicators, collect data, and disseminate information on the comparative performance of NHS providers. For hospitals, the CHI developed a star rating system based on seven components of performance: risk management, clinical audit, research and education, patient involvement, information management, staff involvement, and education, training, and development. The CHI publishes annual hospital ratings.[40] Poor performers (with zero stars) prepare an action plan to correct deficient areas, and the commission monitors and assists hospitals in the implementation of the action plan.[41]

Annex 8D
Hospital Report Cards: Motivating Hospitals to Perform?

Indicator-based evaluation forms the basis of report cards on hospital quality. These are often benchmarking systems that compare quality performance against standards, average performers, and high performers. Although many countries publish quality and outcome data on hospitals, the impact of these efforts on quality performance is unclear (WHO 2003b).

Recent research shows that public release of information on quality can represent a reputational incentive for hospitals (Dudley et al. 2004). This appears to be what happened in New York and Wisconsin, where low-scoring hospitals made quality improvements (Chassin 2002; Hibbard, Stockard, and Tusler 2003). The Wisconsin study, a randomized controlled trial, showed that quality increased in low-performing hospitals after a large purchaser of hospital services published a report on quality in regional hospitals.[42] In the United Kingdom, however, public reporting of clinical outcomes did not result in quality improvements (Mannion and Goddard 2001).

In the United States comparative performance data are becoming increasingly available through a range of institutions. The Leapfrog Group, a nonprofit organization representing large employers and private purchasers, has developed a scorecard for evaluating hospitals. Indicators includes safe, appropriate staffing of intensive care units; referral systems that direct patients needing complex procedures to the hospitals with the most experience, greatest volume, and the best survival rates;[43] the use of computerized systems for physician prescriptions for medications, tests, and procedures; and "safe practice" scores on 27 procedures to reduce preventable mistakes. According to the Leapfrog Group, universal compliance with the first three indicators in the United States would save more than 65,000 lives, prevent 907,000 medication errors, and save US$41.5 billion in corrective treatment costs. The National Quality Forum (NQF), a U.S. public-private partnership whose objective is to develop standards and measures for public reporting of health care performance data, is developing a comparative quality reporting system to foster greater accountability and consumer choice.[44] The safe practice scores used by Leapfrog were developed by the NQF.

Annex 8E

Quality-Based Purchasing in OECD Countries

Quality-based purchasing is most advanced in the United States but has been gaining momentum among European public and social insurance purchasers.[45] The following is a review of how quality is specified in purchaser-provider contracts in OECD countries.[46]

- *Specification of quality "threshold" requirements* by selecting only providers that meet established structural and process standards, through prior accreditation or certification by an external agency. In Europe accreditation is increasingly used as an "extra licensing" system to determine the eligibility of hospitals to receive public or social insurance funding (Figueras, Robinson, and Jakubowski 2005: 226). In the United States only accredited hospitals are eligible for Medicaid and Medicare funds. Many private insurers also require accreditation.
- *Specification (in the contract) of the types of quality information* to be collected and reported (e.g., "tracer" process and outcome indicators for specific high-volume procedures and treatments).[47] For example, government contracts with hospitals in France include percentage reductions in the rate of nosocomial infections. Systems for managing quality at the organizational level, as well as systems for collecting and documenting such data, may have to be developed first. For example, in 1997 the Council of Europe recommended that purchasers require providers to establish quality improvement management systems (see below) in all purchasing contracts. Italy and Germany are two countries that require implementation of such systems. Other structural mandates used in European hospitals include establishment of adverse effects registers (France), specification of maximum waiting times (United Kingdom, Italy, and others), and use of standardized data collection and reporting systems (Germany and Italy). Finally, several European countries specify process indicators in hospital contracts, including establishment of and adherence to clinical protocols.
- *Inclusion in the contract of financial incentives to improve quality.* Quality can be rewarded through payment mechanisms. Quality-based purchasing involves the use of incentives for hospitals to modify behaviors so as to improve quality.[48] Any payment system (global budget, diagnosis-related groups, Brazil's Authorization for Hospitalization) can be structured to better reward quality. Rewarding performance requires robust information systems to ensure that the rewards are allocated to providers that really do achieve the desired improvements. Purchasers in the United States are probably the farthest along in terms of using incentives to improve quality, but implementation is irregular, and evaluations are just getting under way.

Recent research demonstrates that incentives work, but research is inconclusive regarding the most effective quality-based purchasing strategies (Dudley et al. 2004). Several initiatives, however, are worth examining.

The Leapfrog Group has implemented a program involving purchasers and hospitals that awards bonus payments or higher reimbursement rates to hospitals that meet quality and efficiency targets in five clinical areas representing about a third of all admissions.[49] For each area, weighted scores are generated that contribute to a composite index. The table shows the weighting and scoring for one area, community-acquired pneumonia.

Measure	Weight (%)	Scoring
Initial antibiotic received within four hours of hospital arrival	5.5	% rank (0% = worst, 100% = best) multiplied by weight
Influenza vaccination	7.5	% compliance multiplied by weight
Pneumococcal vaccination	12.0	% compliance multiplied by weight
Adult smoking cessation advice and counseling	7.5	% compliance multiplied by weight
Intensive care unit (ICU) staffing	13.5	Fully implemented: full credit (13.5%) Good progress: 2/3 credit (9.0%) Good early-stage effort: 1/3 credit (4.5%) Anything else: no credit
Oxygenation assessment	14.5	% compliance multiplied by weight
Blood cultures (collected prior to antibiotic administration)	14.5	% compliance multiplied by weight

Source: Authors' elaboration from Leapfrog Group data.

As mentioned above, the United Kingdom applies performance indicators to performance agreements between regional health authorities and National Health Service (NHS) Hospital Trusts. These indicators are monitored by the National Health Commission.

As has been seen, promoting quality through purchasing is still in its infancy in Brazil, but two recent initiatives are worth noting. In the public sector, in São Paulo state health social organization (*organizações sociais de saúde*, OSS) hospitals include quality targets and indicators in the management contract with government purchasers. A portion of financing is linked to compliance with these indicators. In the private sector, UNIMED in Belo Horizonte has linked reimbursement rates of contracted hospitals to achievement of accreditation by the National Accreditation Organization (Organização Nacional de Acreditação, ONA). The insurer increases the reimbursement by defined percentages according to the accreditation levels attained. The quality-financing links of the OSSs and UNIMED are absent in nearly all other purchasers in Brazil.

During contract implementation, systematic efforts are required to collect and validate quality measures (e.g., quality indicators, compliance with standards, adverse events, and patient satisfaction). Depending on the results, financial incentives (application or withholding of payments) can be applied. Cancellation of payments may, however, not be indicated because the purchaser may want to work with the hospital to correct the problems. Upon presentation of evidence of corrective action, the purchaser can reconsider and authorize payment. Finally, during the annual contract review process, purchasers can review performance quality and adjust contractual terms and financial incentives to improve quality. In case of continual failure to meet targets specified in the contract, the purchaser can cancel the contract, if alternative providers are available.

Notes

1. Currently, eight such institutions, known as accreditation institutions (IACs), have been credentialed by the ONA. In addition to conducting assessment surveys, IACs provide educational programs to hospitals seeking accreditation.
2. This accreditation program is sometimes known by its Portuguese abbreviation as the JCI/CBA program. JCI (Joint Commission International) refers to the international subsidiary of the JCAHO.
3. UNIMED/Belo Horizonte, discussed below, is an important exception.
4. The survey was commissioned for this report. All hospitals were medium size, with an average of about 170 beds.
5. According to the ONA, the average fee for medium-size hospitals charged by ONA-certified assessment institutions ranges from R$12,000 to R$14,000. For very large hospitals, the fee can be much higher.
6. Barbosa et al. (2002) found that the average budget of nonprofit medium-size hospitals ranges from R$6.1 million to R$35 million. Budgets of smaller facilities (fewer than 100 beds) range from R$700,000 to R$6.1 million.
7. MS annual ledgers on investment financing do not specify investment type or destination.
8. There are exceptions to this general rule. France and Italy recently mandated accreditation for all hospitals. Canada mandates it for teaching hospitals.
9. For a review of research on the costs of poor quality, see IOM (2000).
10. Examples include Hospital Israelita Albert Einstein (São Paulo), Hospital Moinhos de Vento (Porto Alegre), and Hospital Samaritano (São Paulo).
11. Facilities can also opt for ISO certification, but the ISO system is more appropriate for laboratory and diagnostic units (see table 8.4).
12. The CQH study compared an average of 13 hospitals possessing the Seal of Quality over a five-year period (1999–2003) with an average of 133 facilities that had participated in the CQH program over this same period but that had not yet earned the seal. Nearly all the facilities in the sample were located in São Paulo state. Most were large—nearly half (47) operated between 151 and 500 beds, 41 had between 51 and 150 beds, and only 12 had fewer than 50 beds. The breakdown by ownership was as follows: 50 private for-profit, 29 private nonprofit, and 21 public facilities. The research focused on a subset of indicators that were regularly reported by the hospitals over this period. The facilities included in the analysis were selected because they regularly contributed to the CQH database. This may bias the results in that facilities interested in collecting and monitoring data may display better quality and efficiency than other program participants. Also, no attempt was made to match the hospitals by size, budget, or level of complexity.
13. Data collection and analysis are increasingly part of accreditation systems (Scrivens 2002; Shaw 2004a, 2004b).
14. The analysis of hospitals with and without the CQH Seal of Quality discussed earlier was based on the database of benchmarking indicators. CQH benchmarks were included in the efficiency analysis in chapter 3.
15. Kisil (2004) reports that under the CQH program data gathering and dissemination are not always reliable or consistent. Although over 150 hospitals were part of the program in 2004, only about 100 regularly provided data to a central unit, and the information was often archived within hospitals using different systems and databases.
16. Areas included clinical organization and management, diagnostics, supply management, human resource management, administrative support, public relations, and client focus.
17. Indicators include occupation rates, production data, LOS, and a subset of disease- and treatment-specific mortality rates.
18. About two-thirds of Brazil's disease burden is attributable to NCDs, and treatment cost is estimated at nearly half the cost of hospital admissions (see table 2.2). Demand will only increase as the

demographic transition continues. In 2000 an estimated 15 percent of the Brazilian population was age 50 and over. This group is projected to increase to 42 percent by 2050 (World Bank 2005a).

19. There is increasing evidence that coordinated care results in better outcomes and improved efficiency. This is true for chronic conditions (IOM 2001: 134). The health and quality of life of asthmatic children, for example, greatly improves when they are cared for by well-organized and well-supported teams of clinicians instead of by doctors acting independently (Lawrence 2003).

20. See, for example, the following regulations: NOAS 01/02; Portaria GM 1101 (June 12, 2002); Portaria GM 2309 (December 19, 2001); Portaria SAS 494 (June 30, 1996); Portaria SAS 39 (February 6, 2006).

21. According to Schilling et al. (2006), most large cities reported that the vast majority of referrals were for municipal residents rather than residents of other municipalities.

22. The recently approved (2006) Health Management Covenant (Pacto de Gestão) aims to cofinance, strengthen, and enforce intergovernmental agreements related to referral systems.

23. As explained in chapter 2, about half of state and municipal health financing comes from the federal government, generally in the form of grants deposited directly in their accounts. Nearly all municipalities manage spending for primary care, while those under full system management *(gestão plena do sistema)* manage spending for all services. Nearly all large and medium-size urban municipalities are under full system management.

24. This is slowly changing with the adoption of the Family Health Program, but there has been considerable variation in the program's implementation across municipalities.

25. The guidelines were the instruments used to induce providers to coordinate across organizations (e.g., primary care, specialty ambulatory centers, diagnostic units, and hospitals).

26. These consist of preventable and easily treatable conditions that can be resolved at the primary care or ambulatory level if patients have access to quality care (Starfield 1998).

27. The plan was based on analyses that examined the spatial, supply, and demand characteristics of hospital care in the state.

28. Clinical pathways across medical care organizations are under development to serve as a basis for clinical integration within these territories.

29. Primary care facilities have yet to be incorporated into the CR-managed referral system.

30. This is not to suggest that the issue is being ignored. In a series of interviews with senior management staff in several São Paulo hospitals, Kisil (2004) found that many managers were concerned about measuring results but did not have the know-how, support, or wherewithal to take a system forward.

31. Although these features are applied at the organizational level, they require systemwide support (Category 1) and accountability arrangements (Category 2) to achieve sustained quality improvement. In other words, national performance standards, benchmark indicators, and quality targets—usually established and monitored by statutory bodies, regulatory agencies, purchaser groups, and other institutions—provide the expectations, guidelines, and goals that enable hospitals to assess, monitor, and improve care delivery.

32. According to Dlugacz, Restifo, and Greenwood (2004: 28, 62), "the best way to assert [the] notion that the care [your facility] delivers is quality care is to quantify your processes, services and outcomes. With data, a manager can know if the staff is effective and efficient, and if patient outcomes meet expectations . . . Having data allows the manager to clearly communicate information about the delivery of care . . . In other words, you can't manage until you measure. The analysis should lead to the development of a [quality improvement] program, and measurements should be developed to assess the effectiveness of the improvement."

33. Here, the accountability mechanisms are assumed to be sufficiently strong to drive data collection and analysis at the facility level. However, collecting data to fulfill regulatory requirements is qualitatively different from the data collection, analysis, and feedback approach for CQI.

34. Technical assistance and training for data management are available in Brazil as well as on the Web. Joint Commission International publishes several manuals and Web-based training courses

on data measurement, collection, and analysis in hospitals; see http://www.jointcommission international.com/international.

35. See IOM (2001) and Lighter and Fair (2004) for a review of the literature.

36. As in nearly all middle-income and many high-income countries, in Brazil most clinical information is still stored in paper form that is inefficiently managed. It is not uncommon for hospitals to possess multiple (paper) records for the same patient.

37. A number of hospitals analyzed in this volume had information systems, but basic information was unavailable.

38. Echoing best practice in chronic care, Lawrence (2003: 21) states, "Chronic-disease care must be provided continuously, throughout the patient's life, rather than in interrupted visits when conditions flare up or acute complications rise. Care must be coordinated among the many professionals and institutions involved with such patients during the long course of these illnesses . . . Medical professionals with different backgrounds (*and usually in different settings*) must work together to give the patient what he needs" (italics added).

39. The report cites the National Committee on Vital and Health Statistics, Working Group on Computerization of Patient Records (2000).

40. See Commission for Health Improvement, http://www.chi.nhs.uk/Ratings/Search/SearchResults. asp?TrustType=A.

41. See Lawrence (2003: 96) on the Institute for Healthcare Improvement.

42. The report compared quality performance indicators of adverse events (deaths and complications from surgical and nonsurgical care) in 24 hospitals in the Madison, Wisconsin, area.

43. For example, for coronary artery bypass graft, more than 450 procedures per year (http://www. leapfroggroup.org).

44. According to the NQF mission statement, "Consumers and purchasers need reliable, comparative data to buy value in health care and to generate market demand for quality. Providers also need comparative data to design improvement programs and compare their performance against regional and national benchmarks" (http//:www.qualityforum.org).

45. As in Brazil, in Europe there exists an array of purchasing arrangements: private purchasing of private provision, public purchasing of public provision, and public purchasing of private provision (Figueras, Robinson, and Jakubowski 2005; Preker and Langenbrunner 2005).

46. This section draws on Figueras, Robinson, and Jakubowski 2005; Preker and Langenbrunner 2005.

47. Quality-based purchasing can be greatly enhanced through consensus on the definition, specification, and measurement of quality (Category 1 elements).

48. Incentives can also be directed to individual physicians, but this is beyond the scope of this review. For further information on incentive systems, see Dudley et al. (2004).

49. The clinical areas are coronary artery bypass graft (CABG), percutaneous coronary intervention (PCI), acute myocardial infarction (AMI), community-acquired pneumonia, and deliveries and newborn care. The core quality measures are drawn from accreditation and quality evaluation indicators developed by the Joint Commission. Efficiency indicators include average length of stay (LOS), readmission rates, and severity-adjusted risk factors. See Leapfrog Group (2006).

9

Conclusions and Recommendations

Hospitals are critical to the health of the Brazilian people, many of whom, when ill, first seek care at a hospital. Hospitals are just as critical to the health of the government's budget, absorbing nearly 70 percent of public spending on health. Hospitals influence the ebb and flow of politicians' careers, when shocking news of hospital mishaps hits the headlines, or when news of high-performing hospitals puts the politicians in the limelight. Hospitals are also at the forefront of policy discussions in Brazil. The discussions reflect their promise as centers of technological innovation and medical advances, as well as widespread concern about their cost and performance. In short, Brazilian hospitals are important to many people, and for many different reasons. What makes hospitals important is easy to understand. What makes hospitals deliver quality care efficiently—or fail to meet performance expectations—is much harder to grasp.

The findings and recommendations presented in this volume are based on available evidence culled from a mix of sources and analyses: systematic review of research on the efficiency, quality, and equity of hospital care; analysis of national facility databases; original research comparing the performance of small samples of facilities; and case studies of specific initiatives and innovative programs for assessing and improving hospital performance. Limitations related to the availability and quality of data, the quality of available research on hospital performance, the cost of securing primary data, and small sample sizes restricted the breadth and depth of some analyses reported here.

Most of the preceding chapters contain recommendations related to that chapter's subject. Together, these recommendations constitute a large, and potentially overwhelming, agenda for hospital improvement. This chapter therefore attempts to synthesize the priorities that are integral to improving hospital performance and that should be considered for implementation in the near and medium term. Many of the actions are linked; they will not work as intended on their own. The linkages among policies are highlighted in this chapter.

Brazil's challenge is not unique. Implementing hospital reform policies is notoriously difficult, and it is more difficult still when hospital ownership, governance, and payment mechanisms take as many different forms as they do in a federal state like Brazil. Yet the pluralistic nature of these arrangements is also a strength of the Brazilian hospital sector. As revealed throughout this report, experiments and initiatives abound that can set the stage for broader systemic reform.

A 2004 publication by the Ministry of Health (Ministério da Saúde, MS) on hospital reform opened a national discussion on the problems, potential, and performance of hospitals (MS 2004c). It was the first MS document to focus entirely on the hospital sector. The study presented conclusions from a series of workshops on hospitals held in late 2003 and early 2004 and was not intended to be an in-depth assessment of issues or to make policy recommendations. Rather, the MS viewed the document "as a step toward organizing ideas" (MS 2004c: 68) on hospital

---

April Harding coauthored this chapter.   **345**

reform for future policy making.[1] The broad policy directions outlined in the MS report are aligned with a subset of the policy recommendations specified in this volume. Noteworthy are recommendations to reform payment mechanisms, develop autonomous management in public facilities, strengthen contracting by both public and private hospitals, and rationalize the number of small facilities.[2] The authors of the MS study also called on the broader research and hospital communities to collaborate with the MS in strengthening the analyses and to contribute to the development of vision and strategy for hospital reform. It is in this spirit of collaboration that the recommendations which follow are made.[3]

This summary chapter has four parts. The first synthesizes this volume's findings regarding the salient challenges to improving the performance of Brazilian hospitals. The second describes selected best practices and promising innovations highlighted in the volume that are based on Brazilian experience and can serve as building blocks for change. The third section sets forth the main policy recommendations, and the fourth and concluding section presents insights into actions to foster their implementation.

Problems in Brazil's Hospital Sector

Many middle- and upper-income countries still struggle to ensure predictable access to hospital services for all their people—a goal that Brazil, to its credit, has largely achieved. Yet serious problems remain in Brazil's hospital sector. Considering the constantly growing demand for more, and more technologically advanced, services facing all hospital systems and the resultant calls for additional resources to meet that demand, it is distressing that funding for Brazilian hospitals is not getting "value for money." Overall spending on hospital care is high, yet many hospitals funded by the Unified Health System (Sistema Único de Saúde, SUS) and an undetermined number of privately financed facilities are plagued by low quality and efficiency. The inefficiency of Brazilian hospitals reported in this volume, as measured by data envelopment analysis (DEA) and benchmark analysis, is noteworthy. There can be little doubt that success in dealing with inefficiencies (in, e.g., scale of operations, distribution of infrastructure and technologies, clinical and nonclinical management, and resource use) would enable Brazil to spend more wisely on hospital care.

Efficiency and quality are intricately linked. Improving efficiency through, for example, greater standardization and control of treatment practices reduces undesirable variation in both quality and cost. Hospitals performing a high volume of complex procedures achieve economies of scale while reducing mortality and the risk of adverse events. Furthermore, disparities in quality are increasingly a major cause of inequity, as is evident from the two-tier nature of hospital care in Brazil, where world-class facilities, generally catering to the well-off, coexist with substandard facilities, generally frequented by the poor. Enhancing efficiency can create a virtuous circle, resulting in broader quality and equity gains. Similarly, many quality improvements lead to lower resource use by reducing medical errors, adverse events, and overuse.

What are the main drivers of inefficiencies and low quality? Five areas of critical weakness have been identified in these chapters: rigid and unaccountable hospital governance; weak coordination and distorted capacity configuration; passive, distorted, and diluted funding; lack of systematic and continuous programs to enforce standards and to measure and ensure quality; and lack of information for decision making. Each is discussed below.

Rigid and Unaccountable Hospital Governance

Nearly all Brazilian public hospitals display a rigidity that is inherently at odds with modern hospital management. Under the existing organizational rules, even motivated and committed managers can make only limited improvements. Hospital managers who lack the authority to manage staff, reorganize departments, or reconfigure services cannot make the kinds of changes that could substantially improve their operations. Many managerial functions are rule based and are centralized in higher administrative levels located in municipal and state health, finance, and administrative secretariats. In addition to being far removed from the front line of service provision, most central-level managers lack the know-how, motivation, or information to manage hospitals. Excessive centralization of managerial functions, combined with rigid civil service rules, political interference, and lack of information, create an organizational environment that deprives facility managers of the means of managing and improving performance. In part because of this distorted organizational environment, public facilities under direct administration are, on average, the lowest-performing hospitals in Brazil.

Deficient governance practices and organizational arrangements contribute to low performance in many private hospitals, but their problems are qualitatively different from those facing public facilities. Because information is lacking, the relation between performance and governance arrangements in private facilities remains unknown, but it is evident that overlapping and informal governance and management functions, together with lax monitoring and a weak information environment, may compromise these hospitals' performance. This is especially true in the small, nonprofit facilities that account for most of the SUS-financed private hospitals. The weakness of contract pressures and lack of competition mean that few incentives exist to perform and therefore to address organizational shortcomings.

For many years, the costs of these inefficiencies have been passed on to funding agencies through demands for increased budgetary allocations by public facilities and for higher reimbursement rates and special bailouts by private facilities. This situation is no longer tenable because of already high public and private spending, low macroeconomic growth, and a high tax burden.

Passive, Distorted, and Diluted Funding

Payment mechanisms remain a relatively unused policy instrument for supporting policy priorities and stimulating performance. In fact, some payment mechanisms such as line-item budgets (the dominant form in public hospitals) contribute to inefficiencies and higher costs. Line-item budget allocations are based on historical input and spending patterns, with no rewards for quality or cost-consciousness.

The Authorization for Hospitalization (Autorização de Internação Hospitalar, AIH) payment mechanism, consisting of a predefined fee schedule linked to outputs (in the form of procedures), is used to pay private hospitals under contract with SUS and theoretically can contribute to more efficient resource use. But as currently applied, it contributes only modestly to cost control because the payment rates are seriously distorted. For most inpatient care, AIH payment rates are much below cost, and they are substantially over cost for a few treatments and procedures, mostly high-complexity care. The result is overemphasis on a few "profitable" services and not enough provision of money-losing but high-volume services. This imbalance seriously undermines patient access to needed services and cost-effective use of public resources. It is also a major driver of the well-publicized financial crisis in the nonprofit hospital sector, which is heavily dependent on SUS funding. Moreover, it may drive hospitals to provide overlapping services or submit fraudulent coding in order to raise revenues, to specialize in lucrative treatments, and to seek (and depend on) lump-sum bailouts from local governments to make ends meet.

SUS-imposed expenditure ceilings set an overall limit on spending but do not drive behaviors that result in efficient resource use at the facility level. The ceilings themselves are based on historical trends and therefore harbor embedded inefficiencies that have accumulated over the years. They are also moving targets, dependent on government tax revenues during the course of the fiscal year. Moreover, hospitals often reduce service supply near the end of the fiscal year, as they approach their assigned ceilings, and then exert political pressure for extrabudgetary transfers, or they may reduce planned outlays for equipment maintenance and material inputs. In general, financial planning and management, and efforts to improve the efficiency of resource use so as to stay within expenditure limits, are rare. This passive and nonstrategic utilization of SUS funds for hospital care is striking because in pluralistic hospital systems, public funding can be a powerful instrument for stimulating efficiency and quality improvements.

Most private insurers and health plans pay for hospital care through a predefined fee schedule negotiated between the plans and hospitals. Although fee schedule–based payment systems used by private insurers are associated with more efficient use of resources, the reason may be that private facilities usually treat less complex and severe cases than do many public facilities and enjoy far more managerial autonomy. Rate setting also has little to do with costs or with resource use, partly because of the absence of reliable information on costs and the lack of cost-consciousness among providers and insurers alike. As with the SUS, discrepancies between rates and costs in the private sector are evident but have not been systematically analyzed. However, the disputes over rates between insurers and providers (e.g., hospitals and physicians) that are often aired in the press suggest that fee schedules are not aligned with costs. As in the case of the SUS-AIH mechanism, the impact of discounted fee schedules on cost containment appears modest at best because private facilities, too, have an incentive to overprovide more generously reimbursed treatments.

The multiplicity of payment systems confronting the typical hospital manager dilutes the impact of the incentives associated with any single mechanism. Incentives to improve efficiency and quality or to control costs in any one mechanism may be offset by disincentives in another system. In addition, discrepancies in payment rates may contribute to systemwide distortions. For example, lower-rate payers such as the SUS may drive hospitals to skimp on quality, shift costs to higher-rate payers, or transfer complex cases to public facilities, which do not depend on production-based payment but are bound to treat everyone. An increasing number of private hospitals cater to patients covered by private health plans, which pay higher rates than the SUS and cover higher-income patients. This contributes to stratification in the hospital system.

Finally, contracts accompany many payment mechanisms because they specify the terms and conditions of the payment. Although the SUS has a long history of contracting private hospitals to deliver hospital services, purchasing is a passive and often poorly managed activity. The contracting instruments (*convenios*) are essentially legal instruments for distributing budget to private providers traditionally linked to the public system. The convenio, as a contracting tool, is devoid of accountability and is not used to create incentives to improve the production, quality, and efficiency of hospital services.

Weak Coordination and Distorted Capacity Configuration

Publicly funded hospital services are delivered by different types of public and private hospitals in Brazil. Public hospitals may be federally, state, or municipally owned. Private hospitals are owned by individuals, philanthropic organizations and charitable groups, and corporations. Some private facilities belong to conglomerates, but most are stand-alone organizations. The various hospital owners make decisions largely in isolation from other hospitals. Pluralism in hospital ownership by itself does not preclude coordination, but it does demand strong mechanisms that ensure coordination both in the delivery of care and in the expansion of capacity.

By and large, Brazilian publicly funded hospitals do not coordinate with one another or with other care providers with regard to patient care, referral, and follow-up. Even hospitals and other providers controlled or financed by the same entity (e.g., a municipality) do not coordinate effectively, and coordination between SUS and non-SUS private hospitals is nonexistent. This is not because the people involved do not care but because no mechanisms are in place to motivate and enable coordination. And, even in the best of circumstances, coordination is hard to accomplish, in part because of Brazil's federal structure, which grants state and municipal governments considerable independence. Furthermore, most municipalities—which directly administer more health care delivery than other actors—cover too small a catchment area. In the absence of regional or intermunicipal coordination, scale economies are missed, and cost shifting takes place.

Many hospitals in Brazil are in the wrong places and are too small to operate efficiently or to ensure quality. Distribution of expensive, complex technologies is another area of concern. Oversupply, underuse, misplaced small, low-volume hospitals, and inequitable concentration of medical equipment contribute to inefficient and distorted resource use and are themselves related to the shortcomings in resource allocation mechanisms discussed above. This distortion of hospital capacity makes services much costlier than necessary and compromises quality. All levels of government own hospitals in Brazil and so do many nongovernmental entities. Currently, all these hospital "owners" make important decisions about capital investment largely in isolation from one another. In contrast to other systems with pluralistic hospital sectors (e.g., Germany and France), no roadmap guides the development of independent hospital capacity to meet the people's needs and demands.

As is true elsewhere, coordination of care across clinical and organizational settings is in its infancy in Brazil. Despite the high and increasing incidence of chronic diseases, which are best prevented and treated through integrated and continuous treatment arrangements across provider settings, the health system, particularly the hospital sector, is organized mostly to provide acute care through stand-alone facilities. Networks, in which different providers come together to formalize arrangements to manage and provide health care, are rare.

Lack of Systematic and Continuous Programs to Enforce Standards and to Measure and Ensure Quality

In contrast to many middle-income countries, Brazil has an adequate regulatory (licensing) framework for ensuring minimal quality standards related to structure and, to a lesser degree, processes (e.g., reporting requirements for hospital-acquired infections). Brazil is also ahead of many countries in the region in the development of accreditation programs. The critical problem is that these standards are not applied, or enforced, in most hospitals. Brazil is unusual, too, in that it has established regulations and institutional mechanisms to protect its citizens from physician malpractice. Partly because of physician self-interest, however, the mechanisms seem ineffective. Brazil is one of the few middle-income countries with a well-established biomedical and clinical research industry, resulting in pioneering medical advances and technological innovations in a number of areas. Yet treatment and technological advances, whether achieved in Brazil or elsewhere, do not always make their way into clinical practice in Brazilian hospitals except at a few prestigious centers of excellence. Equally troubling are the large discrepancies in the quality of care between and within Brazilian hospitals.

Few systematic and continuous efforts have been made to measure and improve the quality of care in Brazilian hospitals. Generally absent are national policies, programs, and systems to support measurement and evaluation of quality, quality performance review and comparison, capacity building for quality improvement, dissemination of evidence-based research, and public disclosure. Moreover, the institutional infrastructure to develop, coordinate, and implement such policies is lacking. (These shortcomings are not confined to Brazil.) A few promising MS and regional initiatives, as well as organizationwide and continuous facility-based quality improvement programs exist, but because they have not been evaluated, their suitability for replication is unknown. Without a more concerted policy and institutional effort, any real progress toward addressing quality concerns will remain elusive.

Lack of Information for Decision Making

The absence of useful information about the quality, efficiency, and cost of hospital services underlies all issues. At every level, critical information for informing decisions is absent or incomplete, even though relatively large amounts of data are collected. For example, the quality of care provided in most Brazilian hospitals is unknown and is nearly impossible to assess because information is not available. The absence of systematic and reliable information on costs, volume, outcomes, and patient characteristics impedes the design of more effective hospital payment mechanisms. Without systematic data collection, it is impossible to monitor, analyze, and compare progress on quality outcomes, efficiency, and costs. Limited data availability and the cost of collecting primary data at the facility level drive Brazilian researchers to focus on small-scale and often ungeneralizable studies. Moreover, when data are available, they are often unreliable or not comparable because of variations in the definition and measurement of variables. This situation limits the volume and usefulness of policy-relevant research on hospital performance.

Policy makers at every level of government are forced to make key decisions about resource allocation without having minimal information about the quality, cost, or value of services. Hospital managers, likewise, rarely have the information needed to identify pressing quality problems or to reconfigure staff or other resources to improve quality or productivity. In essence, decision makers are flying blind as they seek to take steps to improve Brazil's hospitals.

Building on Brazilian Innovations and Experience

A number of home-grown innovations and initiatives that can serve as foundations for change have been reviewed in this volume. Some were the subject of in-depth analysis; others were highlighted in case studies. Several would require more in-depth evaluation to ascertain their replicability in Brazil's institutional and ownership contexts.

Improvement of hospital performance initiatives should build on these foundations while taking into account lessons from international experience. Box 9.1 suggests the formation of partnerships with other countries that are seeking to reform their hospital sectors. Policy makers should seek to capture the momentum and knowledge of these initiatives so that policy design and implementation are grounded in the contemporary context of Brazil.

These experiences in Brazil provide valuable knowledge and a foundation for improving hospital policy, but continued incremental and uncoordinated efforts will not achieve the performance improvements needed. Although the purview of this volume did not permit a comprehensive review of all efforts, the initiatives discussed next are the most promising for addressing some of the problems outlined in the previous section.

Organizational Arrangements and Governance

The hospitals in São Paulo state managed by health social organizations (*organizações sociais de saúde*, OSSs) represent a successful example of an alternative organizational arrangement for public hospitals. Considerable information exists on the OSS experience from evaluations, case studies, and doctoral dissertations. Although the OSS hospitals were set up in new facilities and thus had no existing organizational infrastructure, the evidence suggests

---

Box 9.1
Building on International Innovations and Experience

Many high- and middle-income countries are struggling with the same challenges outlined in this volume as they seek to improve hospital performance. Relevant international experience has been cited throughout the volume. As with Brazilian experience, lessons from initiatives taken elsewhere can serve as building blocks for change. To date, government efforts to identify and learn from these experiences have been timid. Establishing partnerships with governments and institutions dealing with hospital reform and quality improvement can create the conditions for information exchange and comparative analysis of what works, and how and why.

The partnership between the MS's Health Surveillance Secretariat (Secretaria de Vigilância em Saúde, SVS) and the U.S. Centers for Disease Control (CDC) provides an example of such a partnership. Activities include joint research, training sessions, staff exchanges, study tours, and policy discussions, benefiting both institutions. The SVS-CDC venture can serve as a model for similar partnerships with institutions in other countries dealing with the complex issues of hospital reform.

Source: Authors' elaboration.

that the regime has a sound accountability arrangement, consisting of managerial autonomy, flexible human resource management, and strategic purchasing through performance-based contracts. Vigorous monitoring, as well as contract management and enforcement, by the state health secretariat is another feature of the OSS model as practiced in São Paulo state. These are important elements that should be part of any reform model.

Although Brazilian experience is limited, recent state and municipal initiatives in São Paulo with converting hospitals from direct administration to OSS organizational forms highlight the potential for performance gains, especially in efficiency and quality. The experience to date also suggests the need for transitional strategies to address complex human resource and financial issues and to garner political and community support.

Importantly, the MS has taken initial steps to reform and strengthen contracting arrangements in both public and SUS-funded private hospitals. Currently, the MS has signed management contracts with 86 teaching hospitals specifying services and defining performance indicators. The challenge is to apply these innovations to the majority of public and SUS-funded private hospitals.

Coordination

The regionalization initiative in Minas Gerais state is a promising endeavor that aims to rationalize the supply of hospital services while strengthening care coordination among hospitals and between hospitals and other providers within defined territories. The state has developed a regional network model based on the spatial, demand, and supply characteristics of hospital and ambulatory care. Small management units have been established in 75 microregions, and investment financing is directed only to large facilities with the technical and volume capacity to serve as regional referral centers. Most hospitals—small facilities with fewer than 50 beds—will be converted to ambulatory or emergency care centers. Some will be closed as the state gradually eliminates financing for hospitals too small to serve as referral centers or achieve minimal economies of scale. The state is developing logistical support and care coordination arrangements for the nascent networks.

Curitiba city has also introduced network arrangements, including the development of electronic medical records that are used by hospital and ambulatory providers; distribution of electronic ID cards (linked to medical records) to all users, which enable information sharing on patient conditions; and establishment of a central laboratory that has raised the quality and efficiency of diagnostic services. Importantly, the network formation efforts in both Minas Gerais state and Curitiba city were accompanied by initiatives to extend primary care coverage.

Most states and large municipalities are implementing referral systems (*centros de regulação*, CRs) to screen and manage requests for higher-level services. These systems can contribute to greater vertical and horizontal coordination among health care providers.

With the support of the World Bank, the MS QUALISUS-REDE Investment Program has recently commissioned a series of studies analyzing care coordination and network arrangements in Brazil. The results will serve as the basis for an investment program to encourage hospital rationalization, care coordination, and network formation.

The establishment of municipal consortia, as specified in recent Brazilian legislation (Law 11.107/2005), offers as a mechanism for resource pooling and management for coordinating service delivery across municipalities in defined regions. The MS has also mandated the formation of regional management councils that can serve as a governance structure for configuring health care networks (Portaria 699/GM of 2006).

Finally, the MS Policy for Small Hospitals, issued in 2004, attempts to clarify what is meant by the term "hospital" and indicates that small, underutilized facilities are not really hospitals. Although the policy is limited in scope, it has initiated a debate questioning the raison d'être of small facilities and has set the stage for comprehensive policies that would define their role within the broader delivery system. An important issue is how to balance the realization of scale efficiencies against the goal of ensuring access to hospital care in remote areas.

Payment Mechanisms

The MS AIH/SIA systems used for paying private hospitals can provide significant information on hospital care and serve as a basis for developing a payment system similar to the diagnosis-related group (DRG) mechanism. Further study of the strengths and weaknesses of diagnostic data, service groupings, input standardization, and costs can provide the SUS with solid foundations for configuring a DRG-based hospital payment mechanism and an information system to support it. The contract-based global budget model used by São Paulo state to pay OSS hospitals and, more recently, nonprofit facilities can also provide lessons for public and private payers interested in linking payment to performance. A similar model is under MS consideration for funding services in teaching hospitals and private hospitals. Finally, a private prepayment plan in the city of Belo Horizonte (the UNIMED Cooperative Health Plan) recently launched a quality-based purchasing arrangement in which affiliated hospitals are paid at differentiated reimbursement rates linked with their compliance with facility licensure requirements and accreditation standards. This effort shows promise in stimulating quality improvement in hospitals and could be a model for other public and private payers.

Quality of Care

Unlike most middle-income countries, Brazil has a robust facility licensing framework and possesses three rigorous hospital accreditation and certification programs.[4] Strengthening licensing enforcement and expanding accreditation are important building blocks for improving quality of care in hospitals. Participation in accreditation and certification programs also is a key driver for development by facilities of continuous quality improvement (CQI) programs. Although an undetermined but increasing number of Brazilian hospitals has launched such programs, it is estimated that only a minority has collected the relevant data and documented the impact of these initiatives. Evaluation of these experiences would bring to light the knowledge of CQI already present in Brazilian hospitals. Considerable know-how also exists on the change processes required to support quality improvement in hospitals.

This volume has demonstrated that Brazilian hospitals seeking accreditation programs have adopted an array of internationally recognized management tools to facilitate organizational change in support of quality enhancement. Finding out how these tools were applied and soliciting facilities' assessment of their effectiveness would make valuable information available to hospitals contemplating CQI programs. Recent MS quality enhancement programs such as HumanizaSUS and CartaSUS have the potential to stimulate significant quality improvements in hospitals. More information on their impact, systematic analysis of available data, and stronger follow-up on results are required if these programs are to meet their stated quality enhancement objectives.

Information and Performance Assessment

The MS AIH/SIA hospital payment and information system can serve as a means for improving patient and service information systems. AIH/SIA systems contain considerable data on service production and diagnostics and, once updated to eliminate distortions, can provide useful information for establishing global budgets and assessing performance. The CHQ benchmarking systems, the ONA capacity-building program on quality performance indicators, and the National Agency for Sanitary Surveillance (Agência Nacional de Vigilância Sanitária, ANVISA) hospital surveillance system are important starting points for developing and expanding standardized data collection, measurement, and tracking systems in all Brazilian hospitals.

Finally, São Paulo state has implemented information and cost accounting systems in all OSS and some nonprofit hospitals to facilitate budget negotiations, contract management, and performance monitoring. Both facility managers and state authorities enjoy a rich information environment that includes the exchange of timely information on service production, quality, and costs. This exchange is supported by processes and capacity in the oversight agency (the State Health Secretariat) as well as in the reporting hospitals. The information environment facilitates regular feedback on results and problem identification while enabling the design of corrective actions.

What Can be Done? Key Policy Priorities

This volume has covered a broad range of performance issues and diagnoses, while focusing on information and analytical gaps related to the policy dimensions identified in the framework presented in chapter 1 (see figure 1.1).[5] Drawing on these policy dimensions, as well as on the findings that emerged from the analyses, the main recommendations are grouped into five policy areas: enhancing hospital autonomy, accountability, and governance; leveraging financial flows and payment mechanisms; systematically pursuing service and investment coordination and capacity configuration; raising quality standards in all hospitals; and strengthening the institutional environment for resource use and performance management. The need to set a strategic framework for hospital reform constitutes another policy dimension and gives rise to recommendations on taking the first steps toward generating commitment and building societal and institutional support for change. Annex 9A summarizes the main policy recommendations and lists suggested short- and medium-term actions to implement them, along with the agencies responsible for each action.

Enhance Hospital Autonomy and Accountability

> RECOMMENDATION 1: Develop a strategy, regulatory framework, and implementation plan to convert direct and indirect administration facilities to alternative organizational arrangements that offer autonomous authority and flexible human resource management.

> RECOMMENDATION 2: Formulate an investment policy that promotes the application of autonomous organizational arrangements in any new public hospital.

> RECOMMENDATION 3: Establish public-private program mechanisms to strengthen governance arrangements in private hospitals under contract with the SUS, including regulatory reform and enforcement, strengthening of contracting, and stimulation of competition.

Improving governance arrangements for public hospitals is a priority for the Brazilian government. The organization of these hospitals seriously constrains management and operational decisions—often locating key decisions entirely outside the hospital. Such rigid constraints on management undermine efforts to increase accountability. When managers do not control important decisions, they can rightly point to such constraints to explain hospital performance problems. Just as a football coach needs to be able to select and manage his players and reorganize them to carry out his strategy, hospital managers must have adequate control of their "teams" if they are to be able to ensure good performance.

Virtually any effort to enhance hospital quality or efficiency will rely on increasing the motivation and proactivity of public hospital managers. And managerial motivation depends critically on the hospitals' organizational arrangements. Autonomy-enhancing reforms can give public hospital managers the ability to undertake needed changes, but other actions are needed to motivate them to use this autonomy to improve quality and contain costs. In particular, the basis of hospital funding must change to reward these positive steps. This issue is described in the next section.

Policies to enhance the autonomy of public hospital management are a prerequisite for addressing most of the performance issues in public hospitals discussed in this volume. Many of the current policy discussions focus on expanding resources and improving skills. None of these changes will have their desired effect, however, if hospital managers are not given adequate flexibility to make needed changes. Various implementation strategies can be explored. Some countries have implemented sectorwide organizational changes in public hospital governance; others have phased in governance reforms.[6] Mandating organizational changes in new hospitals is an important first step, but it leaves untouched the hospitals where most patients are treated. It seems clear that a strategy must be developed that can apply to existing hospitals. Actions are needed to develop and test hospital conversion strategies against Brazilian and international experience. Because of the human resource issues involved, conversion will require leadership and a strong policy push. Tinkering at the margins is unlikely to result in substantive improvements in organizational arrangements.

The 2007 MS policy and legislative proposal to convert public hospitals under direct administration to fully autonomous state foundations (*fundações estatais*, FSs) represents a promising step forward with strong potential for improving public hospital performance. The model contains many of the features included in the OSS arrangement, including managerial autonomy, performance-based contracting, performance-based financing, and flexible human resource management (under private law). Importantly, the proposal mandates the constitution of governance boards to oversee and monitor performance. The model also involves the conversion of civil servants to the private labor regime (Consolidação das Leis do Trabalho, CLT) and the professionalization of hospital management.

Once legislative approval is achieved, the MS needs to work on an effective implementation strategy involving the gradual conversion of civil servants to the private labor regime—or their replacement—and the development at all levels of government of contract management units with the capacity to monitor, evaluate, and enforce contractual provisions. Evaluative research of Brazilian hospital conversion experiences, as well as in-depth analyses of international experience, would facilitate preparation of an implementation strategy.

Applying hospital autonomy reforms to individual hospitals can undermine service coordination. Hence, it is important that any design for reforming hospital governance take into account the need to affirm, or elevate, the responsibilities that hospitals have with respect to coordination with other providers. The drive to improve governance of public hospitals will need to be linked closely with efforts to improve service coordination via the creation of network arrangements. These are discussed below.[7]

Weak governance is not limited to the public sector. Most nonprofit hospitals, especially the many small ones, manifest very weak oversight and management. Although they do not suffer from the rigidities and lack of decision-making authority seen in public facilities, informality and the absence of clear lines of authority contribute to their weak performance. Action is needed to strengthen both the regulations specifying governance arrangements and functions in nonprofit hospitals and the enforcement of those regulations. Additional measures include strengthening contracting and promoting competition for public contracts. These measures will increase pressure to perform, which would stimulate efforts to address governance shortcomings.

Enhance the Leverage of Funding Flows to Increase Efficiency, Cost Consciousness, and Quality

RECOMMENDATION 4: Enhance the leverage of public funding (SUS) flows by

- Implementing alternative payment systems, such as global budgets linked to performance, for public hospitals to replace line-item budgets and build in strong incentives for quality and efficiency enhancement
- Improving contractual arrangements by applying instruments that specify volume and type of services and priority targets, linking a proportion of payment to performance, and enforcing compliance with agreed targets
- Upgrading the AIH/SIA system, aligning payment with costs, and gradually converting to a DRG-like system.

RECOMMENDATION 5: Initiate regulatory reform that will improve private funding flows (to constrain cost shifting and enhance cost containment and fiscal discipline), foster payment system consistency, and generate incentives for efficiency for hospitals and managers.

A sizable portion of most hospitals' operations in Brazil is funded by the SUS. This funding is a powerful potential lever for influencing hospital behavior, but currently it is not being used to its fullest potential—some SUS hospital funding arrangements even hamper performance. Changes are needed on several critical fronts: eliminating line-item budgets in public hospitals and substituting alternative methods such as global budgets; modifying the content of contracts and the process for making and implementing them; introducing policy-based investment financing; aligning the AIH/SIA payment systems with costs; and consolidating the multiple hospital payment mechanisms currently in use.

Most funding flows to public hospitals are line-item allocations. Such funding arrangements are not tied to performance and preclude cost consciousness because cost savings in one category cannot be allocated to other categories. These budget structures diminish the ability of management to link hospital activities to the needs and demands of the communities they serve. The input basis of most public funding critically hampers flexibility and effective management in Brazilian hospitals. Budgets do not relate to performance or promote efficiency. Budget-related information flows do not generate information on the cost of outputs or on quality.

A global budgeting system would address these problems. A few states and municipalities have introduced global budgeting systems that feature resource ceilings and link a portion of payment to performance. Equally important, these funding arrangements leave hospital managers sufficient flexibility to allocate funding across expenditure categories in ways that will improve productivity and quality. Evidence suggests that when combined with other measures such as greater autonomy and strategic contracting (discussed below), global budgets would improve accountability and performance. Expansion of global budgeting to all public hospitals would go a long way toward improving their performance.

True accountability for hospitals requires more than governance arrangements and performance-based funding; it requires that the roles and responsibilities of public hospitals and their managers be clearly specified so that what constitutes meeting those obligations is clearly understood.

Similarly, clarity in communication about performance expectations makes it easier to identify shortcomings and to come to consensus on corrective actions. This clarity can best be achieved through strong contractual arrangements that define the content of funding agreements. Such arrangements with SUS-funded public and private hospitals should establish clear goals related to performance, including the specification of outputs and results, as well as the resources for achieving them. Contracts should also specify the portion of funding linked to the achievement of the goals, as suggested above.

Changing the content of the funding agreements between the SUS and hospitals is necessary but not sufficient. The process of the relationship must also change. As demonstrated by experience with the OSSs, and in many member countries of the Organisation for Economic

Co-operation and Development (OECD), the funder's capacity to manage the contracting process, and monitor the contracts contributes critically to outcomes (den Exter 2005). Most successful hospital contracting initiatives have included a contract management capacity-building program in the initial phase.

It is also critical that the contractual relationship minimize opportunities for bias in public contracting with public facilities. In organizational arrangements such as direct administration, facilities are essentially budgetary arms of the funding agency. This creates a conflict of interest. Some countries have achieved an "arm's-length" relationship by implementing reforms that separate public payer and providers. In others, external bodies have been established to oversee the contracting process and fulfillment of the contracted provisions. The latter option was used in Sao Paulo state to ensure transparency and fairness in the implementation of the OSS contracts.

If the payment system is to motivate better performance by all hospitals, the method of paying nonprofit hospitals under the SUS must also be changed. Currently, private hospitals receive from the SUS mostly activity-based payments that are passively allocated. This reimbursement does not cover the cost of most services. Nonprofits are strongly motivated to overprovide the few services for which the activity-based payment exceeds cost, or to specialize in highly reimbursed services. It is critical that the funding arrangements provide reimbursement that covers costs, to ensure the financial stability of private hospitals and minimal levels of quality. Once reimbursement rates are adjusted to cover costs, it is equally important to move toward using contracts to motivate improvements in quality and efficiency. Where capacity is sufficient to permit delivery of certain services by multiple hospitals, the introduction of selective contracting and competition for these services should be explored. In a more competitive environment where hospitals face the loss of money-generating services, they would naturally shift toward a more proactive strategy for quality enhancement and cost containment.

Although no payment system is perfect in terms of its usefulness for achieving performance objectives, many countries have adopted case-adjustment methods such as DRGs to pay hospitals directly or to strengthen global budgeting systems. The main rationale for adopting DRGs has been to improve the efficiency of hospital care and to control costs. Though not without problems, DRGs have an established track record of stimulating efficiency and cost containment in hospital services. Unlike the AIH system, which is based mainly on procedures (services provided) and hospital characteristics (teaching vs. non-teaching), DRGs also reflect patient characteristics, such as diagnoses and age, and costs (relative use of resources). Thus, a DRG-based system is more effective than some others in linking resource allocation to disease patterns, risks, and costs. The AIH system represents a building block for developing DRGs. In addition to eliminating distortions in available AIH data on procedures, DRG development would require the strengthening of data collection on diagnostics, to facilitate case adjustment, as well as the introduction of systematic and standardized collection of cost data. Recommendations for improving the information environment are outlined later in this section.

Development of a DRG-based payment mechanism would contribute to another policy recommendation—reducing fragmentation in the payment systems—if private payers can be motivated through regulation or other means to utilize the same payment basis. In the current situation of multiple and often poorly designed payment systems, hospital managers face a mix of often contradictory incentives and inequities in payment, resulting in under- or overfunding of certain services, depending on the payer and mechanism applied. A system in which all hospital payers apply the same payment mechanism and rates would reduce the distortions (e.g., the practice of shifting care from low-paid to high-paid services) that result from the multiplicity of rates for the same service. Application of such a system would entail first studying international experience with efforts to achieve uniformity of payment across different payers. Without a solidly designed payment mechanism, such as DRGs, that both the SUS and private payers can adopt, uniform payments will be impossible.

Systematically Pursue Service Coordination and Capacity Configuration

> RECOMMENDATION 6: Develop and implement state-level master plans for care coordination and establishment of regional networks.

> RECOMMENDATION 7: Strengthen the national strategy for rationalizing hospital supply, including the transformation or closure of inefficiently small hospitals and improvement of primary care coverage and quality.

> RECOMMENDATION 8: Strengthen policy-based investment financing for hospitals on the basis of regulatory approval or investment master plans.

> RECOMMENDATION 9: Develop a national system for technology assessment and allocation.

Hospital service delivery requires close coordination, within the hospital and with other providers (specialists, diagnostics, and primary care services). For health systems to work well and for people to receive good care, providers need to coordinate in myriad ways: with each other (e.g., sharing patient information to ensure quality of care and follow up); with the public health system (e.g., regarding reportable diseases for surveillance); with regulatory and self-regulatory bodies, for quality (e.g., reporting medical errors, adverse events, and practice statistics to identify problems); and with funders, as well as planning and regulatory bodies (e.g., securing approval to buy high-cost equipment or expand capacity).

Difficulties emerge in coordinating across political jurisdictions in highly decentralized systems where hospitals are owned by local governments.[8] In these instances, where the political jurisdiction is much smaller than the catchment population served by the facility, local governments must establish coordination mechanisms with each other, as well as with private providers. In Brazil this means that hospital planning and operation must be coordinated across multiple government levels and providers.

Coordination in Brazil is, however, handicapped by the decision-making and financial independence granted states and municipalities under the decentralized federal (and SUS) structure, in which the federal government remains an important financier of health services.

For example, the federal government is expected to bail out states and municipalities during financial crises, but these lower-level entities often resist federal demands to increase local financing, link federal financing to performance, rationalize provision, and improve efficiency. Coordination is further compromised at the subnational level by often fragile public administration, weak capacity to manage public hospitals, ill-defined responsibilities across subnational levels, precarious referral systems, and the absence of ties with non-SUS private providers. The situation has resulted in a blame game between federal, state, and municipal authorities over financing, responsibilities, and results that is often played out in the hospital sector. In addition, many SUS-funded patients are treated in private facilities under contract with the SUS. Currently, little coordination takes place among this wide array of decision makers and care providers, and coordination mechanisms within the SUS are poorly designed and ineffectual. Instruments already in place such as Integrated and Negotiated Programming (Programação Pactuada e Integrada, PPI) have yet to achieve strong coordination because of these underlying problems. Balancing responsibilities among different hierarchical levels is a challenge in any federal system. Box 9.2 highlights recent health reforms in highly decentralized Scandinavian countries.

Service coordination is achieved in at least three ways. One is through joint ownership of providers, and therefore administrative links among them, as in hospital networks in Victoria (Australia) and in the U.S. Veterans Administration hospitals. Provider behavior is coordinated on the basis of hierarchical or employment relations and in the public sector usually involves some regulatory provisions or service norms. (This is the current modus operandi for SUS-

---

Box 9.2
Recentralization in Scandinavia? Achieving Coordination across Political Jurisdictions

---

The challenge of coordinating across political jurisdictions has been addressed in the heavily decentralized Scandinavian countries. Recent reforms show a tendency toward regionalization and the creation of organizational structures. In Sweden this is achieved through the operation of associations of county councils, which establish binding legal and funding agreements to ensure coordination among providers owned by different counties and to provide for reimbursement for services rendered to noncounty residents. The associations also undertake capacity planning. In addition, a number of counties have merged into microregions, partly to improve efficiency and contain costs.

In Norway dissatisfaction with county coordination of hospital services led to centralization (e.g., regionalization) of administrative authority at the national level. For example, five regional health enterprises with executive boards were established and were made responsible for service delivery in specific geographic regions Hospital ownership was transferred from the counties to the central health ministry. These reforms were intended in part to counteract the proliferation of duplicate or unnecessary county hospitals, hospital budgetary deficits, county micromanagement of hospital operations, and the diffuse accountability and lack of transparency of the "shared responsibility" governance arrangement between the central government and counties for care coordination.

Denmark is also merging county council health agencies into regional health authorities to improve coordination, quality of care, and cost containment. There, counties have been grouped into five regions with between 0.6 and 1.6 million inhabitants. Recent reforms have merged a large number of municipalities, introduced a block grant financing system for the regions, and redefined subnational roles and responsibilities.

Source: Bibbee and Padrini 2006; Strandberg-Larsen et al. 2006; Hagen and Kaarbøe 2004.

funded providers, and it has been unsuccessful, partly because of the constraints discussed above.) Corporations that own a wide network of providers, such as Kaiser Permanente in the United States, are another example of ownership-administrative coordination. A second mechanism is funding-based contractual coordination, as in the Canadian regional health authorities and U.S. health plans. In this setting, the funders pursue coordination through their contracting procedures and coordination-related requirements for contracted providers. The third is regulatory-based coordination. Although this method is more appropriate for coordination of capital investment to prevent proliferation of medical technologies, in the United States such an arrangement regulated new hospital construction (see below).

Considering the monetary and quality costs of continued fragmentation, Brazil should expand and strengthen one or more of the mechanisms described above to enhance coordination of hospital services. Since in Brazil government bodies do not directly control private hospitals, and given the constraints on norm-based coordination, administrative approaches to enhancing coordination cannot be applied. Instead, funding-based coordination through contractual arrangements may offer the best possibility of success.

Funding-based coordination can be enhanced by pooling funding and authority across municipalities, as in Sweden. Such pooled funding could support expanded political and administrative coordination. This pooling of resources may reduce the problems associated with the too-small catchment populations served by municipally owned hospitals.[9]

Coordination across providers will be impossible if there is not a command structure with real decision-making authority over a defined catchment area and a network of SUS-funded primary care units, diagnostic centers, and hospitals, including nonprofit facilities. Such a coordinating body would probably require a governance structure involving municipal consortiums, public but independent holding companies, or state-affiliated but autonomous foundations to enable oversight, financial pooling, and accountability for results. An executive arm would manage the network. For example, public hospitals and specialty units could be transferred to a regional enterprise in which the municipalities that compose the region (and the state) are shareholders. Both the municipalities and the state could then purchase services from the regional enterprise, and in turn, the regional enterprise would purchase services from public and private facilities through contracts.

Although governance and management arrangements can be highly context-specific, there are some basic principles:

- Coordinating bodies must be at the right territorial (regional) level, with authority over, or ability to offer incentives to, a sufficient breadth of providers (primary care, diagnostic centers, and hospitals).
- Coordinating bodies must have sufficient authority over resource allocation within the network—for example, over distribution of pooled funds to providers within a specified region that includes multiple municipalities.
- Coordinating bodies must have authority over, or ability to offer incentives for, a minimum bundle of decisions regarding such subjects as capital investment, service configuration, and technology acquisition.
- Coordinating bodies must have sufficient authority to substantially direct or motivate hospital strategic development (but not day-to-day activities).
- Coordinating authority must encompass private SUS-funded facilities.

Much more needs to done regarding the oversupply of small hospitals and the inequitable distribution of technological resources. The current MS strategy regarding small hospitals does not go far enough toward reducing the unnecessary waste of scarce resources in these facilities. A more comprehensive policy is required, one that addresses the need for and role of any facility with fewer than 100 beds. This ties in with the recommendation regarding policy-based investment financing. Although some small facilities are clearly warranted in remote rural areas, over the last 20 years road networks have improved considerably in Brazil, expanding people's access to larger and higher-quality facilities.

The location, scale, and service configuration of hospitals in a country strongly influence the cost of services. For this reason, governments throughout the world guide the development of hospital capacity. In Brazil funding mechanisms for capital replacement are deficient because of their susceptibility to political pressure. The current system sets priorities for public investments, but they are not based on a rigorous needs assessment and are ineffective in influencing additional, often politically driven, investments unrelated to stated priorities. In countries where publicly funded hospital services are delivered mostly via public hospitals, this is done directly through the allocation of public funds for capital investments. In these instances, policy-based (and enforced) allocation of investment funds precludes construction of unneeded hospitals or hospital wings or indiscriminate procurement of high-cost equipment. Similarly, these allocations can be used to ensure that new capacity is located in areas where population is growing. In systems with pluralistic delivery, such as Germany, a master plan is developed (and enforced) indicating medium-term plans for hospital capacity development.[10] Only facilities and departments whose capacities are included in this master plan are reimbursed with public funds. Hence, if a municipal government builds a facility that is not provided for in the master plan, there is no assurance that any services will be paid for with public funds.

Hospital capacity can also be directly regulated through a mandate that all new facilities receive regulatory approval. The United States used this approach for many years, requiring all new hospitals or hospital departments to obtain a certificate of need before embarking on construction. The certificate was required of all new facilities, not just those which were to be eligible for public reimbursement, and so the program succeeded in constraining capacity expansion sectorwide.

The cost of having the wrong hospitals in the wrong places is an expense Brazil cannot afford for much longer, in terms of both cost and quality. Significant gains can be made by guiding the capacity of the hospital sector toward a better geographic distribution, more economical scale, and better configuration of services across facilities. Either the sectorwide direct regulatory constraint via a certificate of need or the enforced master plan approach linked to public funding could work for Brazil. Both approaches have proven workable in pluralistic hospital systems, with capital investments being undertaken by a wide range of actors, governmental and nongovernmental.

The cost of treating in hospitals cases that can be resolved more efficiently and effectively at a primary level is another expense that Brazil can no longer afford. Extending the coverage and improving the quality of primary care services must therefore remain government policy priorities for the foreseeable future.

This volume has presented evidence of inefficiencies and inequities in allocation and use of medical—especially hospital—technology. Although the MS has been discussing mechanisms to foster vigorous technological assessment, these initiatives have been timid. To reduce duplication, waste, and inefficiency, a strong national system is needed for assessment of technology and decisions on its allocation. Such a system requires not only the design and implementation of a methodology for technology assessment but also the training of sufficient specialists to apply and interpret assessment results.[11] Above all, it requires mechanisms for enforcing its recommendations or decisions. Enforcement can be achieved through funding mechanisms (allocation of public funding only to technologies proven cost-effective—the preferred approach in the SUS sector); through regulation (the feasible approach in the private sector); or by both means. Internationally, many of the successful initiatives in this area established strong national independent bodies with broad stakeholder participation.

Raise Quality Standards in All Hospitals

> RECOMMENDATION 10: Develop and implement a three-pronged national strategy for quality assessment and improvement consisting of three building blocks: system support, accountability mechanisms, and organizational development (see figure 8.1 in chapter 8).

> RECOMMENDATION 11: Institute a rigorous national licensing exam for medical school graduates.

No citizen should face unnecessary risks associated with receiving hospital treatment in Brazil. Yet although isolated efforts to improve quality abound, they have yet to coalesce into a national movement for quality improvement. National leadership is sorely needed to establish the policies and institutional arrangements that will support quality improvement systemwide, but particularly in hospitals. Broad stakeholder involvement will be required to formulate a national strategy for improving quality and establishing the institutional infrastructure for measuring and monitoring quality; to conduct quality-based evaluation research; and to provide technical support to facilities seeking to develop continuous quality improvement programs.

Another priority is to rapidly raise all hospitals operating in Brazil to minimum standards of quality. The standards already exist in the form of licensure requirements, and action should be taken urgently to ensure that all hospitals meet them. In most countries compliance with minimum standards is usually achieved through regulation (e.g., withholding or revoking permission for noncompliant hospitals to operate). In Brazil such regulatory provisions are already in place but are not enforced. An alternative strategy is clearly necessary.

Most licensing standards are related to structural quality, and hence compliance alone is unlikely to have a sufficient impact on quality of care. Brazil therefore simultaneously needs to expand accreditation to ensure that hospitals are increasingly motivated to monitor and improve care processes and outcomes. The country possesses well-designed accreditation programs, but uptake is limited to a small number of mostly elite hospitals.

In modern hospital systems, quality is pursued through a range of mechanisms—administrative (norm-based), regulatory, funding, and contracting—and through information dissemination strategies such as benchmarking. Government, however, has a responsibility to ensure quality in both public and private hospitals. Improving the effectiveness of the regulatory framework and the capacity of regulatory bodies is important in the medium term. More promising in the short term is use of the power of SUS funding to expand licensing and accreditation.

Probably the best implementation strategy is to reduce over time reimbursement rates for unlicensed hospitals while shifting funds to increase reimbursement to hospitals that do comply with licensure standards. This should be part of a strategic purchasing framework in both the SUS and the private sector aimed at fostering compliance with licensing requirements and promoting accreditation. In several countries accreditation is also broadly implemented via public funding criteria. For example, in the United States the Medicare program does not reimburse unaccredited hospitals, and accreditation is required for hospitals to receive public funding in Spain (Catalonia) and Belgium. The funding reforms discussed above should incorporate financial incentives for achieving accreditation. Some hospitals, however, are the only providers in their catchment areas, so withdrawing SUS-funding is not an option (or a viable threat) in every situation. Bonuses or higher reimbursement rates should therefore be considered to motivate hospitals to become accredited.

Many critical actions for improving the quality of hospital services must take place at the hospital level under the leadership of hospital management. These actions span a broad range, entailing assessment of performance, effective teamwork, use of information technologies, incorporation of evidence into practice, and coordination of care within the hospital, as well as with providers at other levels. A range of policies is needed to motivate such changes. To begin with, managers need to be highly motivated to improve quality. Such motivation can be enhanced in Brazil via management hiring practices, incentives in hospital funding arrangements, and clear delineation of management responsibility and performance expectations in contracts. But, as was shown above, even if such policies lead managers to be highly motivated, public hospital managers must also be allowed latitude to act. Moreover, hospital managers will need significant technical and capacity-building support from national-level structures to acquire the know-how to develop, introduce, and maintain quality improvement programs.

Brazilian hospitals make little use of clinical guidelines, even when these do exist. A strong effort is needed to promote the development and standardization of clinical guidelines and their gradual adoption by all hospitals, public and private. Again, a mix of regulation and economic incentives is likely to be the best approach for expanding the use of guidelines.

The quality of education is weak in a number of medical schools. Voluntary assessments of recent graduates suggest that some medical schools do not adequately train their students for medical practice. Although an exam alone will not improve the quality of new physicians, it may put pressure on medical schools to raise their quality of instruction. Publishing each medical school's results will also enable future students to choose wisely among schools, thereby exerting pressure on the low performers.

Strengthen the Institutional Environment for Efficient Resource Use and Effective Performance Management

> RECOMMENDATION 12: Promote the effective use of information technologies to support performance and outcome measurement, cost collection and analysis, access to clinical information, clinical decision making, and coordination across medical care organizations and teams.

> RECOMMENDATION 13: Support modernization of management practices in public and SUS-financed private hospitals.

> RECOMMENDATION 14: Develop a nationwide benchmarking and public report card system trained on efficiency and quality.

Brazilian hospitals, with few exceptions, do not collect, analyze, or share critical information on costs or quality. Hospitals need information systems that allow them to assess quality, identify problems, and take remedial actions. These systems need to generate both quality-related information and cost- and efficiency-related information. To be useful for policy makers, the systems must be standardized across all SUS-funded hospitals. Standardization of information reporting, analysis, and presentation will also enable insurers and patients to make informed decisions about where to seek care. Such choices, based on good information, can put valuable pressure on hospitals to make improvements. The federal government should develop standards to allow cross-hospital and cross-state benchmarking, similar to those for U.S. Medicare. Establishment of conditionality for receiving SUS funding or bonuses should be used to motivate the introduction of standardized information systems.

Global budgeting systems were recommended above as a mechanism for funding public hospitals. These systems, however, do not always generate good information, so critically needed in Brazil, about the cost of services. It is important that the global budgeting system support the establishment of a meaningful cost information base. In this way, over time hospital payment can be based on realistically and reliably priced services.

For any of the foregoing initiatives to have an effect, hospital managers in Brazil need modern hospital management skills—which few now have. The current system in which hospital directors function largely as passive administrators does not involve management skills. A significant effort is critically needed to build the capacity of new and current managers to function as proactive, strategic leaders of their facilities.

Three additional and desirable features of these information systems should be considered. First, they need to be selective and to focus on essential information useful for decision making. Currently, considerable data are routinely collected in the SUS, but they are often irrelevant and are not used for decision making. Second, information systems should be designed with the needs of the local manager in mind, so that he or she can actually use the information to monitor and evaluate the services managed. Third, cost information systems should be designed taking into account recommendation 6, above: that is, they should enable the costing of specific treatment procedures or cases and thus provide input for the creation of a DRG-like payment system.

Moving Forward with Implementation

Can Brazil improve the performance of its hospitals? The evidence presented in this volume suggests that the answer is, yes. But it will take strong and constant leadership, coordinated efforts by federal, state, and municipal governments, direct engagement with the private health sector, systematic but continuous vision, evolving policies, and consistent actions. The weakness or absence of such enabling factors in the Brazilian health system has brought about an implementation gap in which promising initiatives die with the outgoing government. Given the autonomy of subnational governments, fragmented and uneven implementation is always a threat.

Nevertheless, the policy and institutional contexts suggest that chances for implementation are good. The Health Management Covenants (*Pactos pela Saúde*) of 2006 are oriented toward using federal financing to tighten accountability for results. The 2004 MS publication on hospital reform placed hospitals squarely on the policy agenda. Further evidence of a fledgling movement to improve hospital performance is seen in the 2007 MS legislative proposal to reform public hospital governance, in MS measures to improve contracting of private hospitals, and in state-led initiatives to establish organized care networks and reform organizational arrangements in public hospitals. Fiscal constraints and calls from financial authorities to contain costs are additional enabling factors.

The challenge will be to coordinate these efforts, generate and maintain dialogue among public and private stakeholders, and allow flexibility to accommodate Brazil's diverse regional circumstances. Of equal importance, this should be accomplished within a coherent and consistent vision of a reformed hospital sector. In keeping with the time-tested incremental nature of SUS-led reforms, hospital reform should be rolled out incrementally, anchored in a comprehensive policy, and linked to time-bound implementation benchmarks.

The actions discussed here are urgently needed, but they are complex. They require active and coordinated efforts by federal, state, and municipal governments and government agencies. They also require engagement of private hospitals, which deliver a large portion of hospital services in Brazil. Such engagement will not happen unless all actors first reach consensus on problems and priority actions. The creation of a comprehensive vision will help guide the actions of all the actors. It is hoped that this document will contribute to laying a foundation for the process. One important strategic advantage Brazil has, and should exploit, is its reservoir of experience from the initiatives already in place, with its relevance to the policy priorities discussed.

Brazilian policy makers have focused on raising financing for hospitals while leaving decision making on resource allocation and use to managers, both in individual facilities and in government and corporate administrative hierarchies. Hospital managers, however, often become fixated on the immediate tasks of meeting demand by securing material inputs and administering human and financial resources. Most lack the time, training, authority, or information to reflect on how well they use resources, assess the performance obtained with those resources, define future directions and needs, or examine their facility's changing role within the broader health system. Spending decisions require a partnership between health policy makers, hospital managers, consumer groups, and representatives of nonhospital providers. Governments and governance institutions have a responsibility to ensure that hospitals use resources efficiently to provide quality services and that they are linked to the broader health care systems. This is best done by ensuring adequate institutional arrangements and embedding appropriate incentives in funding mechanisms.

Crafting long-term hospital master plans, including the specification and sequencing of implementation arrangements, to improve the hospital system was the starting point in most countries for which information is available. In some cases these master plans were anchored in policy white papers that gave overall direction to hospital reform. In each country, conversion of public facilities to autonomous organizations was part of a broader hospital reform or system restructuring effort aimed at improving the efficiency and overall financial sustainability of health services. Nearly all countries formed special commissions or task forces to plan and oversee hospital reform. Although a major element of some plans was to determine capacity and technological needs (based on demographic and epidemiological projections, and including criteria for travel time), the plans also aimed to free hospitals from centralized (often politicized) control.[12] Plan provisions fostered clear separation of purchasing from provision, performance-based financing and contracting, autonomous legal status for heretofore public hospitals, and an output-based prospective payment system such as DRGs. In a sense, the plans also encompassed directly or indirectly the elements of the purchasing and accountability arrangements inherent in the OSS model.

Most countries did not introduce all these measures simultaneously. Once the overall vision and plan was formulated, implementation was an incremental process: some measures were implemented in parallel, and others were introduced sequentially by federal, state, and municipal governments. The key was the prior development of a comprehensive policy that guided plan development and subsequent implementation. Strong and consistent leadership, sometimes supported by unambiguous regulations, nurtured the deep rooting of the reforms nationwide.

In Brazil any hospital reform effort will require a comprehensive policy, as well as coordinated policy actions by federal, state, and municipal governments and private stakeholders. The agreed vision and policy must be accompanied by a work plan with agreed actions, and actors must be committed to coordinated implementation and understand how the pieces fit together. The first step, therefore, is to elaborate the vision or policy, and the second step is to develop a coordinated plan of action with an outline of explicit implementation strategies and actions that ensure coordination.

A comprehensive vision and coordinated action plan is the beginning, not the end. Actions must be implemented systematically, and implementation must be motivated and monitored. This is always a challenge in federal states. The Australian Commonwealth has met the challenge by establishing agreements every five years between the commonwealth and state governments concerning hospital policies to be implemented. If the agreed policies are not executed, fund transfers to the state are reduced until implementation takes place. Another approach used in federal states is to establish a special policy-related fund, disbursements from which are contingent on implementation of the specified policy. Whatever path it takes, a federal government must establish a mechanism for motivating and monitoring implementation in the hospital sector, where many policies must be addressed in a coordinated fashion by multiple levels of government. This is certainly the situation in Brazil.

In hospital systems like Brazil's where private provision is extensive, addressing certain policy issues requires substantial involvement by private actors. In Brazil these critical issues are service quality, service coordination and capacity planning, and hospital reimbursement. Increasingly, governments are moving to formalize the involvement of private actors, especially providers, in the formulation, promulgation, and implementation of hospital policies in these areas. Such engagement improves the quality of policy design and can help mobilize implementation and the desired behavioral changes by private providers.

To foster sectorwide efficiency and quality improvement, strong collaboration between the SUS and the private sector is needed. Some principles of collaboration are as follows:

- Formalization of the mechanisms and scope of private sector involvement can help make the process more predictable and transparent.
- Engagement should be focused on policies of strong interest and relevance to the private actors. (Formal consultative mechanisms are most commonly focused on rate setting.)
- Consultations should be well run and productive, to motivate continued private participation.

A final question is whether more resources are needed to accomplish the steps outlined here. Additional resources will be required to support the design and implementation of a number of the policies discussed in this chapter. Certain activities, such as information systems, are underfunded, and more resources will need to be targeted to them. In addition, AIH payments for low- and medium-complexity care will have to be raised to bring them into alignment with costs. Overall, however, the hospital sector is not underfunded. Given the need for fiscal constraint, the program to improve Brazilian hospitals could be implemented by raising productivity and efficiency and rationalizing hospital supply to free up resources that are already in the system but are being wasted. Any new resources for hospital care should be tied to improvements in productivity, efficiency, and quality. Without such a link, mobilization of additional resources for hospitals might prove counterproductive by relieving existing pressures to enhance performance.

Annex 9A
Recommended Policies and Actions

Policy objective or area	Policy recommendations	Actions to implement recommended policies (short-term priority actions are highlighted in gray)	Who does what
Precondition: set strategic framework for hospital reform.	• Develop a comprehensive hospital reform policy and strategy that address the main quality, efficiency, and equity problems facing the sector. • Prepare a time-bound action plan with implementation benchmarks to execute the strategy. Plan should include provisions for the policy areas listed below. • Prepare a regulatory framework to facilitate implementation of hospital reform.	• Create an independent commission with participation of major opinion leaders and representatives of major stakeholders to produce a hospital reform strategy. • Plan and implement formal consultations with major stakeholders in public and private sectors, including representatives from health plans, medical and nursing schools, professional organizations, consumer groups, and trade associations. • Conduct study tours and assess experience in countries that have launched hospital reform efforts.	Federal government, with congressional support, takes lead with strong stakeholder participation.
Enhance hospital autonomy, accountability, and governance.	1. Develop a strategy, regulatory framework, and implementation plan to convert direct and indirect administration facilities to alternative organizational arrangements that offer autonomous authority and flexible human resource management.	• Support demonstration pilots for public hospital conversion, starting in facilities under indirect administration. • Conduct in-depth evaluation of human resource conversion and costs in Brazilian health and nonhealth institutions converted to autonomous organizations.	Federal and state governments.
	2. Formulate an investment policy that promotes the application of autonomous organizational arrangement in any new public hospital.	• Review lessons from international experience in public hospital conversion, including human resource management reform. • Strengthen contract mechanisms and promote competition for public contracts, increasing pressure for performance and thereby providing incentives to address governance shortcomings in private hospitals.	Nonprofit hospital trade associations in collaboration with federal government.
	3. Establish public-private program mechanisms to strengthen governance arrangements in private hospitals under contract with the SUS, including regulatory reform and enforcement, strengthening of contracting, and stimulation of competition.	• Approve legislation enabling government to convert public hospitals to alternative organizational arrangements that, among other things, allow for flexible resource management and give hospital managers authority to manage human resources.	All government levels.
		• Strengthen regulations and their enforcement regarding governance arrangements in the nonprofit hospital sector, with special focus on defining governance arrangements and responsibilities, separating governance and managerial structures, specifying reporting requirements, and taking actions to verify regulatory compliance. • Undertake a large-scale study to analyze key features of performance-enhancing organizational arrangements in public and private facilities.	Federal government in collaboration with universities, research institutions and private hospital trade associations.

(continued)

Policy objective or area	Policy recommendations	Actions to implement recommended policies (short-term priority actions are highlighted in gray)	Who does what
Enhance the leverage of funding flows to increase efficiency, cost consciousness, and quality.	4. Enhance the leverage of public funding (SUS) flows by (a) implementing alternative payment systems, such as global budgets linked to performance, for public hospitals to replace line-item budgets and build in strong incentives for quality and efficiency enhancement; (b) improving contractual arrangements by applying instruments that specify volume and type of services and priority targets, linking a proportion of payment to performance, and enforcing compliance with agreed targets; and (c) upgrading the AIH/SIA system, aligning payment with costs, and gradually converting to a DRG-like system. 5. Initiate regulatory reform that will improve private funding flows (to constrain cost shifting and enhance cost containment and fiscal discipline), foster payment system consistency, and generate incentives for efficiency for hospitals and managers.	• Establish standardized cost accounting systems in all SUS-financed hospitals and train managers to use them. • Eliminate distortions in AIH/SIA procedures list and payment levels, converting AIH/SIA into solid information systems to define and monitor global budgets and treatment costs. • Develop research agenda to identify and evaluate hospital payment mechanisms that stimulate improvements in quality, efficiency, and equity; agenda to include evaluation of global budget initiatives in university and other federal hospitals and effects of provider payment systems in the private sector (e.g., impact of costs on the SUS). • Develop and test a diagnosis-based group (DRG) information and payment system for measuring, and adjusting for, patient case mix. • Initiate implementation of a comprehensive regulatory framework for all (public and private) hospital payers, gradually moving toward comprehensive standardization of hospital service reimbursement rates and reporting systems. • Introduce selective contracting for a portion of privately provided services where sufficient capacity enables provision of services by multiple hospitals. Such services should be tendered following the highest standards of transparency and oversight to ensure effective contracting and to avoid all perceptions of politicization.	Federal government sets framework and standards for cost systems. Investments are financed by any level of government and private sector. Federal government in collaboration with universities, research institutions, and trade associations representing private hospitals and health plans.

Systematically pursue service coordination and capacity configuration.	6. Develop and implement state-level master plans for care coordination and establishment of regional networks. 7. Strengthen the national strategy for rationalizing hospital supply, including the transformation or closure of inefficiently small hospitals and improvement of primary care coverage and quality. 8. Strengthen policy-based investment financing for hospitals on the basis of regulatory approval or investment master plans. 9. Develop a national system for technology assessment and allocation.	• Analyze impact of initiatives that have established regional hospital networks in Brazil and elsewhere. • Prepare federal guidelines for drawing up state master plans for care coordination and regional network formation, based on agreed principles for service reconfiguration, hospital rationalization, network design, and strengthening of primary care. • Pilot regional networks with a clear role for and active participation of hospitals.	Federal government takes lead but with strong participation of state and municipal governments, together with the private sector.
		• Evaluate impact of MS policy for small hospitals. as well as state initiatives to reduce their number; based on those results, prepare policy guidelines for states and municipalities to convert or close unneeded small facilities. • Develop regulatory, institutional, and financial environment to enable pooled funding and establish viable coordinating bodies across municipalities.	Federal government in collaboration with state and municipal governments.
		• Legislate the requirement of a certificate of need for investments in new hospitals and establish capacity to undertake review of applications for investment under a certificate of need program. • Approve legislation setting parameters for allocation of hospital technology and resources according to demand and policy priorities, optimizing their utilization; establish responsible authority to review and make decisions on applications. • Strengthen the existing investment master plan framework and establish mechanisms for its enforcement	Federal government in collaboration with private hospital trade associations.

(continued)

Policy objective or area	Policy recommendations	Actions to implement recommended policies (short-term priority actions are highlighted in gray)	Who does what
Raise quality standards in all hospitals.	10. Develop and implement a three-pronged national strategy for quality assessment and improvement consisting of three building blocks: system support, accountability mechanisms, and organizational development. 11. Institute a rigorous national licensing exam for medical school graduates.	• Establish a high-level commission on quality and conduct broad, participatory, credible quality assessment, revealing quality issues to stakeholders and the general public through substantial dissemination and accessible presentation of information. • Establish a pool of funds to support, disseminate, and evaluate promising quality improvement initiatives in Brazilian hospitals; roll out initiatives that work. • Establish a national institutional infrastructure (agencies, staff, mandate, capability, resources, and leadership) to support (1) quality assessment, measurement, and research; (2) evidence-based medicine, including systematic review and dissemination of scientific evidence and best practices and development and implementation of clinical pathways; and (3) design and introduction of continuous quality improvement programs in hospitals. • Promote. through regulation and financial incentives, expanded development, implementation and use of clinical guidelines. • Create and enforce accountability mechanisms to foster quality assessment and improvement by linking hospital investment financing to compliance with licensure regulations; promoting quality-based purchasing, including accreditation incentives; and establishing a public reporting system on hospital quality performance. • Support continuous quality improvement at the facility level by creating a public–private program to provide training and technical assistance and to promote cross-hospital collaboration on clinical management and data-driven assessment. • Strengthen medical school curricula to support evidence-based practices, quality measurement and assessment, and use of information technologies.	Federal government takes lead, with strong stakeholder participation by professional associations, medical and nursing schools, research institutions, accreditation and quality certification organizations such as the ONA and the CQH, state licensure bodies, medical councils, and hospital associations.

| Strengthen the institutional environment for efficient resource use and effective performance management. | 12. Promote the effective use of information technologies to support performance and outcome measurement, cost collection and analysis, access to clinical information, clinical decision making, and coordination across medical care organizations and teams.
13. Support modernization of management structures and practices in public and SUS-financed private hospitals.
14. Develop a nationwide benchmarking and public report card system trained on efficiency and quality. | • Evaluate the impact and cost of information technologies used in public and private hospitals.
• Establish an information technology development policy and investment plan with the initial focus on provision of consistent and robust information on costs, quality, and case mix in hospitals; include investments in capacity building for information management and use, data collection, and analysis.
• Evaluate effects of promising managerial initiatives in public and private hospitals.
• Establish a pool of funds to support a public-private program to improve hospital management.
• Develop guidelines for use and allocation of human resources in hospital care.
• Develop and implement a national hospital benchmarking and report card system, preferably through an independent institute. | Collaborative effort, with participation by all levels of government, as well as universities (including management schools), research institutions, and private hospital associations. |

Source: Chapter 9 text.
Note: AIH, Autorização de Internação Hospitalar (Authorization for Hospitalization); CQH, Controle de Qualidade Hospitalar (Control of Hospital Quality); MS, Ministério da Saúde (Ministry of Health); ONA, Organização Nacional de Acreditação (National Accreditation Organization); SIA, Sistema de Informação Ambulatorial, (Ambulatory Care Information System); SUS, Sistema Único de Saúde (Unified Health System).

Notes

1. The authors were technical staff and consultants of the MS General Coordination for Hospital Care.
2. As described in this volume, the MS has followed up with policies and actions related to contracting and conversion of small hospitals.
3. The research for the current volume commenced in 2003 and was completed in December 2005. Preliminary results and policy recommendations were presented to the Minister of Health and his cabinet in June 2005.
4. These organizations are the National Accreditation Organization (Organização Nacional de Acreditação, ONA), the Brazilian Accreditation Consortium (Consórcio Brasileiro de Acreditação, CBA) and the Control of Hospital Quality (Controle de Qualidade Hospitalar, CQH) program.
5. Policy dimensions include structure and trends of the hospital system, resource allocation and utilization within hospitals, allocation of financial resources within the hospital sector, organizational and governance arrangements, management practices, and regulation and quality.
6. For example, policies in the United Kingdom endowed hospitals with more autonomous foundation trust status, based on explicit criteria related to management performance and information systems. This approach has come to be called "earned autonomy."
7. Similarly, the network design initiative should take into account the implications of any planned hospital governance reforms.
8. Among OECD countries, only the Scandinavian countries have such decentralized hospital ownership.
9. Hospitals serve patients from multiple municipalities, and this encourages duplication of capacity.
10. A master plan documents existing hospital sector supply, broken down by service lines or departments, as well as the planned evolution of supply. In social insurance health systems, reimbursement of services is usually limited to hospitals or departments included in the master plan. In Brazil, although each state is required to produce a master investment plan, the plans are often wish lists and are not based on analysis of future needs. Furthermore, investments that are not part of the plan often receive funding as a result of political pressure.
11. Examples are the systems used by the Canadian Agency for Drugs and Technology in Health and the National Institute for Health and Clinical Excellence (NICE) in the United Kingdom.
12. In Australia, Estonia, and Austria, plans also entailed reconfiguration of the hospital system, reducing the supply of hospitals and beds.

Bibliography

ACSQHC (Australian Council for Safety and Quality in Health Care). 2000. "Safety First: Report to the Australian Health Ministers' Conference." ACSQHC, Canberra. http://www.health.gov.au/internet/safety/publishing.nsf/Content/84DB8F909972B098CA2571C600154A80/$File/safetyfirst.pdf.

AHAMAC (Australian Health Ministers' Advisory Council). 1996. *The Final Report of the Taskforce on Quality in Australian Health Care.* Canberra: AHAMAC.

AHRQ (Agency for Healthcare Research and Quality). 2006. "Inpatient Quality Indicators Overview." AHRQ, Rockville, MD. http://www.qualityindicators.ahrq.gov/iqi_overview.htm.

Aiken, Linda H., Sean P. Clarke, and Douglas M. Sloane. 2002. "Hospital Staffing, Organization, and Quality of Care: Cross-National Findings." *International Journal for Quality in Health Care* 14 (1): 5–13.

Aiken, Linda H., J. Sochalski, and E. T. Lake. 1997. "Studying Outcomes of Organizational Change in Health Services." *Medical Care* 35 (11 Supp.): NS6–18.

Akashi, Daniela, Flávia K. Issa, Alexandre C. Pereira, Anna C. Tannuri, Daniele Q. Fucciolo, Maurício L. Lobato, Tatiana G. Galvão, Isabela M. Benseñor, and Paulo A. Lotufo. 1998. "Tratamento Anti-Hipertensivo. Prescrição e Custo Medicamentos. Pesquisa em Hospital Terciário." *Arquivos Brasileiros de Cardiologia.* 71 (1): 55–57.

Akhavan, Dariush. 2001. "Decentralization in the Administration of SUS—Strategic Issues in Northeastern Brazil." Consultant report for the World Bank, Brasília, DF.

Alba, T., J. Souders, and G. McGhee. 1994. "How Hospitals Can Use Internal Benchmark Data to Create Effective Managed Care Arrangements." *Managed Care Quarterly* 2 (2): 79–89.

Allsop, Judith, and Kathryn Jones. 2005. *Quality Assurance in Medical Regulation in an International Context.* Brayford Pool, Lincoln, UK: University of Lincoln, Department of Health. http://www.lincoln.ac.uk/policystudies/.

Almeida, P. G. 2001. "Estudo da Mortalidade Materna no Hospital das Clínicas da Faculdade de Medicina da Universidade São Paulo no período de 1986 a 1998." Master's thesis, University of São Paulo.

AMB (Associação Médica Brasileira). 2005. "Classificação Brasileira Hierarquizada de Procedimentos Médicos." AMB, São Paulo, SP. http://www.ramb.org.br/CBHPM_4_Edicao.pdf.

ANS (Agência Nacional de Saúde Suplementar). 2006a. "Caderno de Informação da Saúde Suplementar." ANS, Brasília, DF. http://www.ans.gov.br/portal/upload/informacoesss/caderno/informaca_06_2006.pdf (accessed October 8, 2006).

———. 2006b. "Caderno de Informação de Ressarcimento e Integração como o SUS." ANS, Brasília, DF. http://www.ans.gov.br/portal/upload/informacoesss/Caderno_Ressarcimento_Junho_2006.pdf (accessed October 8, 2006).

———. 2005. "Qualificação da Saúde Suplementar—Nova perspectiva no processo de regulação." ANS, Brasília, DF. http://www.ans.gov.br/portal/site/_qualificacao/pdf/texto_base.pdf (accessed December 12, 2005).

Arieta, C. E. L., M. A. Nascimento, R. P. C. Lira, et al. 2004. "Desperdício de exames complementares na avaliação pré-operatória em cirurgias de catarata". *Cadernos de Saúde Pública* 20 (1, January–February): 303–10.

Associação Paulista de Medicina and Conselho Regional de Medicina. 2001. *Programa de Controle da Qualidade do Atendimento Médico-Hospitalar: Manual de Orientação aos Hospitais Participantes.* São Paulo, SP; Rio de Janeiro, RJ; and Belo Horizonte, MG.

Audit Commission. 2000. "Getting Better All the Time: Making Benchmarking Work." Management Paper. Audit Commission, London. http://www.audit-commission.gov.uk/products/guidance/ 80DDA381-E506-4769-9ED2-7E9DDD4D7C4B/archive_mpgettin.pdf.

Auton, G. M. 1994. "Using Benchmarking Techniques to Improve Efficiency and Quality in Cardiology Services, Part One." *Journal of Cardiovascular Management* 5 (2): 16–18, 20–21.

Axene, D. V., and Susan J. McQuillian. 1999. *Analysis of Potentially Avoidable Inpatient Services.* Research Paper, Milliman and Robertson, Radnor, PA.

Banker, R. D., Abraham Charnes, and William Cooper. 1984. "Models for Estimating Technical and Scale Efficiencies in Data Envelopment Analysis." *Management Science* 30 (9): 1078–92.

Barbosa, Pedro R. 2007. "Fundações Estatais: Um Novo Modelo de Gestão para as Organizações Públicas de Saúde." Presented at QUALIHSAP, São Paulo, SP, May 4.

Barbosa, Pedro R., Margareth Crisóstomo Portela, Maria Alicia Dominguez Ugá, Migule Murat Vasconcellos, Sheyla Maria Lemos Lima, and Silvia Victoria Gerschman. 2002. Hospitais Filantrópicos no Brasil, vols. 1, 2, and 3. Rio de Janeiro: Banco Nacional de Desenvolvimento Econômico e Social.

Barboza, Denise Beretta, and Zaida Aurora Sperli Geraldes Soler. 2003. "Nursing Absenteeism: Occurrences at a University Hospital." *Revista Latino-Americana de Enfermagem* 11(2, March–April): 177–183.

Barclay, T. S., and K. S. Patterson. 1998. "An Introduction to Diagnosis-Based Risk Adjusters." Research Report, Milliman and Robertson, Radnor, PA.

Barnum, H., and Joseph Kutzin. 1993. *Public Hospitals in Developing Countries: Resource Use, Cost, Financing.* Baltimore, MD: Johns Hopkins University Press for the World Bank.

Barnum, H., Joseph Kutzin, and Helen Saxenian. 1995. "Incentives and Provider Payment Methods." Human Resources Development and Operations Policy Working Paper 51, World Bank, Washington, DC.

Barros, Fernando C., Cesar G. Victora, and Bernardo L. Horta. 2001. "Ethnicity and Infant Health in Southern Brazil: A Birth Cohort Study." *International Journal of Epidemiology* 30: 1001–8.

Berman, B., Lisa Arellanes, Pamela Henderson, and Alessandro Magnoli. 1999. "Health Care Financing in Eight Latin American and Caribbean Nations: The First Regional National Health Accounts Network." In *Partnerships for Health Reform.* Bethesda, MD: Abt Associates, Partnerships for Health Reform. http://www.phrproject.com.

Bibbee, Alexandra, and Flavio Padrini. 2006. "Balancing Health Care Quality and Cost Containment: The Case of Norway." Economics Department Working Paper 482, Organization for Economic Cooperation and Development, Paris.

Birkmeyer, John D., Therese A. Stukel, Andrea E. Siewers, Philip P. Goodney, David E. Wennberg, and F. Lee Lucas. 2003. "Surgeon Volume and Operative Mortality in the United States." *New England Journal of Medicine* 349: 2117–27.

Bitrán, R., and Winnie C. Yip. 1998. "A Review of Health Care Provider Payment Reform in Selected Countries in Asia and Latin America." Major Applied Research 2, Working Paper 1, Partnerships for Health Reform, Abt Associates, Bethesda, MD.

Bitrán, R., C. Má, and P. Gómez. 2005. "The San Miguelito Hospital Reform in Panama: Evaluation and Lessons." In *Health System Innovations in Central America*, ed. Gerard M. La Forgia, 89–108. Washington, DC: World Bank.

Bloom, Abby L., and Annette Achimiede. 2004. "The International Experience with Hospital Services Conversion, Australia." Draft, Karolinska Institutet, Stockholm.

Blumen, Abrão. 2004. "Difilculdades e Benefícios dos Programas de Qualidade Implementados em Hospitais Selados pelo Controle de Qualidade Hospitalar—CQH." In *Hospitais—Administração da Qualidade e Acreditação de Orgazanições Complexas*, ed. Antônio Quinto Neto and Olímpio J. N. V. Bittar, 81–98. Porto Alegre, RS: Dacasa Editora.

Bogan, Christopher E., and Michael J. English. 1994. *Benchmarking for Best Practices: Winning through Innovative Adaptation.* New York: McGraw-Hill.

Bogue, Richard, Claude H. Hall, and Gerard M. La Forgia. 2007. "Hospital Governance in Latin America: Results from a Four Nation Survey." HNP Discussion Paper, World Bank, Washington, DC.

Bohomol, E. 2003. "Erros de medicação: causas e fatores desencadeantes sob a ótica da equipe de enfermagem." Master's thesis, Universidade Federal de São Paulo, Escola Paulista de Medicina, Enfermagem, São Paulo, SP.

Boland, Tony, and Alan Fowler. "A Systems Perspective of Performance Management in Public Sector Organizations." *International Journal of Public Sector Management* 13 (5): 417–46. http://www.emerald-library.com.

Borba, Amariles de Souza, Maria Rosália Ribeiro, and Nadir do Nascimento Nogueira. 2001. "Análise Situacional da Assistência Obstétrica e Perinatal em Maternidades de Teresina." Consultant report, United Nations Children's Fund (UNICEF), Brasília, DF.

Bowlin, W. F., Abraham Charnes, William Cooper, and H. David Sherman. 1985. "Data Development Analysis and Regression Approaches to Efficiency Estimation and Evaluation." *Annals of Operations Research* 2: 113–38.

Boyce, N., J. McNeil, D. Graves, and D. Dunt. 1997. *Quality & Outcome Indicators for Acute Healthcare Services.* Report for the Department of Health and Family Services, Canberra: Australian Government Publishing Service.

Bresser-Pereira, Luiz Carlos. 2003. "The 1995 Public Management Reforms in Brazil: Reflections of a Reformer." In *Reinventing Leviathan: The Politics of Administrative Reform in Developing Countries*, ed. Ben Ross Schneider and Blanca Heredia, 89–109. Miami, FL: North-South Center Press.

———. 1998. "As Organizações Sociais." *Reforma do Estado para a Cidadania*. São Paulo, SP: Editora 34.

Brosi, J., Rachel Portelli, Joanne Williams, Brian T. Collopy, and L. Reti. 1997. *Measurement of Care in Australian Hospitals.* Vol. 3. Sydney: Australian Council on Healthcare Standards.

Bueno, Ronaldo, R. Loures, and M. C. Pieruccini. 2004. *Abertura de Escolas de Medicina no Brasil. Relatório de um Cenário Sombrio.* Diretoria da Associação Médica Brasileira and Diretoria do Conselho Federal de Medicina. São Paulo: Associação Médica Brasileira.

Bullivant, R. 1996. "Benchmarking in the UK National Health Service." *International Journal of Health Care Quality Assurance* 9 (2): 9–14.

Burgess J. F., Jr., and Paul W. Wilson. 1996. "Hospital Ownership and Technical Inefficiency." *Management Science* 42 (1): 110.

———. 1993. "Technical Efficiency in Veterans Administration Hospitals." In *The Measurement of Productive Efficiency—Techniques and Applications*, eds. H. Fried, K. Lovell, and S. Schmidt, 335–51. New York: University Press.

CAHSA (Comissão de Avaliação dos HH SA). 2006."Resultados da Avaliação dos Hospitais S.A." Presentation, Ministério de Saúde, Lisbon. http://www.min-saude.pt/portal/conteudos/a+saude+em+portugal/publicacoes/estudos/cahsa.htm.

Calil, Jorge Said. 2004. "Situação dos hospitais brasileiros—Panorama da distribuição e dos custos de e manutenção de (alguns) equipamentos médicos para diagnóstico." Prepared for presentation at Centro de Engenharia Biomédica (CEB)/UNICAMP, Campinas, SP.

Calvo, M. F. 2002. "Hospitais Públicos e Privados no Sistema Único de Saúde do Brasil: O Mito da Eficiência Privada no Estado de Mato Grosso em 1998." PhD dissertation, Universidade Federal de Santa Catarina, Florianópolis, Brazil.

Caminal, J., Barbara Starfield, Emilia Sánchez, et al. 2004. "The Role of Primary Care in Preventing Ambulatory Care Sensitive Conditions." *European Journal of Public Health* 14: 246–51.

Caminal, J., Emilia Sánchez, Mariângela Morales, Rosana Peiró, and Soledad Márquez. 2002. "Avances en España en la Investigación con el Indicador 'Hospitalización por Enfermedades Sensibles a Cuidados de Atención Primaria.'" *Revista Española de Salud Pública* 76: 189–96.

Carvalho, F. M., M. R. Widmer, M. Cruz, V. Palomo, and C. Cruz. 1991. "Diagnóstico Clínico Versus Autopsia." *Boletin de la Oficina Sanitaria Panamericana* 110 (3): 213–18.

Cashin, C., Yevgenyi Samyshkin, and Sheila O'Dougherty. 2005. "Case-Based Hospital Payment Systems: A Step-By-Step Guide for Design and Implementation in Low- and Middle-Income Countries." Consultant report for United States Agency for International Development (USAID), Abt Associates, Bethesda, MD.

Castaño, Ramón, Ricardo Bitrán, and Ursula Giedion. 2004. "Monitoring and Evaluating Hospital Autonomization and Its Effects on Priority Health Services." Consultant report, Partners for Health Reform*plus* (PHR*plus*), Abt Associates, Bethesda. MD.

Castelar, R. M., Patrick Mordelet, and Victor Grabois. 1995. "Gestão hospitalar: um desafio para o hospital brasileiro." Escola Nacional de Saúde Pública (ENSP), Rio de Janeiro.

Castro, M. S. M., Claudia Travassos, and Marilia S. Carvalho. 2002. "Fatores associados às internações hospitalares no Brasil." *Ciência & Saúde Coletiva* 7 (4): 795–811.

CDC (Centers for Disease Control and Prevention). 2000. "Hospital Infections Cost U.S. Billions of Dollars Annually." CDC, Atlanta, GA. http://www.cdc.gov/od/oc/media/pressrel/r2k0306b.htm.

Cecílio, Luiz Carlos de Oliveira, ed. 1994. *Inventando a mudança na saúde.* São Paulo: Hucitec.

Charlson, M. E., P. Pompei, K. L. Ales, and C. R. McKenzie. 1987. "A New Method of Classifying Prognostic Comorbity in Longitudinal Studies: Development and Validation." *Journal of Chronic Diseases* 40: 373–83.

Charnes, A., William Cooper, and E. Rhodes. 1978. "Measuring Efficiency of Decision Making Units." *European Journal of Operational Research* 3: 429–44.

Chassin, Mark R. 2002. "Achieving and Sustaining Improved Quality: Lessons from New York State and Cardiac Surgery." *Health Affairs* 21 (4): 40–51.

———. 1997. "Assessing Strategies for Quality Improvement." *Health Affairs* 16 (3): 151–61.

Chaudhury, Nazmul, Jeffrey Hammer, Michael Kremer, Karthik Muralidharan, and Halsey Rogers. 2006. "Missing in Action: Teacher and Health Worker Absence in Developing Countries." *Journal of Economic Perspectives* 20 (1): 91–116.

Chawla, Mukesh, Ramesh Govindaraj, Peter Berman, and Jack Needleman. 1996. "Improving Hospital Performance through Policies to Increase Hospital Autonomy." Consultant report for United States Agency for International Development (USAID), Harvard University, Cambridge, MA.

CHC (Consorci Hospitlalari de Catalunha). n.d. "La reinvención del Hospital." Consultant report for CHC, Barcelona.

Chiyoshi, F. Y. 1989. "O Sistema de Assistencia Medico-Hospitalar da Previdencia Social." Presented at II Congresso Brasileiro de Saúde Coletiva, São Paulo, July 3–7.

Chiyoshi, F., and A. Moura. 1989. "O Sistema de Assistência Médico-Hospitalar da Prevedência Social (SAMHPS)—Sistema AIH." Informally published.

CIHI (Canadian Institute for Health Information). 2005. *Health Care in Canada 2005.* Ottawa: CIHI.

Coelli, T., D. S. Prasada Rao, and George E. Battese. 1999. *An Introduction to Efficiency and Productivity Analysis.* Boston,. MA: Kluwer Academic Publishers.

Cohn, A., and P. Elias. 1999. *O Público e o Privado na Saúde.* São Paulo, SP: Pan American Health Organization.

Coile, R. 1994. *The New Governance: Strategies for an Era of Health Reform.* Ann Arbor, MI: Health Administration Press.

Collins, David, Grace Njeru, and Julius Meme. 1996. "Hospital Autonomy in Kenya: The Experience of Kenyatta National Hospital." Consultant report for United States Agency for International Development (USAID), Management Sciences for Health, Boston, MA.

CMS (Centers for Medicare and Medicaid Services). 2002. "Cost of Caring: Key Drivers of Growth in Spending on Hospital Care." PriceWaterhouseCoopers for American Hospital Association, Washington, DC.

Comissão de Seguridade Social e Familia (Congressional Commission on Social Security and Family Affairs). 2004. "Relatório 2004," 33–34. http://www2.camara.gov.br/internet/comissoes/cssf/relatorio.html/relatoriofinal2004.pdf.

Commonwealth Department of Health and Aged Care, National Expert Advisory Group on Safety and Quality in Australian Health Care. 1999. *Implementing Safety and Quality Enhancement in Health Care: National Actions to Support Quality and Safety Improvement in Australian Health Care.* Canberra: Commonwealth Department of Health and Aged Care.

CONASS (Conselho Nacional de Secretários de Saúde). 2006. *SUS: Avanços e Desafios.* Brasília, DF: CONASS.

———. 2005. "Programa de Reestruturação e Contratualização dos Hospitais Filantrópicos do SUS." Technical Note, CONASS, Brasília, DF.

———. 2003a. *A Saúde na Opinião dos Brasileiros.* Brasília, DF: CONASS.

———. 2003b. *Legislação do SUS.* Brasília, DF: CONASS.

Conselho Federal de Medicina. 2006. "Sistema de Processos Ético Profissional." Brasília, DF. http://www.portalmedico.org.br (accessed April 27, 2006).

Considera, C. M., Heloíza Valverde Filgueiras, Antonio Braz Oliveira e Silva, Carlos César B. Sobral, and Adriene Zaeyen. 1995. *Economia Política da Saúde: Uma Perspectiva Quantitativa*. Série Economia e Financiamento 5. Brasília, DF: Pan American Health Organization, Brazil Representation Office.

Cooper, W. W., Lawrence M. Seiford, and Kaoru Tone. 2002. *Data Envelopment Analysis—A Comprehensive Text with Models, Applications, References and DEA-Solver Software*. Boston, MA; Dordrect, Netherlands: Kluwer Academic Publishers.

Corden, Simon. 2003. "Autonomous Hospitals Become a Commercial Network: Hospital Rationalization in Victoria, Australia." In *Innovations in Health Service Delivery: The Corporatization of Public Hospitals*, ed. Alexander Preker and April Harding, 345–90. Washington, DC: World Bank.

Costa, I. C., S. Hinrichsen, J. L. Alves, M. Batista Jucá, B. Alves da Silva, and S. da Costa Albuquerque. 2003. "Prevalência e Custos de Processos Infecciosos em Unidade de Terapia Intensiva." *Revista de Administração em Saúde* 5 (20): 7–16.

Costa, José Orleans, César Coelho Xavier, Fernando Augusto Proietti, and Margarida S. Delgado. 2004. "Avaliação dos Recursos Hospitalares para Assistência Perinatal em Belo Horizonte, Minas Gerais." *Saúde Publica* 38 (5): 701–8.

Costa, Nilson do Rosário, and José Mendes R. 2005. "Estudo Comparativo do Desempenho de Hospitais em Regime de Organização Social." FIOCRUZ/ENSP, consultant report for World Bank, Rio de Janeiro, RJ.

Couttolenc, B. F., Alexandre C. Nicolella, Carlos A. Machado, Paulo Zapparoli, and Leni H. de S. Dias. 2005. "Estudo sobre gasto hospitalar no Brazil. Em busca da excelência: Fortalecendo o desempenho hospitalar no Brasil." Consultant report for World Bank, São Paulo, SP.

Couttolenc, B. F., Leni H. de S. Dias, Alexandre C. Nicolella, Shahbaz Fatheazam, and Carlos A. Machado. 2004. "Estudo de custos, eficiência e mecanismos de pagamento, Fase II: eficiência e mecanismos de pagamento. Em busca da excelência: Fortalecendo o desempenho hospitalar no Brasil." Consultant report for World Bank, São Paulo, SP.

CQH (Controle de Qualidade Hospitalar). 2003. *Manual de Gestão Hospitalar do CQH: Livro de Casos Práticos*. São Paulo, SP; Rio de Janeiro, RJ; Belo Horizonte, MG: CQH.

CREMESP (Conselho Regional de Medicina do Estado de São Paulo). 2007. "Exame do CRESMESP, 2007." *Jornal do CREMESP*. http://www.cremesp.org.br/?siteAcao=salaimprensa&id=190. (accessed December 7, 2007)

———. 2005. "Série SUS: A crise nas santas casas do Estado de São Paulo." *Jornal do CREMESP*. http://www.cremesp.org.br (accessed April 10, 2006).

———. 2004a. "Avaliação das Condições de Funcionamento dos Hospitais e Prontos-Socorros. 2001–2003." CREMESP, São Paulo.

———. 2004b. "Médicos Denunciados Segundo Número de Denúncias." *Jornal do CREMESP*. http://www.cremesp.org.br/?siteAcao=JornalCremesp2&pag=grafico05&req=sim.

———. 2002 "Mercado de Trabalho Médico no Estado de São Paulo." CREMESP, São Paulo.

———. 2000. "Avaliação dos Serviços de Assistência ao Parto e ao Neonato no Estado de São Paulo." CREMESP, São Paulo.

Dalmau-Matarrodona, E., and J. Puig-Junoy. 1996. "Market Structure and Hospital Efficiency: Evaluating Potential Effects of Deregulation in a National Health Service." Presented at the International Health Economics Association Conference, Vancouver, BC, Canada, May.

Das, Jishnu, and Jeffrey Hammer. 2005. "Money for Nothing: The Dire Straits of Medical Practice in Delhi, India." Policy Research Working Paper 3669, World Bank, Washington, DC.

Daucourt, Valentin, and Philippe Michel. 2003. "Results of the First 100 Accreditation Procedures in France." *International Journal for Quality in Health Care* 15 (6): 463–71.

De Matos, A. 2002. "Apuração dos custos de Procedimentos hospitalares: Alta e média complexidade." Relatório do projeto REFORSUS 003/99. Consultant report for Ministério da Saúde, PLANISA, São Paulo, SP.

den Exter, Andre P. 2005. "Purchasers as the Public's Agent." In *Purchasing to Improve Health Systems Performance*, ed. Josep Figueras, Ray Robinson, and Elke Jabubowski, 122–39. Buckingham, UK: Open University Press.

Department of Health. 2000. "An Organization with Memory: Report of an Expert Group on Learning from Adverse Events in the NHS." Stationery Office, London.

———. 1998. "A First Class Service: Quality in the National Health Service." Stationery Office, London.

———. 1997. "The New National Health Service: Modern and Dependable." Stationery Office, London.

Department of Human Services. 1997. "Performance Indicators: Paper prepared for Acute Health Quality Committee." Department of Human Services, Victoria, Australia.

Desai, J., P. J. O'Connor, and D. B. Bishop. 1997. "Variation in Process and Outcomes of Diabetes Care in HMO Owned and Controlled Clinics." *Proceedings*, Centers for Disease Control (CDC) Diabetes Translation Conference, Atlanta, GA, February. Atlanta, GA: CDC.

Dias, L. H. de S., Bernard F. Couttolenc, and Afonso J. De Matos. 2004. "Estudo de custos, eficiência e mecanismos de pagamento, Fase I: Análise de custos de procedimentos hospitalares. Em busca da excelência: Fortalecendo o desempenho hospitalar no Brasil." Consultant report for World Bank, São Paulo, SP.

D'Innocenzo, M. 2001. "Indicativo de qualidade dos recursos humanos de enfermagem das unidades de clínica médica de hospitais de ensino e universidades." PhD dissertation, Universidade Federal de São Paulo, Escola Paulista de Medicina, Enfermagem, São Paulo.

Dlugacz, Yosef D., Andrea Restifo, and Alice Greenwood. 2004. *The Quality Handbook for Health Care Organizations*. San Francisco, CA: Jossey-Bass.

Docteur, E., and Howard Oxley. 2003. "Health Care Systems: Lessons from the Reform Experience." Economics Department Working Papers 374, OECD, Paris.

Donabedian, A. 1980. *Explorations in Quality Assessment and Monitoring*. Vol. 1: *The Definition of Quality and Approaches to Its Assessment*. Ann Arbor, MI: Health Administration Press.

Donahue, K. Tina, and Paul van Ostenberg. 2000. "Joint Commission International Accreditation: Relationship to Four Models of Evaluation." *International Journal for Quality in Health Care* 12 (3): 243–46.

DREES (Direction de la recherche, des études, de l'évaluation et des statistiques)/Ministère de l'Emploi, du travail et de la cohésion sociale/Ministère de la Santé et de la protection sociale. 2005. "Données sur la Situation Sanitaire et Sociale en France en 2004—Annexe A au projet de loi de financement de la Sécurité Sociale en 2005." Paris.

Dubois, Carl-Ardy, Martin McKee, and Ellen Nolte. 2006. *Human Resources for Health in Europe*. Berkshire, UK: Open University Press.

Dudley, R. A., A. Frolich, D. L. Robinowitz, J. A. Talavera, P. Broadhead, and H. S. Luft. 2004. *Strategies to Support Quality-Based Purchasing: A Review of the Evidence*. Technical Review 10. AHRQ Pub. 04-P024. Rockville, MD: Agency for Healthcare Research and Quality.

Eid, F. 2003. "Understanding Good Institutional Design in Hospital Corporatization: A Decision Rights Approach." Working Paper 2028, American University of Beirut. http://www.erf.org.eg/uploadpath/pdf/2028.pdf.

Englert, Jan, Kenneth M. Davis, and Karen E. Koch. 2001. "Using Clinical Practice Analysis to Improve Care." *Joint Commission Journal on Quality and Patient Safety* 27 (6): 291–301.

Eriksson, Pär, Vinod Diwan, and Ingvar Karlberg. 2001. *Health Sector Reforms: What about Hospitals?* Göteborg, Sweden: World Health Organization.

Ersoy, K., S. Kavuncubasi, Y. A. Ozcan, and J. M. Harris II. 1997. "Technical Efficiencies of Turkish Hospitals: DEA Approach." *Journal of Medical Systems* 21 (2): 67–74.

Farrell, M. J. 1957. "The Measure of Productive Efficiency." *Journal of the Royal Statistical Society* 120 (III): 243–81.

Federation of State Medical Boards. 2006. "Trends in Physician Regulation." Federation of State Medical Boards, Dallas, TX. http://www.fsmb.org.

Federighi, Waldomiro, and J. Pedroso. 2002. "Absenteísmo em Hospitais." *O Mundo da Saúde* 1: 283–94.

FEHOSP (Federação das Santas Casas e Hospitais Beneficentes do Estado de São Paulo). n.d. "Panorama das Santas Casas e Hospitais Beneficentes." FEHOSP, São Paulo, SP. http://www.fehosp.com.br/index.php?option=com_content&task=view&id=/38&Itemid=27.

Ferraz, Marcos Bosi. 2006. "Reconciling 21st Century Temptations with 20th Century Resources and Problems." *British Medical Journal* 332 (April 8): 861.

Ferreira, Regina Moreira. 1999. "Tumores do sistema nervoso central: fatores prognósticos relacionados a sobrevida em crianças e adolescentes em duas coortes hospitalares". PhD dissertation, Fundação Oswaldo Cruz, Escola Nacional de Saúde Pública, Rio de Janeiro, RJ.

Ferreira, Walter Cintra, Jr. 2004. "Gerenciamento de Hospitais Estaduais Paulistas: Estudo comparativo entre a administração direta e as organizações sociais de saúde." Master's thesis, Fundação Getúlio Vargas, Escola de Administração de Empresas de São Paulo.

Fidler, Armin H., Reinhard R. Haslinger, Maria M. Hofmarcher, Maris Jesse, and Tomas Palu. 2007. "Incorporation of Public Hospitals: A 'Silver Bullet' against Overcapacity, Managerial Bottlenecks and Resource Constraints? Case Studies from Austria and Estonia." *Health Policy* 81: 328–38.

Fiedler, John, and Gerard La Forgia. 2005. "The Nicaraguan Social Security Health Insurance Scheme—A Promising Work in Progress." In *Health System Innovations in Central America: Lessons and Impact of New Approaches*, ed. Gerard La Forgia, 135–72. Washington, DC: World Bank.

Figueras, Josep, Ray Robinson, and Elke Jakubowski, eds. 2005. *Purchasing to Improve Health System Performance.* Buckingham, UK: Open University Press.

Finkler, M. D., and D. D. Wirtschafter. 1993. "Cost-Effectiveness and Data Envelopment Analysis." *Health Care Management Review* 18 (3): 81–88.

FIPE (Fundação Instituto de Pesquisas Econômicas da USP). 1994. "Proposta de um novo modelo para a saúde." FIPE/Universidade de São Paulo.

Garcia Rosa, Maria Luiza Garcia, and Virginia Alonso Hortale. 2000. "Óbitos Perinatais Evitáveis e Estrutura de Atendimento Obstétrico na Rede Pública: Estudo de Caso de um Município da Região Metropolitana do Rio de Janeiro." *Cadernos de Saúde Pública* 16 (3): 773–83.

Gastal, Fábio Leite, Gerard La Forgia, Jaqueline K. Gonçalves, Juliana C. Melo, Laura P. Siqueira, and Tany M. Soares. 2005a. "Qualidade em Saúde e Acreditação no Brasil—Experiências Acumuladas, Análise Crítica e Resultados." Consultant report for World Bank and Organização Nacional de Acreditação, Brasília, DF.

———. 2005b. "O Cenário da Acreditação e da Gestão da Qualidade nos Hospitais Brasileiros: Avanços, Experiências, Resultados, Problemas e Perspectivas." Consultant report for World Bank and Organização Nacional de Acreditação, Brasília, DF.

Gaynor, M., and Gerard F. Anderson. 1991. "Hospital Costs and the Cost of Empty Hospital Beds." NBER Working Paper 3872, National Bureau of Economic Research, Cambridge, MA.

Giardi, Sabado Nicolau, and Maria Elizabeth Barros. 2001. "Rede Hospitalar Filantrópica no Brasil: Perfil Histórico-Institucional e Oferta de Serviços." Consultant report for Ministerio de Saúde (REFORSUS Project), Brasília, DF.

Gift, Robert G., and Doug Mosel. 1994. *Benchmarking in Health Care: A Collaborative Approach.* Chicago, IL: American Hospital Association (AHA).

Gittell, J. H., K. M. Fairfield, B. Bierbaum, W. Head, R. Jackson, M. Kelly, R, Laskin, S. Lipson, J. Siliki, T. Thornhill, and J. Zukerman. 2000. "Impact of Relational Coordination on Quality of Care, Postoperative Pain and Functioning, and Length of Stay: A Nine-Hospital Study of Surgical Patients." *Medical Care* 38 (8): 807–19.

Gohlke, A. 1997. "Benchmark for Strategic Performance Improvement." *Information Outlook* 1 (8): 22–24.

Gomes, U.A., A. A Silva, H. Bettiol, and M.A Barbieri. 1999. "Risk Factors for the Increasing Caesarean Section Rate in Southeast Brazil: A Comparison of Two Birth Cohorts, 1978–1979 and 1994." *International Journal of Epidemiology* 28 (4, August): 687–94.

Gouveia, C. S. D. 1996. "Tendências recentes na assistência hospitalar no estado do RJ 1992–1995." Master's thesis, Fundação Oswaldo Cruz (FIOCRUZ). Rio de Janeiro.

Govindaraj, Ramesh, and Mukesh Chawla. 1996. "Recent Experiences with Hospital Autonomy in Developing Countries—What Can We Learn?" Consultant report for United States Agency for International Development (USAID), Data for Decision-Making Project, Harvard University, Cambridge, MA.

Govindaraj, Ramesh, A. A. D. Obuobi, N. K. A. Enymayew, P. Atwi, and S. Ofosu-Amaah. 1996. "Hospital Autonomy in Ghana: The Experience of Korle Bu and Komfo Anokye Teaching Hospitals." Consultant report for United States Agency for International Development (USAID), Data for Decision-Making Project, Harvard University, Cambridge, MA.

Grassetti, L., E. Gori, and R. Bellio. 2003. "Efficiency Estimation of Hospital Services: A Survey and Multilevel Developments." University of Naples, Department of Mathematics and Statistics. Paper presented at Intermedio SIS, 2001, Plenary Session on Multivariate Statistical Analysis for Social, Economic, and Natural Science and Technology, Naples, November.

Griffin, S., and A. L. Kinmouth. 1998. *Diabetes Care: The Effectiveness of Systems for Routine Surveillance for People with Diabetes.* Oxford, UK: Cochrane Library.

Grosskopf, S., and Vivian Valdmanis. 1987. "Measuring Hospital Performance. A Non-Parametric Approach." *Journal of Health Economics* 6 (2): 89–107.

Grosskopf, S., Dimitris Margaritis, and Vivian Valdmanis. 2001. "The Effects of Teaching on Hospital Productivity." *Socio-Economic Planning Sciences* 35: 189–204.

Gruca, T. S., and Deepika Nath. 2001. "The Technical Efficiency of Hospitals under a Single Payer System: The Case of Ontario Community Hospitals." *Health Care Management Science* 4 (2): 91–101.

Guichard, Stéphanie. 2004. *The Reform of the Health Care System in Portugal.* Economics Department Working Paper 405, Organisation for Economic Co-operation and Development, Paris. http://www.oecd.org/eco.

Hagen, Terje P., and Oddvar M. Kaarbøe. 2004. "The Norwegian Hospital Reform of 2002: Central Government Takes Over Ownership of Public Hospitals." Health Organization Research Norway (HORN) Working Paper 2004: 1, University of Oslo.

Halm, Ethan A., Clara Lee, and Mark R. Chassin. 2002. "Is Volume Related to Outcome in Health Care? A Systematic Review and Methodologic Critique of the Literature." *Annals of Internal Medicine* 137: 511–20.

Ham, Chris, and Loraine Hawkins. 2003. "Implementing Organizational Reforms to Hospitals in the Public Sector." In *Innovations in Health Service Delivery: The Corporatization of Public Hospitals*, ed. Alexander Preker and April Harding, 79–104. Washington, DC: World Bank.

Harding, April, and Alexander Preker. 2003. "A Conceptual Framework for the Organizational Reforms of Hospitals." In *Innovations in Health Service Delivery: The Corporatization of Public Hospitals*, ed. Alexander Preker and April Harding, 23–78. Washington, DC: World Bank.

Harvard Medical International. 1998. "Health Reform in the Municipality of São Paulo, Brazil: Public Finance and Private Provision." Consultant report to Municipality of São Paulo, Harvard Medical International, Brookline, MA.

Hay, J. 2002. "Hospital Cost Drivers: An Evaluation of State-Level Data." Report for the National Association of Health Underwriters, Arlington, VA.

Heerey, M., and E. Necochea. 2005. "An Overview of Accreditation and Certification for Improving Health Service Quality." Johns Hopkins University, Baltimore, MD. http://www.jhuccp.org/quality/accredit.shtm1.

Hewitt, Maria, and Joseph V. Simone, eds. 1999. *Ensuring Quality Cancer Care.* Washington, DC: National Academy Press. http://www.nap.edu/catalog.php?record_id=6467#toc.

Hibbard, J. H., J. Stockard, and M. Tusler. 2003. "Does Publicizing Hospital Performance Stimulate Quality Improvement Efforts?" *Health Affairs* 22 (2): 84–94.

Higgins, I. 1997. "Benchmarking in Health Care: A Review of the Literature." *Australian Health Review* 20 (4): 60–69.

Holanda, M. C., Francis C. Petterini, and André G. Nogueira. 2004. "O SUS no Ceará: avaliação de eficiência técnica nos municípios." Texto para Discussão 13, Governo do Estado do Ceará/SEPLAN/IPECE, Fortalellza, CE.

Hsia, C. D., W. Mark Krushat, A. B. Fagan, J. A. Tebbut, and R. P. Kusserow. 1988. "Accuracy of Diagnostic Coding for Medicare Patients under the Prospective-Payment System." *New England Journal of Medicine* 318: 352–55.

Hurst, Jeremy, and Melissa Jee-Hughes. 2001. "Performance Measurement and Performance Management in OECD Health Systems." OECD Directorate for Employment, Labour, and Social Affairs, OECD Labour Market and Social Policy Occasional Paper 47, Organisation for Economic Co-operation and Development, Paris.

Huskamp, H. A., and Joseph P. Newhouse. 1999. "Future Directions for the National Health Accounts." *Health Care Financing Review* 21 (2): 5–13.

Ibern, Pere. 1998. "Innovation in Organization of Health Service Delivery: Case Study: Spain." Consultant report, National Economic Research Associates, Madrid.

IBGE (Instituto Brasileiro de Geografia e Estatística). 2005. *Pesquisa Nacional por Amostra de Domicílios: Acesso e Utilização de Serviços de Saúde 2003.* Rio de Janeiro: IBGE.

——. 2004a. *Pesquisa de Orçamentos Familiares 2002–2003.* Rio de Janeiro: IBGE.

——. 2004b. *Projeção da População do Brasil por Sexo e Idade para o Período 1980–2050, Revisão 2004.* Rio de Janeiro: IBGE, Diretoria de Pesquisas, Coordenação de População e Indicadores Sociais, Gerência de Estudos e Análises da Dinâmica Demográfica.

——. 2004c. *Pesquisa Nacional por Amostragem de Domicílios 2003.* Rio de Janeiro: IBGE.

——. 2003. *Estatísticas da Saúde—Assistência Médico Sanitária 2002.* Rio de Janeiro: IBGE.

——. 2000a. *Estatísticas da Saúde—Assistêncioa Médica-Sanitária 1998.* Rio de Janeiro: IBGE.

——. 2000b. *Pesquisa Nacional por Amostra de Domicílios (PNAD): Acesso e Utilização de Serviços de Saúde 1998.* Rio de Janeiro: IBGE.

Ichnose, R. M., and R. T. Almeida. 2001. "Desmistificando a Certificação e a Acreditação de Hospitais." Presented at II Congresso Latinoamericano de Engenharia Biomédica, Havana, May 23–25. http://www.hab2001.sld.cu/.

IHBF (International Hospital Benchmarking Forum). 2005. "International Hospital Benchmarking Forum," Centrum für Krankenhaus-Management, Münster, Germany. http://www.hospital-benchmarking.de/conpresso/ihbf_start/index.php (accessed May 15, 2005).

IHI (Institute for Healthcare Improvement). 2007. "Getting Started Kit: Prevent Surgical Site Infections: How-To Guide." IHI, Cambridge, MA.

——. 2006. "Patient Safety." IHI, Cambridge, MA. http://www.ihi.org/IHI/Topicos/PatientSafety/SurgicalSiteINfections/Changes/.

Ingenix. 2007. "HospitalBenchmarks.com." http://www.hospitalbenchmarks.com.

IOM (Institute of Medicine). 2001. *Crossing the Quality Chasm: A New Health System for the 21st Century.* Washington, DC: National Academy Press.

——. 2000. *To Err is Human: Building a Safer Health System,* eds. Linda T. Kohn, Janet M. Corrigan, and Molla S. Donaldson. Washington, DC: National Academy Press.

——. 1999. *Ensuring Quality Cancer Care,* eds. Maria Hewitt and Joseph V. Simone. Washington, DC: National Academy Press.

IPEA (Instituto de Pesquisas Econômicas Aplicadas). 2001. *Tendências do Sistema de Saúde Brasileiro.* Estudo Delpi. Brasília, DF: IPEA.

IPEA (Instituto de Pesquisas Econômicas Aplicadas) and PNUD (Programa das Nações Unidas para o Desenvolvimento). 2000. *Atlas do Desenvolvimento Humano no Brasil.* Brasília, DF: IPEA.

Jacobs, R. 2001. "Alternative Methods to Examine Hospital Efficiency: Data Envelopment Analysis and Stochastic Frontier Analysis." In *Health Care Management Science* 4: 103–15.

Jakab, M., A. S. Preker, A. Harding, and L. Hawkins. 2002. "The Introduction of Market Forces in the Public Hospital Sector." HNP Discussion Paper, World Bank, Washington, DC.

JCAHO (Joint Commission on Accreditation of Healthcare Organizations). 2005. *Comprehensive Accreditation Manual for Integrated Delivery Systems.* Oakbrook Terrace, IL: JCAHO.

——. 1990. *Primer on Indicator Development & Application.* Oakbrook Terrace, IL: JCAHO.

Kamwanga, J., K. Hanson, B. McPake, and O. Mungule. 2003. "Autonomous Hospitals in Zambia and the Equity Implications of the Market for Hospital Services." Consultant report to Ministry of Health, Republic of Zambia. London School of Hygiene and Tropical Medicine, London.

Kanamura, Alberto H. 2006. "Organizações Sociais e Parcerias Público Privadas." *Debates GV (Gertulio Vargas) Saúde* 1 (1). São Paulo, SP: Gertulio Vargas Foundation.

Kazandjian, V., Parnell Wood, and Jane Lawthers. 1995. "Balancing Science and Practice in Indicator Development: The Maryland Hospital Association Quality Indicator Project." *International Journal for Quality in Health Care* 7 (1): 39–46.

Kisil, Marcos. 2004. "Qualidade Hospitalar." Consultant report for World Bank, Brasília, DF.

——. 2003. "Qualidade e Performance Hospitalar no Brasil: Revisão Analítica da Literatura." Consultant report for World Bank, Brasília, DF.

Kizer, Kenneth W. 2003. "The Volume-Outcome Conundrum." *New England Journal of Medicine* 349: 2159–61.

Knaus, W. A., E. A. Draper, D. P. Wagner, and J. E. Zimmerman. 1986. "An Evaluation of Outcome from Intensive Care in Major Medical Centers." *Annals of Internal Medicine* 104 (3, March): 410–18.

Kohn, Linda. 2000. "Organizing and Managing Care in a Changing Health System." *Health Services Research* 35 (Part I): 37–52.

Kowalski-Dickow Associates, Inc., in cooperation with the Association for Healthcare Resource & Materials Management. 1997. *Managing Hospital Materials Management*. Milwaukee, WI: Kowalski-Dickow Associates, Inc.

Krauss da Silva, L., T. P. Costa, A. F. Reis, N. O. Iamada, A. P. Azevedo, and C. P. Albuquerque, 1999. "Avaliação da qualidade da assistênca hospitalar obstétrica: uso de corticóides no trabalho de parto prematuro [Assessment of quality of obstetric care and corticoid use in preterm labor]." *Cadernos de saúde pública* 15 (4): 817–29.

La Forgia, Gerard Martin, ed. 2005. *Health System Innovations in Central America: Lessons and Impact of New Approaches*. Washington, DC: World Bank.

———. 1990. "Challenging Health Service Stratification: Social Security—Health Ministry Integration in Panama." Doctoral dissertation, University of Pittsburgh, School of Public Health.

Langenbrunner, J. C., and Miriam M. Wiley. 2002. "Hospital Payment Mechanisms: Theory and Practice in Transition Countries." In *Hospitals in a Changing Europe*, ed. Martin McKee and Judith Healy, 150–76. European Observatory on Health Care Systems Series. Buckingham, UK: Open University Press.

Lansky, Sônia, Elizabeth França, and Ichiro Kawachi. 2007. "Social Inequalities in Perinatal Mortality in Belo Horizonte, Brazil: The Role of Hospital Care." *American Journal of Public Health* 97 (5): 867–73.

Lansky, Sônia, Elizabeth França, Cibele Comini Césear, Luiz Costa Monteiro Neto, and Maria do Carmo Leal. 2006. "Mortes Perinatales e Avaliação da Assistência ao Parto em Maternidades do Sistema Único de Saúde em Belo Horizonte, Minas Gerais, Brasil, 1999." *Cadernos de Saúde Pública* 22 (1): 117–28.

Lawrence, David. 2003. *From Chaos to Care: The Promise of Team-Based Medicine*. Cambridge, MA: Da Capo Press.

Leal, Maria do Carmo, Silvana Granado Nogueira da Gama, and Cynthia Braga da Cunha. 2005. "Desigualidades Raciais, sociodemográficas e na asistência ao pré-natal e ao Parto, 1999–2001." *Revista de Saúde Pública* 31 (1): 100–107.

Leapfrog Group. 2006. "Leapfrog Hospital Rewards Program." Leapfrog Group and Thomson Medstat, Washington, DC. https://leapfrog.medstat.com/rewards/.

Lebrão, M. L. 1999. "Determinantes da morbidade hospitalar em região do Estado de São Paulo (Brasil)." *Revista de Saúde Pública* 33 (1): 55–63.

Leonard, L. Kenneth, Melkiory C. Masatu, and Alex Vialou. 2005. "Getting Clinicians to Do Their Best: Ability, Altruism and Incentives." Consultant report to World Bank and National Science Foundation, Washington, DC.

Levcovitz, E., and T. R. C. Pereira. 1993. "SIH/SUS (Sistema AIH): uma análise do sistema público de remuneração de internação hospitalar no Brasil, 1983–1991." Universidade Estadual do Rio de Janeiro/Instituto de Medicina Social, Rio de Janeiro, RJ.

Levit, K., Helen C. Lazenby, and Bradley R. Braden. 1996. "National Health Spending Trends." *Health Affairs* 17(1): 35–51.

Lighter, Donald E., and Douglas C. Fair. 2004. *Quality Management in Health Care. Principles and Methods*. Dubery, MA: Jones and Bartlett Publishers.

Lohr, K. N., ed. 1990. *Medicare: A Strategy for Quality Assurance*. Washington, DC: National Academy Press.

Maarse, Hans, Thomas A. Rathwell, Tamas Evetovits, Alexander Preker, and Elke Jakubowski. 2005. "Responding to Purchasing: Provide Perspectives." In *Purchasing to Improve Health Systems Performance*, ed. Josep Figueras, Ray Robinson, and Elke Jabubowski, 265–87. Berkshire, UK: Open University Press.

Macinko, J., Federico C. Guanais, and Maria de Fatima M. de Souza. 2006. "An Evaluation of the Impact of the Family Health Program on Infant Mortality in Brazil, 1990–2002." Consultant report to Ministério da Saúde. Brasília, DF.

Maniadakis, N., B. Hollingsworth, and E Thanassoulis. 1999. "The Impact of the Internal Market on Hospital Efficiency, Productivity and Service Quality." *Health Care Management Science* 2 (2): 75–85.

Mannion, R., and M. Goddard. 2001. "Impact of Published Clinical Outcome Data: Case Study in HNS Hospital Trusts." *British Medical Journal* 323: 262–63.

Marçal dos Santos, A. A., F. F. de Paula Lopes, R. Alves Cardoso, and J. C. Serufo. 2005. "Diagnóstico do Controle da Infecção Hospitalar no Brasil." Report prepared for Agência Nacional de Vigilância Sanitária (ANVISA), Brasília, DF. http://www.anvisa.gov.br/servicosaude/controle/Infectes%20Hospitalares_diagnostico.pdf.

MARE (Ministério da Administração Federal e Reforma do Estado). 1996. "Projeto organizações sociais." MARE, Brasília, DF.

Marinho, A. 2001a. "Estudo de Eficiência em Alguns Hospitais Públicos e Privados com a geração de *rankings*." Discussion Paper 794, Instituto de Pesquisa Econômica Aplicada, Rio de Janeiro, RJ.

———. 2001b. "Hospitais Universitários: Indicadores de Utilização e Análise de Eficiência." Discussion Paper 833, Instituto de Pesquisa Econômica Aplicada, Rio de Janeiro, RJ.

———. 2001c. "Avaliação da Eficiência Técnica nos Serviços de Saúde nos Municípios do Estado do Rio de Janeiro." Discussion Paper 842, Instituto de Pesquisa Econômica Aplicada, Rio de Janeiro, RJ.

Marinho, A., and L. O. Façanha. 2001. "Hospitais universitários: Avaliação Comparativa de eficiência técnica." Discussion Paper 805, Instituto de Pesquisa Econômica Aplicada, Rio de Janeiro, RJ.

Martín Martín, José Jesús. 2003. "Nuevas Fórmulas de Gestión en las Organizaciones Sanitarias." Working Paper, Fundación Alternativas, Madrid.

Martins, M., and Claudia M. R. Travassos. 1998. "Assessing the Availability of Casemix Information in Hospital Database Systems in Rio de Janeiro." *International Journal for Quality in Health Care* 10 (2): 125–33.

Martins, M., Claudia Travassos, and José C. Noronha. 2001. "Sistema de Informações Hospitalares como ajuste de risco em índices de desempenho." *Revista de Saúde Pública* 35 (2): 185–92.

Mathias, T. A. F., and Maria Lucia Soboll. 1998. "Confiabilidade de diagnósticos nos formulários de autorização de internação hospitalar." *Revista de Saúde Pública* 32 (6): 526–32.

McCaughey, Betsy. n.d. "Hospital Infection Fact Sheet." Committee to Reduce Infection Deaths, New York. www.hospitalinfection.org/infectionfacts.shtml.

McKee, Martin. 1997. "Indicators of Clinical Performance." *British Medical Journal* 315 (July 19): 142.

McKee, Martin, and Judith Healy, eds. 2002. *Hospitals in a Changing Europe.* European Observatory on Health Care Systems Series. Buckingham, UK: Open University Press.

McKillop, Donal G., J. Colin Glass, Christine A. Kerr, and Gillian McCallion. 1999. "Efficiency in Northern Ireland Hospitals: A Non-Parametric Analysis." *Economic and Social Review* 30 (2): 175–96.

McLoughlin, Vivienne, Sheila Letherman, Martins Fletcher, and John Wyn Owen. 2001. "Improving Performance Using Indicators: Recent Experiences in the United States, the United Kingdom, and Australia." *International Journal for Quality in Health Care* 13: 455–62.

McPake, Barbara, Francisco José Yepes, Sally Lake, and Luz Helena Sanchez. 2003. "Is the Colombian Health System Reform Improving the Performance of Public Hospitals in Bogotá?" *Health Policy and Planning* 18 (2): 182–94.

Médici, André C. 2005. "Financiamento Público em Saúde na América Latina e no Caribe: uma Breve ánalise dos anos 1990." Health Technical Note 3, Inter-American Development Bank, Washington, DC.

Mello, J. B., and M. Camargo. 1998. *Qualidade na Saúde: Práticas e Conceitos, Normas ISO nas áreas: Médico-Hospitalar e Laboratorial.* São Paulo, SP: Best Seller.

Mendes, Eugênio V. 2005. "Redes de Atenção a Saúde." Consultant report for World Bank, Brasília, DF.

———. 2002. *A Atenção Primária à Saúde no SUS.* Fortaleza, CE: Escola de Saúde Pública do Ceará.

————. 2001. *Os grandes dilemas do SUS*. 2 vols. Salvador, BA: Casa da Qualidade.

————. 1998. "A Reengenharia do Sistema de Serviços de Saúde no Nível Local." In *A organização da saúde no nível local*, ed. Eugenio V. Mendes, 57–86. São Paulo, SP: Hucitec.

————. 1986. "Reordenamento do Sistema Nacional de Saúde: Visão General." Presented at Conferencia Nacional de Saúde, Brasília, DF, March 17–21.

Mendes R., Jose, and Nilson do Rosário Costa. 2005. "Mecanismos de Governança e Modelos Alternativos de Gestão Hospitalar no Brasil." Osvaldo Cruz Foundation and National School of Public Health (FIOCRUZ/ENSP). Consultant report for World Bank, Rio de Janeiro, RJ.

Mendes, R., Jose, Nílson do Rosário Costa, Pedro Barbosa, Carlos Gadelha, Luiz Felipe Pinto, Antônio Werneck, Pedro Luiz Barros Silva, Daniel Soranz, Monica Chaves Reis, and Victor Grabois. 2002. "Estudo de Novos Modelos de Gerência de Unidades Hospitalares." Consultant report for Ministério da Saúde (REFORSUS Project), Brasília, DF.

MF (Ministério da Fazenda/STF). 2005. *Balanço Geral da União 2004*. Brasília, DF: MF.

————. MF/SIAFI Database. http://www.stn.fazenda.gov.br/siafi/index.asp (accessed March 15, 2005).

Minotto, Ricardo. 2003. *A Estratégia em Organizações Hospitalares*. Porto Alegre, RS: Pontifícia Universidade Católica do RS.

MS (Ministério da Saúde). 2006a. *Saúde da Família no Brasil—Uma análise de indicadores selecionados 1998–2004*. Brasília, DF: MS.

————. 2006b. "Diretrizes Para a Implantação de Complexos Reguladores." Serie Pactos Pela Sáude. Vol. 6. MS, Brasília, DF.

————. 2006c. "Manual de Orientações: Central Nacional de Regulação da Alta Complexidade." MS, Brasília, DF.

————. 2006d. "Preliminary Report, Programa de Nacional de Avaliação de Serviços de Saúde (PNASS)." MS, Brazilia.

————. 2005. *Saúde Brasil 2005: Uma análise da situação de saúde no Brasil*. Brasília, DF: MS, Secretaria de Vigilancia em Saúde.

————. 2004a. *Política Nacional de Humanização*. Documento base para Gestores e Trabalhadores do SUS. Brasília, DF: MS.

————. 2004b. *Reduzindo as desigualdades e ampliando o acesso à assistência à saúde no Brasil 1998–2002*. Brasília, DF: MS.

————. 2004c. *Reforma do Sistema da Atenção Hospitalar Brasileira*. Brasília, DF: MS.

————. 2004d. *PNASS—Programa Nacional de Avaliação de Serviços de Saúde*. Brasília, DF: MS, Secretaria de Atenção à Saúde.

————. 2004e. "HumanizaSUS—Politica Nacional de Humanização." Brasília, DF: MS, Secretaria Executiva.

————. 2004f. *Hospitais de Pequeno Porte—Uma estratégia alternativa de organização e financiamento*. Brasília, DF: MS, Secretaria de Atenção à Saúde.

————. 2003. *Gestão Financeira do Sistema Único de Saúde: Manual Básico*. 3rd ed. Brasília, DF: MS.

————. Various years, 1998–2006. "Sistema de Orçamentos Públicos em Saúde (SIOPS)." MS, Brasília, DF.

MS (Ministério da Saúde)/Datasus. 2007. "Informações de Saúde." MS, Brasília, DF. http://w3.datasus.gov.br/datasus/datasus.php?area=359A1B378C5D0E0F359G22HIJd5L25M0N&VInclude=../site/infsaude.php&VObj=http://tabnet.datasus.gov.br/cgi/deftohtm.exe?sim/cnv/mat (accessed March 15, 2007).

————. 2005a. "Indicadores e Dados Básicos 2005 (IDB)." MS, Brasília, DF. http://tabnet.datasus.gov.br/cgi/idb2005/matriz.htm.

————. 2005b. "Cadastro Nacional de Estabelecimento de Saúde (CNES)." MS, Brasília, DF. http://cnes.datasus.gov.br.

————. Various years, 1990–2006. "Sistema de Informações Hospitalares (SIH/AIH)." MS, Brasília, DF.

MS (Ministério da Saúde)/REFORSUS. Various years, 1998—2002. "Pilotos de Modernização Gerencial dos Grandes Estabelecimentos de Sáude." Consultant report to MS, REFORSUS Project. MS, Brasília, DF.

MS (Ministério da Saúde)/RIPSA. 2000. "Indicadores e Dados Básicos (IDB)." MS. Brasília, DF.

MSPS (Ministère de la Santé et de la Protection Sociale). 2004. *Bilan Social 2002.* Paris: MSPS, Direction de l´Hospitalisation et de l´Organisation des Soins.

Murray, Michael D., and Kaveh G. Shojania. 2001. "Unit-Dose Drug Distribution Systems." In "Making Health Care Safer: A Critical Analysis of Patient Safety Practices," ed. K. Shojania, B. Duncan, K. McDonald, and R. Wachter, 101–9. Evidence Report/Technology Assessment 43, Agency for Healthcare Research and Quality, Rockville, MD. http://www.ncbi.nlm.nih.gov/books/bv.fcgi?rid=hstat1.chapter.59276.

Murray, Robert. 2006. Presentation, Human Development Week, September 9, 2006, World Bank, Washington. DC. http://info.worldbank.org/etools/BSPAN/PresentationView.asp?PID=1906andEID=883.

Nakao, J. R. S., Y. D. M. Evora, N. Fávero, and E. Laus. 1986. "Análise de fatores que contribuem para que funcionários do serviço de enfermagem trabalhem em duas instituições hospitalares." *Revista Paulista de enfermagem* 6 (2): 78–82.

NCSL (National Conference of State Legislators). 2003. *A Framework for Considering Health Care Cost Containment.* Washington, DC: NCSL.

Neto, Antonio Quinto. 2004. "Acreditação de Organizações de Saúde: A importância dos Médicos na Segurança da Assistência e dos Consumidores." In *Hospitais: Administração da Qualidade e Acreditação de Organizações Complex*as, ed. Antônio Quinto Neto and Olímpio J. N. V. Bittar, 107–14. Porto Alegre, RS.

Neto, Antonio Quinto, and Olímpio J. Nogueira V. Bittar. 2004. *Administração da Qualidade e Acreditação de Organizações Complexas.* Porto Alegre, RS: Dacasa Editora.

———. 2003. *Hospitais: Administração da Qualidade e Acreditação de Organizações Complexas.* Porto Alegre, RS: Dacasa Editora.

Neto, A. Q., and F. L. Gastal. 1997a. *Acreditação Hospitalar.* Porto Alegre, RS: Escola Superior de Gestão e Ciências da Saúde.

———. 1997b. *Acreditação Hospitalar: Proteção dos Usuários, dos Profissionais e das Instituições de Saúde.* Porto Alegre, RS: Dacasa Editora.

Newble, David, Neil Paget, and Belinda Mclaren. 1999. "Revalidation in Australia and New Zealand: Approach of Royal Australasian College of Physicians." *British Medical Journal* 319: 1185–88.

Nishikuni, Yasuko Y., and Elaine Garcia Minuci. 2006. "Comparação das Médias dos Indicadores: Hospitais Selados e os Gerais." Report prepared for Controle de Qualidade Hospitalar and World Bank, São Paulo, SP.

Norcini, John J. 1999. "Recertification in the United States." *British Medical Journal* 319: 1183–85.

Noronha, José Carvalho, and M. L. Garcia Rosa. 1999. "Quality of Health Care—Growing Awareness in Brazil." *International Journal for Quality in Health Care* 11 (5): 437–41.

Noronha, José Carvalho, and Telma Ruth da Silva Pereira. 1998. "Health Care Reform and Quality Initiatives in Brazil." *Journal on Quality Improvement* 24 (5): 251–63.

Noronha, J. C., C. Travassos, M. C. Martins, M. R. Campos, P. Maia, and R. Panezzuti. 2003. "Avaliação da relação entre volume de procedimentos e a qualidade do cuidado: O caso de cirurgia coronariana no Brasil." *Cadernos de Saúde Pública* 19 (6): 1781–89.

Novaes, Humberto. 1999. *Manual Brasileiro de Acreditação Hospitalar.* Brasília, DF: Ministério da Saúde/Secretaria de Políticas de Saúde.

Novaes, H. M., and D. Neuhauser. 2000. "Hospital Accreditation in Latin America." *Pan American Journal of Public Health* 7 (6): 425–30.

Nunes, E. 1999. *Gramática Política do Brasil: Clientelismo e Insulamento Burocrático.* Rio de Janeiro, RJ: Jorge Zahar.

OECD (Organisation for Economic Co-operation and Development). 2005. *OECD Health Data.* Paris: OECD.

Oliveira, E. X. G., Claudia Travassos, and Marília S. Carvalho. 2004. "Acesso à Internação Hospitalar nos Municípios Brasileiros em 2000: Territórios do Sistema Único de Saúde." *Cadernos de Saúde Pública* 20 (Supp. 2): 5298–5309.

ONA (Organização Nacional de Acreditação). 2006. *Introdução a Indicadores de Desempenho—Treinamento por Educação á Distancia.* Brasília, DF: ONA. http://www.ona.org.br.

———. 2005. *DOS—Diagnóstico Organizacional Simplificado*. Brasília, DF: ONA.

———. 2004. *Manual das Organizações Prestadoras de Serviços Hospitalares*. Brasília, DF: ONA.

Over, Mead, and Naolo Watanabe. 2003. "Evaluating the Impact of Organizational Reforms in Hospitals." In *Innovations in Health Service Delivery: The Corporatization of Public Hospitals*, ed. Alexander Preker and April Harding, 105–51. Washington, DC: World Bank.

Ozcan, Y. A., and R. D. Luke. 1993. "A National Study of the Efficiency of Hospitals in Urban Markets." *Health Services Research* 27 (6): 719–39.

Ozcan Y. A., Roice D. Luke, and Cengiz Haksever. 1992. "Ownership and Organizational Performance: A Comparison of Technical Efficiency across Hospital Types." *Medical Care* 30: 781–94.

Palu, Toomas, and Reet Kadakmaa. 2001. "Estonian Hospital Sector Transition." *Eurohealth* 7 (3, special issue, Autumn): 61–64.

Partnerships for Health Reform Project. 1998. *Cuentas Nacionales de Salude: Mexico*. Informe sobre Iniciativas Especiales 11. Bethesda, MD: Abt Associates.

Peabody, John W., Mario M. Taguiwalo, David A. Robalino, and Julio Frenk. 2006. "Improving the Quality of Care in Developing Countries." In *Disease Control Priorities in Developing Countries*, ed. Dean T. Jamison, Joel G. Breman, Anthony R. Measham, George Alleyne, Mariam Claeson, David B. Evans, Prabhat Jha, Anne Mills, and Philip Musgrove, 1293–1308. 2nd ed. New York: Oxford University Press.

Pereira, A. C., R. A. Franken, and S. R. S. Sprovieri. 2000. "Iatrogenia em Cardiologia." *Arquivos Brasileiros de Cardiologia* 75 (1): 75–78.

Pereira, Marcelo Farid, J. S. Tusi da Silveira, and Edgar Augusto Lanzer. 1995. "Análise da Eficiência Produtiva de Unidades Hospitalares Utilizando Análise de Envelopamento de Dados (DEA)." In *Anais do II Encontro de Economistas de Língua Portuguesa* (conference proceedings). Rio de Janeiro: Instituto de Economia Industrial da UFRJ.

Pestana, Marcus, and Eugênio V. Mendes. 2004. *Pacto de Gestão: da Municipalização Autárquica à Regionalização Cooperativa*. Belo Horizonte, MG: Secretaria de Estado de Saúde de Minas Gerais.

Peterlini, Maria Angélica Sorgini, Massae Noda Chaud, Mavilde da L. G. Pedreira. 2003. "Órfãos de terapia medicamentosa: a administração de medicamentos por via intravenosa em crianças hospitalizadas". *Revista Latino-Americana de Enfermagem* 11 (1, January–February): 88–95.

PHC4 (Pennsylvania Health Care Cost Containment Council). 2005. "Hospital-Acquired Infections in Pennsylvania." *PHC4 Research Briefs* 5 (July): 1–5.

PMSP (Prefeitura Municipal de São Paulo)/Secretaria Municipal da Saúde/CeInfo. 2002. "Índice Saúde por Subprefeitura 2001–02, Painel de Monitoramento das condições de Vida e Saúde e da Situação dos Serviços de Saúde." Fundação SEADE, São Paulo, SP.

PNUD (Programa das Nações Unidas de Desenvolvimento). 2004. *Atlas de Saúde—Brasil*. Brasília, DF: PNUD.

Posnett, J. 2002. "Are Bigger Hospitals Better?" In *Hospitals in a Changing Europe*, ed. Martin McKee and Judith Healy, 100–18. European Observatory on Health Care Systems Series. Buckingham, UK: Open University Press.

Prade, S. S. 2002. "Desenvolvimento e validação de um instrumento de assessoria do programa de controle de infecção para as decisões do dirigente hospitalar." In *Experiências Inovadoras no SUS*, 156–207. Produção Científica: Mestrado e Eoutorado, Ministério da Saúde, Série C. Brasília, DF.

Prade, S. S., S. T. Oliveira, R. Rodrigues, and F. A. Nunes. 1995. "Estudo Brasileiro da Magnitude das Infecções Hospitalares em Hospitais Terciários." *Revista do Controle de Infecção Hospitalar* 1995 (2): 11–25.

Prefeitura da Cidade de Rio de Janeiro. 2002. "Avaliando a eficiência dos hospitais gerais do SUS através da metodologia da análise de envoltório de dados—DEA." Coleção Estudos da Cidade. Rio Estudos 44 (January), Rio de Janeiro, RJ.

Preker, Alexander S. 2005. "Managing Scarcity through Strategic Purchasing of Health Care." In *Spending Wisely: Buying Health Services for the Poor*, ed. Alexander S. Preker and John C. Langenbrunner, 23–46. Washington, DC: World Bank.

Preker, Alexander S., and April Harding, eds. 2003. *Innovations in Health Sector Delivery: The Corporatization of Public Hospitals*. Washington, DC: World Bank.

Preker, Alexander S., and John C. Langenbrunner, eds. 2005. *Spending Wisely: Buying Health Services for the Poor.* Washington, DC: World Bank.

President's Advisory Commission on Consumer Protection and Quality in the Health Care Industry. 1998. *Quality First: Better Care for All Americans.* Washington, DC.

Prior, Diego. 2006. "Efficiency and Total Quality Management in Health Care Organizations: A Dynamic Frontier Approach." *Annals of Operations Research* 145 (1): 281–99.

Proite, A., and Maria da Conceição Sampaio de Sousa. 2004. "Eficiência Técnica, Economias de Escala, Estrutura da Propriedade e Tipo de Gestão no Sistema Hospitalar Brasileiro." Presented at Encontro ANPEC, João Pessoa, PB.

Puig-Junoy, J. 1999. "Ineficiencia técnica y asignativa en la producción hospitalaria: Una aplicación AED-AR." Working Paper, Fundación BBV, Madrid.

Pupo, Tânia Regina G. Botelho. 2004. "Análise do Instrumento Vistoria Técnica Hospitalar." Doctoral dissertation, University of São Paulo.

Qualis Health. 2006. "Surgical Infection Prevention (SIP) Collaborative Problem Statement." Seattle, WA. http://www.qualishealth.org/sip.htm.

Rattner, Daphne. 2001. "Quality of Care in Childbirth: Seeking a Comprehensive Approach." PhD dissertation, University of North Carolina, Chapel Hill, NC.

Register, C. A., and Edward R. Bruning. 1987. "Profit Incentives and Technical Efficiency in the Production of Hospital Care." *Southern Economic Journal* 53 (4): 899–914.

Robinson, Ray, Elke Jabubowski, and Josep Figueras. 2005a. "Introduction." In *Purchasing to Improve Health Systems Performance*, ed. Josep Figueras, Ray Robinson, and Elke Jabubowski, 3-10. Buckingham, UK: Open University Press.

———. 2005b. "Organization of Purchasing in Europe." In *Purchasing to Improve Health Systems Performance*, ed. Josep Figueras, Ray Robinson, and Elke Jabubowski, 11–43. Buckingham, UK: Open University Press.

Rodrigues, P. S., L. Fonseca, and H. Chaimovich. 2000. "Mapping Cancer, Cardiovascular and Malaria Research in Brazil." *Brazilian Journal of Medical and Biological Research* 33 (8): 853–67.

Rooney, Anne L., and Paul R. van Ostenberg. 1999. "Licensure, Accreditation, and Certification: Approaches to Health Services Quality." Prepared for United States Agency for International Development (USAID), Quality Assurance Project, Bethesda, MD.

Rowland, Howard S., and Beatrice L. Rowland. 1984. *Hospital Management: A Guide to Departments.* Rockville, MD: Aspen.

Saltman, Richard B., and Josep Figueras, eds. 1997. *European Health Care Reform—Analysis of Current Strategies.* European Series 72. Copenhagen: WHO Regional Office for Europe.

Sampaio, Luis Fernando R. 2004. "A Qualidade do Cuidado nas Instituições Hospitalares Brasileiras." Consultant report for World Bank, Brasília, DF.

Sánchez Centurión, Carlos Alberto Segundo. 1993. "Avaliação da qualidade de assistência perinatal, no município de Taboão da Serra, São Paulo." Master's thesis, School of Public Health, University of São Paulo.

Sanigest International. 2005. "Estudio de las Herramientas Contractuales entre el Gobierno del Amazonas y las Cooperativas Prestadoras de Servicios de Salud." Consultant report for Gobierno de la República Federada del Brasil Secretaria de Salud del Estado del Amazonas.

Santos, N. Q. 1996. "Prática assistencial de enfermagem: o resgate da microbiologia como fundamento para o controle da infecção hospitalar." Master's thesis, Universidade Federal de Santa Catarina, Florianópolis, Brazil.

Schiesari, Laura Maria César. 2003. "Resultados de Iniciativas de Qualidade em Hospitais Brasileiros." Doctoral dissertation, Universidade de São Paulo.

Schilling, Claunara, Afonso Teixeira dos Reis, and José Carlos de Moraies. 2006. "A Política de Regulação do Brasil." Série Técnica: Desenvolvimento de Sistemas e Serviços de Saúde, 12, Pan American Health Organization and MS, Brasília, DF.

Schneider, Pia. 2007. "Provider Payment Reforms: Lessons from Europe and America for South Eastern Europe." Policy Note, HNP Discussion Paper, World Bank, Washington, DC.

Schneiter, Ellen J., Trish Riley, and Jill Rosenthal. 2002. *Rising Health Care Costs: State Health Cost Containment Approaches.* Portland, OR; Washington, DC: National Academy for State Health Policy. http://www. NASHP.org/Files/GNL56.pdf.

Scrivens, Ellie. 2002. "Accreditation and the Regulation of Quality in Health Services." In *Regulating Entrepreneurial Behaviour in European Health Care Systems,* ed. Richard B. Saltman, Reinhard Busse, and Elias Mossilos, 91–105. Buckingham, UK: Open University Press.

———. 1997a. "Assessing the Value of Accreditation Systems." *European Journal of Public Health* 7: 4–8.

———. 1997b. "Putting Continuous Quality Improvement into Accreditation: Improving Approaches to Quality Assessment." *Quality in Health Care* 6: 212–18.

SES-C (Secretaria da Saúde do Estado do Ceará). 2002a. *A Experiência de Implantação da Microrregião de Saúde de Baturité.* Fortaleza, CE.

———. 2002b. *Sistemas Microrregionais de Serviços de Saúde.* Fortaleza, CE.

SES-MG (Secretaria de Estado de Saúde de Minas Gerais). 2007. "Por um SUS Mais Fácil em Minas Gerais." Presentation, Belo Horizonte, MG, April 17.

———. 2006. "Manual do Pro-Hosp. Programa de Fortalecimento e Melhoria da Qualidade dos Hospitais do SUS/MG." Belo Horizonte, MG.

———. 2005. "Caracterização da Rede Hospitalar do Sistema Único de Saúde em Minas Gerais: Estudos de Políticas de Saúde e de Avaliação Econômica do SUS-MG." Serviços Hospitalares 3, Belo Horizonte, MG.

———. 2003. "O Programa de Fortalecimento e Melhoria da Qualidade dos Hospitais do SUS em Minas Gerais—PROHOSP." Belo Horizonte, MG.

SES-SP (Secretaria de Estado da Saúde de São Paulo). 2007. "Hospitais de Ensino no Estado de São Paulo." Assessoria de Hospitais de Enino, SES, São Paulo, SP.

———. 2006. "Avaliação dos Contratos de Gestão. Coordenadora de Contratação de Serviços de Saúde." Dept. de Gestão e Controle de Contratos, São Paulo, SP.

———. 2004. "Análise das UPS de custos trimestrais dos hospitais administrados por Organizações Sociais." Coordenadoria de Contratação de Serviços de Saúde/DGCC, São Paulo, SP.

———. 2003a. "Relatorio de Execução dos Contratos de Gestão." Commissão de Avaliação, São Paulo, SP.

———. 2003b. "Análize Comparativa entre hospitas de administração Direita e Hospitais Gerenciados por Organizações Sociais de Saúde." Coordenadora de Contratação de Serviços de Saúde, Dept. de Gestão e Controle de Contratos, São Paulo, SP.

Shaw, Charles D. 2004a. *Developing Hospital Accreditation in Europe.* Copenhagen: WHO Regional Office for Europe.

———. 2004b. *Toolkit for Accreditation Programs.* Washington, DC: International Society for Quality in Health Care.

Shen, Y. C., Karen Eggleston, Joseph Lau, and Christopher Schmid. 2005. *Hospital Ownership and Financial Performance: A Quantitative Research Review.* Working Paper Series 11662. Cambridge, MA: National Bureau of Economic Research.

Shepherd, Geoffrey. 2002. "Public Administration in the Federal Government of Brazil: Civil Service and Organization Issues." Consultant report, World Bank, Brasília, DF.

Shortell, Stephen M., Robert H. Jones, Alfred W. Rademaker, et al. 2000a. "Assessing the Impact of Total Quality Management and Organizational Culture on Multiple Outcomes of Care for Coronary Artery Bypass Graft Surgery Patients." *Medical Care* 38 (2): 207–17.

Shortell, Stephen M., Robin R. Gillies, David A. Anderson, Karen M. Erickson and John B. Mitchell. 2000b. *Remaking Health Care in America.* San Francisco, CA: Jossey-Bass.

Shortell, Stephen M., Jack E. Zimmerman, Denise M. Rousseau. Robin R. Gillies, Douglas P. Wagner, Elizabeth A. Draper, William A. Knaus, and Joanne Duffy. 1994. "The Performance of Intensive Care Units: Does Good Management Make a Difference?" *Medical Care* 32 (5): 508–25.

Silva, A. E. B. C. 2003. "Análise do sistema de medicação de um hospital universitário do estado de Goiás." Master's thesis, University of São Paulo, Riberão Preto.

Silver, L. D. 1992. "Quality Assurance in Health Care Issues in Health Care Delivery and Finance in Brazil." Consultant report, World Bank, Washington, DC.

Silver, L. D., Claudia V. Travassos, Marina F. Noronha, Monica S. Martins, and I. C. Leite. 1992. "Estudo da validade dos Diagnosis Related Groups (DRG) para internações hospitalares no Brasil." Relatório final de pesquisa do projeto "Avaliação de métodos alternativos para racionalização e análise de qualidade nos serviços de saúde." Escola Nacional de Saúde Pública, Fundação Oswaldo Cruz, Rio de Janeiro. RJ.

Siqueira, A.A. F., Ana C. d´A. Tanaka, Renato M. Santana, and Pedro A. M. de Almeida. 1984. "Mortalidade Materna no Brasil, 1980." *Revista de Saúde Publica* 18: 448–65.

Solucient. 2004. "Solucient 100 Top Hospitals—National Benchmarks for Success 2003." Thomas Healthcare, Stamford CT. http://www.100tophospitals.com/default.aspx.

Spath, Patrice L., ed. 1999. "Error Reduction in Health Care: A Systems Approach to Improving Patient Safety." San Francisco: Jossey-Bass.

Ssengooba, Freddie, Lynn Atuyambe, Barbara McPake, Kara Hanson, and Sam Okuonzi. 2002. "What Could Be Achieved with Greater Public Hospital Autonomy? Comparison of Public and PNFP Hospitals in Uganda." Wiley InterScience. http://www.interscience.wiley.com.

Starfield, Barbara. 1998. *Primary Care: Balancing Health Needs, Services and Technology.* New York: Oxford University Press.

Starr, Paul. 1982. *The Social Transformation of American Medicine.* New York: Basic Books.

Stevens, Rosemary. 1989. *In Sickness and in Wealth: American Hospitals in the Twentieth Century.* New York: Basic Books.

Strandberg-Larsen, Martin, Mikkel Bernt Nielsen, Allan Krasnik, and Karsten Vrangbæk. 2006. "Is Denmark Prepared to Meet Future Health Care Demands?" *Eurohealth* 12 (4): 7–10.

Swinkels, J. A. 1999. "Reregistration of Medical Specialists in the Netherlands." *British Medical Journal* 319: 1191–92.

Tambour, M., and N. Zethraeus. 1998. "Efficiency in the Treatment of Hip Fractures." Working Paper Series in Economics and Finance 246, Stockholm School of Economics, Department of Economics, Stockholm.

Thomas, Eric J., David M. Studdert, Joseph P. Newhouse, Brett I. W. Zbar, K. Mason Howard, Elliott Williams, and T. Brennan 1999. "Costs of Medical Injuries in Utah and Colorado." *Inquiry* 36: 255–64.

Thompson, C. R., and M. McKee. 2004. "Financing and Planning of Public and Private Not-for-Profit Hospitals in the European Union." *Health Policy* 67: 281–91.

Toro, Teresa M., Enriqueta Cueto, Antonio Giuffrida, Carlos Arango, and Alvaro López. 2007. "Public Hospitals and Health Care Reform in Colombia." Bogotá. Forthcoming, *Lancet.*

UNIDAS (União Nacional das Instituições de Autogestão em Saúde). 2005. *Pesquisa Nacional UNIDAS 2004/2005.* São Paulo, SP.

Valdmanis, V. 1992. "Sensitivity Analysis for DEA Models." *Journal of Public Economics* 48: 85–205.

Vali, F. M. 2001. *Access to Primary Care in New Jersey—Geographic Variation of Hospitalizations for Ambulatory Care Sensitive Conditions in 1995 & 1997.* Princeton, NJ: Health Research & Educational Trust of New Jersey.

Vargas, Alexis. 2006. "Anotações Sobre o contrato de Gestão." *Debates GV Saúde* 1: 32–36. Fundação Gertulio Vargas, Centro de Estudos em Planejamento e Gestão de Saúde, São Paulo, SP.

Veras, C. M. T., and Mônica S. Martins. 1994. "A confiabilidade dos Dados nos Formulários de Autorização de Internação Hospitalar (AIH), Rio de Janeiro, Brasil." *Cadernos de Saúde Pública* 10 (3): 339–55.

Veras, C. M. T., Francisco C. Braga Neto, Marina F. Noronha, and Monica S. Martins. 1990. "Diagnosis Related Groups—DRG's: avaliação do uso de uma metodologia de mensuração do produto hospitalar com utilização de base de dados do SAMHPS/AIH na cidade do Rio de Janeiro." *Cadernos de Saúde Publica* 6 (3): 330–35.

Viacava Francisco, Célia Almeida, Rosangela Caetano, Márcia Fausto, James Macinko, Mônica Martins, José Carvalho de Noronha, Heligonda M. D. Novaes, Eliane dos Santos Oliveira, Silva M. Porto, Liegia M. Vieiria da Silva, and Célia Landmann Szwarcwald. 2004. "Uma metodologia de avaliação do desempenho do Sistema de saúde brasileiro." *Ciência & Saúde Coletiva* 9 (3): 711–24.

Vianna, S. M., ed. 2005. *Atenção de Alta Complexidade no SUS: Desigualdades no Acesso e no Financiamento.* Vol. 1. Brasília, DF: MS/IPEA.

Victora, Cesar G., Patrick Vaughan, Fernando C. Barros, Anamaria C. Silva, and Elaine Tomasi. 2000. "Explaining Trends in Inequities: Evidence from Brazilian Child Health Studies." *Lancet* 356: 1093–98.

Waters, H., and P. Hussey. 2004. "Pricing Health Services for Purchasers: A Review of Methods and Experiences." HNP Working Paper 31590, World Bank, Washington, DC.

Webster, R., Steven Kennedy, and Leanne Johnson. 1998. "Comparing Techniques for Measuring the Efficiency and Productivity of Australian Private Hospitals." Working Paper 98/3, Australian Bureau of Statistics, Canberra.

WHO (World Health Organization). 2005. *World Health Report 2005.* Geneva: WHO.

———. 2003a. *Quality and Accreditation in Health Care Services: A Global Review.* Geneva: WHO.

———. 2003b. *How Can Hospital Performance Be Measured and Monitored?* Copenhagen: WHO Regional Office for Europe. http://www.euro.who.int/document/e82975.pdf.

———. 2000a. *World Health Report 2000.* Geneva: WHO.

———. 2000b. *Health Care Systems in Transition: Germany, European Observatory on Health Care Systems.* Copenhagen: WHO Regional Office for Europe.

———. 2000c. *Health Care Systems in Transition: France, European Observatory on Health Care Systems.* Copenhagen: WHO Regional Office for Europe.

———. 2000d. *Health Care Systems in Transition: Switzerland, European Observatory on Health Care Systems.* Copenhagen: WHO Regional Office for Europe.

———. 2000e. *Health Care Systems in Transition: The Netherlands, European Observatory on Health Care Systems.* Copenhagen: WHO Regional Office for Europe.

———. 2000f. "Equity in Access to Public Health." Working Papers, SEA-HSD-240,. New Delhi: Fifty-Third Regional Committee of the South East Asia Region, New Delhi.

Wiley, Miriam. 2007. "Factors for Consideration When Developing a Case Mix Based Hospital Payment System." Presented at World Bank Global Development Learning Network (GDLN) session, April 11, Economic and Social Research Institute, Dublin.

Work Group on Computerization of Patient Records. 2000. *Toward a National Health Information Infrastructure: Report of the Work Group on Computerization of Patient Records.* Washington, DC: U.S. Department of Health and Human Services.

World Bank. 2007. "Brazil: Governance in Brazil's Unified Health System (SUS): Raising the Quality of Public Spending and Resource Management." Report 36602-BR, World Bank, Washington, DC.

———. 2006a. "Brazil: Enhancing Performance in Brazil's Health Sector: Lessons from Innovations in the State of São Paulo and the City of Curitiba." Report 35671-BR, World Bank, Washington, DC.

———. 2006b. "Brazil: Country Assistance Strategy—Update." World Bank, Brasília, DF.

———. 2006c. *World Development Report 2006: Equity and Development.* Washington, DC: World Bank.

———. 2005a. "Addressing the Challenge of Non-communicable Diseases in Brazil." Report 32576-BR, World Bank, Washington, DC.

———. 2005b. *World Development Indicators 2005.* Washington, DC: World Bank.

———. 2004a. "Implementation Completion Report for Brazil Health Sector Reform Project—REFORSUS." Report 29325, World Bank, Washington, DC.

———. 2004b. "Brazil Country Procurement Assessment Report." Report 28446-BR, World Bank, Washington, DC.

———. 2004c. *Making Services Work for Poor People.* Washington, DC: World Bank.

———. 2002. "Brazil Maternal and Child Health." Report 23811-BR, World Bank, Washington, DC.

———. 1994. "Brazil. The Organization, Delivery and Financing of Health Care in Brazil: Agenda for the 90s." Report 12644-BR, World Bank, Washington, DC.

Wouters, Annemarie, Sara Bennett, and Charlotte Leighton. 1998. "Alternative Provider Payment Methods: Incentives for Improving Health Care Delivery." PHR Primer for Policymakers Series. Bethesda, MD: Partnerships for Health Reform, Abt Associates. http://www.phrplus.org/Pubs/pps1.pdf.

Wrightson, Charles William, Jr. 1990. *HMO Rate Setting and Financial Strategy.* Ann Arbor, MI: Health Administration Press.

Zanetta, S. F. R. n.d. "Uso de DRGs—Diagnosis Related Groups para qualificação das AIHs— Autorizações de Internação Hospitalar como instrumentos de gestão de serviços." São Paulo.

Zere, Eyob. 2000. "Hospital Efficiency in Sub-Saharan Africa. Evidence from South Africa." Working Paper 187, World Institute for Development Economics Research, Helsinki.

Zeribi, K. A., and L. Marquez. 2004. *Approaches to Healthcare Quality Regulation in Latin America and the Caribbean: Regional Experiences and Challenges.* Latin America and Caribbean Regional Health Sector Reform Initiative (LACHSR), Report 63, for United States Agency for International Development (USAID), Quality Assurance Project, Bethesda, MD.

Index

Boxes, figures, notes, and tables are indicated by b, f, n, *and* t, *respectively.*

ECO-AUDIT
Environmental Benefits Statement

The World Bank is committed to preserving endangered forests and natural resources. The Office of the Publisher has chosen to print *Hospital Performance in Brazil: The Search for Excellence* on 50-pound Roland Opaque, a recycled paper made with 30 percent post-consumer waste, in accordance with the recommended standards for paper usage set by the Green Press Initiative, a nonprofit program supporting publishers in using fiber that is not sourced from endangered forests. For more information, visit www.greenpressinitiative.org.

Saved:

- 7 trees
- 340 lbs. of solid waste
- 2,649 gallons of waste water
- 638 lbs. of net greenhouse gases
- 5 million BTUs of total energy

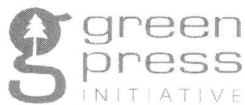